Interventional Endoscopic Ultrasound

Guest Editor

KENNETH J. CHANG, MD

GASTROINTESTINAL ENDOSCOPY CLINICS OF NORTH AMERICA

www.giendo.theclinics.com

Consulting Editor
CHARLES J. LIGHTDALE, MD

April 2012 • Volume 22 • Number 2

SAUNDERS an imprint of ELSEVIER, Inc.

W.B. SAUNDERS COMPANY
A Division of Elsevier Inc.

1600 John F. Kennedy Blvd. ● Suite 1800 ● Philadelphia, Pennsylvania 19103-2899

http://www.giendo.theclinics.com

GASTROINTESTINAL ENDOSCOPY CLINICS OF NORTH AMERICA Volume 22, Number 2
April 2012 ISSN 1052-5157, ISBN-13: 978-1-4557-3866-3

Editor: Kerry Holland

Gastrointestinal Endoscopy Clinics of North America (ISSN 1052-5157) is published quarterly by Elsevier Inc., 360 Park Avenue South, New York, NY 10010-1710. Months of issue are January, April, July, and October. Business and Editorial Offices: 1600 John F. Kennedy Blvd., Suite 1800, Philadelphia, PA, 19103-2899. Periodicals postage paid at New York, NY and additional mailing offices. Subscription prices are $315.00 per year for US individuals, $441.00 per year for US institutions, $168.00 per year for US students and residents, $351.00 per year for Canadian individuals, $538.00 per year for Canadian institutions, $445.00 per year for international individuals, $538.00 per year for international institutions, and $234.00 per year for Canadian and foreign students/residents. To receive student/resident rate, orders must be accompanied by name of affiliated institution, date of term, and the *signature* of program/residency coordinator on institution letterhead. Orders will be billed at individual rate until proof of status is received. Foreign air speed delivery is included in all *Clinics* subscription prices. All prices are subject to change without notice. **POSTMASTER:** Send address change to *Gastrointestinal Endoscopy Clinics of North America*, Elsevier Health Sciences Division, Subscription Customer Service, 3251 Riverport Lane, Maryland Heights, MO 63043. **Customer Service: 1-800-654-2452 (US). From outside the United States, call 1-314-447-8871. Fax: 1-314-447-8029. E-mail: JournalsCustomerService-usa@elsevier.com (for print support) or JournalsOnlineSupport-usa@elsevier.com (for online support).**

Reprints. For copies of 100 or more, of articles in this publication, please contact the Commercial Reprints Department, Elsevier Inc., 360 Park Avenue South, New York, NY 10010-1710. Tel. (212) 633-3812; Fax: (212) 482-1935; E-mail: reprints@elsevier.com.

Gastrointestinal Endoscopy Clinics of North America is covered in *Excerpta Medica, MEDLINE/PubMed (Index Medicus), and MEDLINE/MEDLARS.*

Printed and bound by CPI Group (UK) Ltd, Croydon, CR0 4YY
Transferred to Digital Print 2012

Contributors

CONSULTING EDITOR

CHARLES J. LIGHTDALE, MD
Professor, Department of Medicine, Columbia University Medical Center, New York, New York

GUEST EDITOR

KENNETH J. CHANG, MD, FASGE, FACG
Professor and Chief, Division of Gastroenterology and Hepatology; Director, H.H. Chao Comprehensive Digestive Disease Center, University of California, Irvine, Orange, California

AUTHORS

AMER A. ALKHATIB, MD
Division of Gastroenterology and Hepatology, Mayo Clinic, Scottsdale, Arizona

VIKRAM BHATIA, MD
Department of Medical Hepatology, Institute of Liver and Biliary Sciences, Delhi, India

KENNETH F. BINMOELLER, MD
Paul May and Frank Stein Interventional Endoscopy Services, California Pacific Medical Center, San Francisco, California

WILLIAM R. BRUGGE, MD
Professor of Medicine, Gastrointestinal Unit, Massachusetts General Hospital, Boston, Massachusetts

KENNETH J. CHANG, MD, FASGE, FACG
Professor and Chief, Division of Gastroenterology and Hepatology; Director, H.H. Chao Comprehensive Digestive Disease Center, University of California, Irvine, Orange, California

SURESH T. CHARI, MD
Professor, Division of Gastroenterology and Hepatology, Mayo Clinic, Rochester, Minnesota

JOHN DEWITT, MD, FACG, FACP, FASGE
Associate Professor of Medicine, Division of Gastroenterology and Hepatology, Indiana University Medical Center, Indianapolis, Indiana

J. ENRIQUE DOMÍNGUEZ-MUÑOZ, MD, PhD
Gastroenterology Department, Foundation for Research in Digestive Diseases (FIENAD), University Hospital of Santiago de Compostela, Santiago de Compostela, Spain

DOUGLAS O. FAIGEL, MD, FACG, FASGE, AGAF
Professor of Medicine, Division of Gastroenterology and Hepatology, Mayo Clinic, Scottsdale, Arizona

MARC GIOVANNINI, MD
Chief, Endoscopic Unit, Paoli-Calmettes Institute, Marseille, France

KAZUO HARA, PhD, MD
Department of Gastroenterology, Aichi Cancer Center Hospital, Chikusa-Ku, Nagoya, Japan

MUHAMMAD K. HASAN, MD
Assistant Professor of Medicine, University of Central Florida School of Medicine, Orlando, Florida

ROBERT H. HAWES, MD
Medical Director, Florida Hospital Institute for Minimally Invasive Therapy, Orlando, Florida

SUSUMU HIJIOKA, MD
Department of Gastroenterology, Aichi Cancer Center Hospital, Chikusa-Ku, Nagoya, Japan

JULIO IGLESIAS-GARCIA, MD, PhD
Gastroenterology Department, Foundation for Research in Digestive Diseases (FIENAD), University Hospital of Santiago de Compostela, Santiago de Compostela, Spain

HIROSHI IMAOKA, PhD, MD
Department of Gastroenterology, Aichi Cancer Center Hospital, Chikusa-Ku, Nagoya, Japan

TAKAO ITOI, MD
Department of Gastroenterology and Hepatology, Tokyo Medical University, Tokyo, Japan

TAKUJI IWASHITA, MD, PhD
Clinical Instructor, Division of Gastroenterology and Hepatology, H.H. Chao Comprehensive Digestive Disease Center, University of California, Irvine Medical Center, Orange, California; Project Lecturer, First Department of Internal Medicine, Gifu University Hospital, Gifu, Japan

ZHENDONG JIN, MD
Professor in Gastroenterology, Vice-Director of Gastroenterology Department, Changhai Hospital, Second Military Medical University, Shanghai, China

MASAYUKI KITANO, MD, PhD
Associate Professor, Department of Gastroenterology and Hepatology, Kinki University School of Medicine, Osakasayama, Japan

MASATOSHI KUDO, MD, PhD
Director and Professor, Department of Gastroenterology and Hepatology, Kinki University School of Medicine, Osakasayama, Japan

ALI LANKARANI, MD
Department of Gastroenterology, Mayo Clinic, Jacksonville, Florida

JOHN G. LEE, MD
Professor of Clinical Medicine, Division of Gastroenterology and Hepatology; Associate Director, H.H. Chao Comprehensive Digestive Disease Center, University of California, Irvine Medical Center, Orange, California

MICHAEL J. LEVY, MD
Professor, Division of Gastroenterology and Hepatology, Mayo Clinic, Rochester, Minnesota

NOBUMASA MIZUNO, PhD, MD
Department of Gastroenterology, Aichi Cancer Center Hospital, Chikusa-Ku, Nagoya, Japan

YOUSUKE NAKAI, MD, PhD
Assistant Clinical Professor, Division of Gastroenterology and Hepatology, H. H. Chao Comprehensive Digestive Disease Center, University of California, Irvine, Orange, California; Assistant Professor, Department of Gastroenterology, Graduate School of Medicine, The University of Tokyo, Tokyo, Japan

DO HYUN PARK, MD, PhD
Assistant Professor, Division of Gastroenterology, Department of Internal Medicine, University of Ulsan College of Medicine, Asan Medical Center, Seoul, Korea

GANAPATHY A. PRASAD, MD
Consultant, Associate Professor, Division of Gastroenterology and Hepatology, Mayo Clinic, Rochester, Minnesota

HIROKI SAKAMOTO, MD, PhD
Associate Professor, Department of Gastroenterology and Hepatology, Kinki University School of Medicine, Osakasayama, Japan

JASON B. SAMARASENA, MD
Clinical Instructor, Division of Gastroenterology and Hepatology, H.H.Chao Comprehensive Digestive Disease Center, University of California, Irvine, Orange, California

YASUHIRO SHIMIZU, PhD, MD
Department of Gastrointestinal Surgery, Aichi Cancer Center Hospital, Nagoya, Japan

SHYAM VARADARAJULU, MD
Medical Director of Endoscopy, Division of Gastroenterology, Department of Medicine, Basil I. Hirschowitz Endoscopic Center of Excellence, University of Alabama at Birmingham School of Medicine, Birmingham, Alabama

MICHAEL B. WALLACE, MD, MP
Professor and Chair, Department of Gastroenterology, Mayo Clinic, Jacksonville, Florida

FRANK WEILERT, MD
Peter Stokes Endoscopy Unit, Waikato District Health Board, Waikato Hospital, Hamilton, New Zealand

MAURITS J. WIERSEMA, MD
Private Practice, Lutheran Medical Group, Fort Wayne, Indiana

KENJI YAMAO, PhD, MD
Department of Gastroenterology, Aichi Cancer Center Hospital, Chikusa-Ku, Nagoya, Japan

WON JAE YOON, MD
Research Fellow, Gastrointestinal Unit, Massachusetts General Hospital, Boston, Massachusetts

Contents

Although endoscopic ultrasonography (EUS) is considered superior to MRI and CT in detecting pancreatic masses, it is the ability to target and place a needle into suspicious lesions that has made EUS indispensible in the evaluation of patients with solid pancreatic tumors. Endoscopic ultrasound-guided-fine-needle aspiration (EUS-FNA) is an accurate and safe technique to confirm the diagnosis of pancreatic cancer. EUS-FNA is now the principal technique applied to obtain the diagnosis of malignancy. We have designed this article to address a number of the key technical aspects of EUS-FNA of solid pancreatic masses.

The diagnosis and management of pancreatic cystic lesions remains a challenging area in gastroenterology. Differentiating benign from premalignant or premalignant from malignant cysts is complicated by the large overlap in morphologic, chemical, and clinical characteristics. Imaging alone is insufficient to accurately characterize these lesions. Cyst aspiration and fluid analysis has therefore become a major research focus through which our ability to characterize pancreatic cystic lesions has improved, although accuracy is often still lacking. Future work with molecular analysis of cyst fluid, direct cystoscopy, and confocal laser endomicroscopy will likely further enhance the diagnostic accuracy of these lesions.

Subepithelial lesions are frequently discovered during routine endoscopic examinations. These lesions represent a wide spectrum of heterogeneous benign to malignant conditions. Most of these lesions are asymptomatic. There is no consensus regarding how to manage these lesions. Over the last 2 decades, the approach to these lesions has significantly improved owing to the introduction of endoscopic ultrasonography, fine-needle aspiration, immunohistochemical staining methods, and different treatment options. This article discusses the nature of subepithelial lesions, focusing on the most recent developments that use endoscopic ultrasonography to diagnose and manage these lesions.

and EUS are mandatory in minimizing the potential complications of this procedure.

Endoscopic Ultrasound-Guided Choledochoduodenostomy for Malignant Lower Biliary Tract Obstruction

Kenji Yamao, Kazuo Hara, Nobumasa Mizuno, Susumu Hijioka, Hiroshi Imaoka, Vikram Bhatia, and Yasuhiro Shimizu

Endoscopic ultrasound-guided choledochoduodenostomy (EUS-CDS) is a novel alternative to percutaneous transhepatic biliary drainage, when endoscopic retrograde cholangiopancreatography is unsuccessful in patients with malignant lower biliary obstruction. Some case series and a few prospective studies of EUS-CDS have reported high technical and functional success rates but with the downside of high early complication rates, albeit mostly nonsevere. In addition, the stents placed by EUS-CDS had a longer patency than transpapillary biliary stents.

Endoscopic Ultrasonography-Guided Hepaticogastrostomy

Do Hyun Park

To date, percutaneous transhepatic biliary drainage (PTBD) has been considered as the usual biliary access after failed endoscopic retrograde cholangiopancreatography (ERCP). Since endoscopic ultrasonography (EUS)-guided bile duct puncture was first described in 1996, sporadic case reports of EUS-guided biliary drainage (EUS-BD) have suggested it as an alternative to PTBD after failed ERCP. The potential benefits of EUS-BD include internal drainage, thus avoiding long-term external drainage in cases where external PTBD drainage catheters cannot be internalized. EUS-guided hepaticogastrostomy (EUS-HG) is one form of EUS-BD. This article describes the indications, techniques, and outcomes of published data on EUS-HG.

Endoscopic Ultrasound-Guided Abscess Drainage

Ganapathy A. Prasad and Shyam Varadarajulu

Abdominal and pelvic abscesses have traditionally been drained by percutaneous techniques or surgery. While surgical drainage is associated with considerable morbidity and mortality, percutaneous techniques are associated with the need for multiple interventions, increased length of hospital stay, and an indwelling external catheter for prolonged periods. Endoscopic ultrasound (EUS) is a minimally invasive but highly effective technique that enables internal drainage of the abscess. Although data are limited, evidence supporting its clinical efficacy is increasing rapidly. This article summarizes the current status of EUS-guided approach for drainage of gastrointestinal abscess collections.

Emerging Technologies for Interventional EUS

Endoscopic Ultrasound-Guided Pancreatic Cyst Ablation

John DeWitt

Pancreatic cystic neoplasms represent a wide spectrum of invariably benign to precancerous and malignant tumors. Endoscopic ultrasound-guided

that some diseases, like cancer, lead to a modification in tissue stiffness. Elastography evaluates the elastic properties of tissues and compares images obtained before and after compression to target tissues; differentiating benign from malignant lesions. This article reviews theoretical aspects and the methodology of EUS elastography. Clinical applications, mainly in pancreatic diseases and lymph nodes, are analyzed.

The development of ultrasound contrast agents has allowed for the evaluation of vascularity in digestive organs by contrast-enhanced endoscopic ultrasonography (EUS). Contrast-enhanced Doppler EUS and contrast-enhanced harmonic EUS (CH-EUS) have improved characterization of pancreatic tumors, lymph nodes, and gastrointestinal submucosal tumors and compliment EUS fine-needle aspiration (FNA) in identifying malignant tumors. Moreover, CH-EUS can be used to identify the target for EUS-guided FNA by clearly depicting the outline of the lesions.

With the introduction of curvilinear endosonoscopes, endoscopic ultrasonography (EUS) has achieved the role of a therapeutic modality as well as diagnostic procedure. EUS-guided tumor ablation is one such therapeutic modality. Various techniques of EUS-guided tumor ablation have been described, including radiofrequency ablation, photodynamic therapy, laser ablation, and ethanol injection. Most of the currently described techniques are experimental. Development and continuous improvement of devices, as well as establishment of indications for EUS-guided tumor ablations, are mandatory.

Although some technical challenges in the development of dedicated devices need to be overcome, endoscopic ultrasonography (EUS)-guided anastomosis is promising as a minimally invasive technique for pancreato-biliary diseases.

Recent advances in hepatology have included a new and effective treatment of viral hepatitis, with an increased need for the assessment of liver function and histology. At the same time, there have been a growing number of endoscopic procedures that are pertinent to patients with liver disease. It would be ideal if the assessment and treatment of liver disease and portal hypertension could be performed and assimilated by the liver/gastrointestinal specialist. The authors like to consider this area of integration or overlap of endoscopic procedures within the practice of hepatology as endo-hepatology.

GASTROINTESTINAL ENDOSCOPY CLINICS OF NORTH AMERICA

RELATED INTEREST

Gastroenterology Clinics of North America, March 2012 (Vol. 41, No. 1)
Modern Management of Benign and Malignant Pancreatic Disease
Jacques Van Dam, MD, PhD, *Guest Editor*

NOW AVAILABLE FOR YOUR iPhone and iPad

Foreword

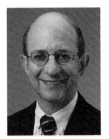

Charles J. Lightdale, MD
Consulting Editor

Almost all endoscopic methods, from EGD and colonoscopy to ERCP, started out primarily with diagnostic intent, but quickly developed therapeutic capabilities that became major factors in their continuing utility, often obtaining results that obviate major surgery. EUS seems now to be following a similar path. Although EUS-guided fine-needle aspiration (FNA) has an "interventional" feel to it, this was strictly a diagnostic method. But then an interesting thing happened. Interventional endoscopists doing ERCP realized that EUS-FNA had a similar focus on the pancreas and biliary tree, and they also learned to do fine-needle injection for celiac neurolysis. Most advanced endoscopy programs began offering training in both ERCP and EUS, and therapeutic applications for EUS blossomed. New devices specifically engineered to facilitate EUS-guided therapies have become available, and more are in the developmental pipeline.

From the beginning, Dr Kenneth J. Chang has been an academic force in the field of therapeutic EUS, and he continues to be at the cutting edge. As Guest Editor for this issue of the *Gastrointestinal Endoscopy Clinics of North America* on "Interventional Endoscopic Ultrasound," he has identified an extraordinary group of experts, who have provided articles on the current state of the art and on EUS-guided therapies under development. Interventional EUS has tremendous potential for growth. I am certain that for all advanced endoscopists and endoscopic ultrasonographers, the "echoes" from this valuable compendium will reverberate far into the future.

Charles J. Lightdale, MD
Department of Medicine
Columbia University Medical Center
161 Fort Washington Avenue, Room 812
New York, NY 10032, USA

E-mail address:
CJL18@columbia.edu

Gastrointest Endoscopy Clin N Am 22 (2012) xiii
doi:10.1016/j.giec.2012.04.022
1052-5157/12/$ – see front matter © 2012 Elsevier Inc. All rights reserved.

Preface

Interventional Endoscopic Ultrasound

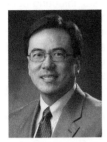

Kenneth J. Chang, MD
Guest Editor

Endoscopic Ultrasound (EUS) has recently turned 30. The previous dedicated volume of the *Gastrointestinal Endoscopy Clinics of North America* to EUS was in 2005 when our fearless consulting editor, Dr Charlie Lightdale, declared EUS as finally "Mainstream!" Now, as a mature adult, EUS is hitting a new stride. EUS images are no longer "Rorschach tests," but quite clear and obvious, even to the novice. EUS-guided fine-needle aspiration (FNA) has gone "viral" across the globe. And as EUS fell into the hands of "therapeutic endoscopists," it became more and more "interventional." Back in 1997, I wrote an article in this series entitled, "Endoscopic ultrasound-guided fine-needle aspiration biopsy and interventional endoscopic ultrasonography: Emerging technologies." At that time, EUS-guided FNA was just beginning to spin off EUS-guided celiac neurolysis, EUS-guided pseudocyst drainage, and the new concept of EUS-guided fine needle injection (FNI).

Dial forward 15 years—previously unimaginable techniques, such as EUS-guided biliary drainage, choledocho-duodenostomy, hepatico-gastrostomy, creation of anastomosis, pancreatico-gastrostomy, pancreatic cyst ablation, abscess drainage, fiducial markers, brachytherapy, vascular access and therapy, tumor ablation, and delivery of antitumor agents, have all emerged within the portfolio of Interventional EUS.

Therefore, Dr Lightdale determined it was high time to dedicate a complete issue to Interventional EUS. To this end, we have assembled world-class endosonographers from Asia, Europe, and the United States, to put in your hands the most concise and authoritative "one-stop-shop" resource for Interventional EUS. The concept of this issue was to devote half of the articles to the current practice of Interventional EUS (including FNA) and the remainder to emerging and future applications. For section one, the authors were challenged to give us evidence-based current "best practice" guidelines for practical issues, such as, which needle should we use for

Disclosures: Dr Chang is consultant for and receives research support from Cook Medical, Inc, Olympus Japan.

Gastrointest Endoscopy Clin N Am 22 (2012) xv–xvi
doi:10.1016/j.giec.2012.04.021
1052-5157/12/$ – see front matter © 2012 Elsevier Inc. All rights reserved.

FNA, how many passes should we make if we don't have a cytologist, which pancreatic cyst should we stick a needle into, what stains should we get for submucosal tumors (SMT), what's our role in lung cancer staging, what are some tricks-of-the-trade for pseudocyst drainage, should we target ganglia during neurolysis, and what is the best EUS approach (or not) after failed ERCP cannulation. Section two, in contrast, focuses on emerging technologies, ie, the more creative side. Here we dive into topics such as instilling chemotherapy into pancreatic cysts, injecting coils and glue into gastric varices, performing needle-based confocal laser induced endomicroscopy (nCLE) and cystoscopy (ie, EUS-guided fine needle imaging), delivering viral "Trojan horses" into cancerous tumors, and presenting a new concept of "Endo-Hepatology." With this blend of practical issues and future prospects, our collective hope is that this volume will become a helpful resource for endosonographers throughout the world. Please join us as we celebrate another milestone for EUS!

Kenneth J. Chang, MD
Division of Gastroenterology and Hepatology
H.H. Chao Comprehensive Digestive Disease Center
University of California, Irvine
101 The City Drive
Orange, CA 92868, USA

E-mail address:
kchang@uci.edu

EUS-Guided FNA of Solid Pancreas Tumors

Muhammad K. Hasan, MD, Robert H. Hawes, MD*

KEYWORDS

- Pancreatic tumors • EUS-FNA • EUS • Pancreatic malignancy

INTRODUCTION

Over the past 2 decades, endoscopic ultrasonography (EUS) has evolved to become an indispensible tool for the evaluation of the pancreas. EUS plays a critical role in the evaluation of the patient with a known or suspected pancreatic mass. Published literature supports the superiority of EUS compared with cross-sectional imaging for tumor detection, with the greatest advantage seen with tumors smaller than 2 to 3 cm.[1] Although the sensitivity for tumor detection is high,[2–4] it is also important to note that it has a very high negative predictive value (NPV).[5,6] This has important implications for the clinician because it means that EUS can reliably exclude pancreatic cancer, especially in the setting of a low or indeterminate pretest probability.[5] Although EUS is not 100% accurate,[7–9] it is the single best choice to detect a pancreatic neoplasm.[2,5,10] It should be noted, however, that cross-sectional imaging techniques (magnetic resonance imaging [MRI] and computed tomography [CT]) are well-standardized procedures, and operator skill is an important factor when performing EUS. As a result, published studies comparing cross-sectional imaging techniques with EUS may not translate into all situations,[11,12] and in clinical practice, the role of CT, MRI, and EUS should be considered complementary.

Although EUS is considered superior to MRI and CT in detecting pancreatic masses, it is the ability to target and place a needle into suspicious lesions (**Fig. 1**) that has made EUS indispensible in the evaluation of patients with solid pancreatic tumors. Endoscopic ultrasound-guided–fine-needle aspiration (EUS-FNA) is an accurate and safe technique to confirm the diagnosis of pancreatic cancer. With the advent of neoadjuvant therapies for pancreatic cancer, most patients with this disease require a tissue diagnosis before initiating treatment. EUS-FNA is now the principal technique applied to obtain the diagnosis of malignancy. We have designed this article to address a number of the key technical aspects of EUS-FNA of solid pancreatic masses.

Center for Interventional Endoscopy, Florida Hospital Orlando, 601 East Rollins Street, Orlando, FL 32803, USA
* Corresponding author.
E-mail address: robert.hawes.md@flhosp.org

Gastrointest Endoscopy Clin N Am 22 (2012) 155–167
doi:10.1016/j.giec.2012.04.016
1052-5157/12/$ – see front matter © 2012 Elsevier Inc. All rights reserved.

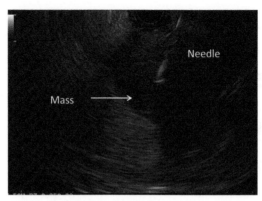

Fig. 1. Endoscopic ultrasound showing a needle in mass.

IS THERE AN OPTIMAL-GAUGE NEEDLE?

EUS-FNA is a well-established modality for cytologic evaluation of solid pancreatic lesions. A principal advantage of EUS compared with CT is the ability to perform FNA at the index examination rather than having to schedule a second examination, as is the case with CT. The precision and safety of EUS-FNA is well established[13–19] and the overall accuracy in establishing a diagnosis of cancer is high.[20–25] In a study by Eloubeidi and colleagues,[26] 101 patients with solid pancreatic masses underwent a median of 4 needle passes with EUS-FNA, resulting in a sensitivity of 95%, specificity of 100%, positive predictive value (PPV) of 100%, and NPV of 85.2%.

EUS-FNA can be performed with 25-gauge, 22-gauge, or 19-gauge needles. Recently, 22-gauge and 19-gauge needles have become available designed with a specially designed side hole, and preliminary studies suggest that they are capable of obtaining a core of tissue suitable for histologic examination (ProCore, Cook Endoscopy, Winston-Salem, NC, USA) (**Fig. 2**). Endosonographers have also had the option of a 19-gauge trucut needle (Cook Endoscopy). This needle is designed with an inner stylet that has a space (tray) cut into it at the distal end. The needle is passed into the mass, the stylet is advanced farther into the mass, and then a spring-fired mechanism is activated that advances the needle over the stylet. The needle is designed to obtain a "core" of tissue, similar to a liver biopsy. Although a larger number of cells are required for certain tests, such as RNA extraction, a diagnosis can usually be made on smears containing fewer than 100 cells. When choosing a particular gauge needle, there are several considerations: (1) which will provide the optimal yield of cells, (2) which will minimize contamination with blood, (3) how much flexibility is required to access the lesion, and (4) which will minimize complications? A smaller-gauge needle may decrease contamination with blood, generally has greater flexibility, and may decrease the potential for bleeding.[27] Historically, the 22-gauge needle has been the needle of choice for FNA of pancreatic lesions. Thinner needles have the disadvantage of not being able to obtain a core specimen for histopathological diagnosis.[25] Having increased flexibility in the needle is particularly important when accessing a lesion in the uncinate process or other positions in the duodenum, when significant tip deflection and maximum elevator are required to pass the needle into the lesion. A prospective study by Sakamoto and colleagues[28] showed that the 25-gauge needle was significantly superior in terms of technical success rate and overall diagnostic accuracy, especially for the lesions in the head and uncinate process of the pancreas, when compared with the standard 22-gauge and the 19-gauge trucut needles. They concluded that the 25-gauge needle was the "best choice" needle for

Procore

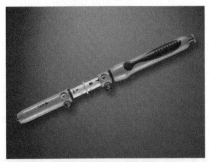

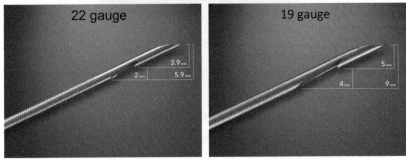

Fig. 2. ProCore needle. (*Courtesy of* ProCore, Cook Endoscopy, Winston-Salem, NC.)

cytologic diagnosis of solid pancreatic lesions. In cases in which a histologic diagnosis is desired, the 22-gauge FNA needle and 19-gauge trucut needle may be at an advantage in head/uncinate and body/tail lesions, respectively. The overall accuracy for the 25-gauge, 22-gauge, and 19-gauge trucut needle in the previously cited study was 91.7%, 79.7%, and 54.1%, respectively. Accuracy for cytologic diagnosis irrespective of the site of lesions with 25-gauge, 22-gauge, and trucut needles was 91.7%, 75.0%, and 45.8%, respectively. For uncinate masses, it was 100.0%, 33.3%, and 0.0%, respectively. With regard to accuracy for histologic diagnosis, the 25-gauge needle was significantly inferior (*P*<.05) to the 22-gauge and trucut needles.

A recently published study[29] compared the rates of diagnostic accuracy, technical success, and complications of EUS-FNA performed with 22-gauge and 25-gauge needles on the same solid pancreatic lesion. Fifty patients underwent EUS-FNA with both 22-gauge and 25-gauge needles with randomization of the needle sequence. The accuracy of the EUS-FNA was determined by comparing the cytologic results with the final surgical pathologic diagnoses or with the results of a clinical follow-up. Technical success was 100% and no complications occurred. Diagnostic accuracy of EUS-FNA was 94% and 86% for the 25-gauge and 22-gauge needles, respectively. Analysis of the cytologic score showed a tendency toward the 25-gauge needle, although the difference was not statistically significant.

In studies that have looked primarily at cytologic yield, some have demonstrated no difference in diagnostic yield, number of passes required, and safety when 25-gauge and 22-gauge needles were compared.[30–32]

In case an on-site cytopathologist is not available, EUS-FNA with a 19-gauge aspiration needle may be a valuable method for the diagnosis of pancreatic/peripancreatic masses. The amount of cellular material obtained by a 19-gauge needle is higher as compared with a smaller-caliber needle.[33] The problem with the use of the standard 19-gauge needle in lesions in the head of the pancreas is that it is often too stiff to allow complete access to the mass. Recently, a new 19-gauge aspiration needle (**Fig. 3**) has been introduced (Flex 19, Boston Scientific, Natick, MA, USA). This needle is made of nitinol and, as a result, is more flexible and does not become distorted after passing over the elevator. More experience will be required to determine its efficacy in accessing lesions in the head of pancreas, safety, and cellular yield, as well as its ability to obtain a core sample for histopathologic analysis.

Given the trade-offs between the different-gauge needles, the clinician's choice of needle should be based on (1) the location of the lesion (head vs body/tail), (2) the nature of the lesion (pancreatic mass vs peripancreatic lymph node), and (3) whether cytology is sufficient or if a core will be needed (solid pancreatic mass vs possible autoimmune pancreatitis). Either 25-gauge or 22-gauge needles can be used for solid masses of the pancreas, but because of its greater flexibility, the 25-gauge needle is the preferred option for lesions in the head of the pancreas, especially the uncinate process. If an on-site cytopathologist is not available or a core specimen may be required, the 22-gauge or 19-gauge Procore or the 19 Flex needle may be better option to obtain a larger sample of tissue.

HOW MANY PASSES DO I MAKE AND IS THERE AN OPTIMAL TECHNIQUE?

The determination of the number of passes to make is dependent on whether or not an experienced cytopathologist is present in the EUS suite to make real-time interpretation

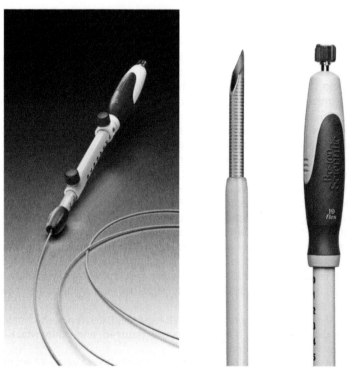

Fig. 3. New 19-gauge aspiration needle. (*Courtesy of* Flex 19, Boston Scientific, Natick, MA.)

of the EUS-FNA specimens.[34–37] If absent, one has to determine the optimal number of samples required to maximize the chance that an accurate diagnosis can be made. LeBlanc and colleagues[38] concluded that 7 is the optimal number of passes for pancreatic masses (sensitivity and specificity of 83% and 100%), whereas 5 passes are optimal for lymph nodes (LNs) (sensitivity and specificity of 77% and 100%). Wallace and colleagues[39] suggested that 3 samples obtained by back-and-forth needle movement for 30 seconds each is sufficient for diagnosis of all malignant LNs. Erickson and colleagues[40] showed that FNA of liver lesions and LNs requires significantly fewer needle passes to obtain adequate diagnostic material as compared with solid tumors of the pancreas. In this study, the investigators suggested that without a cytopathologist in attendance, 5 to 6 passes should be made for pancreatic masses and 2 to 3 for liver metastases or LNs.

There are as many opinions on the optimal technique for EUS-FNA as there are endosonographers. Accurate evaluation of a specific technique is very difficult without introducing bias and, as a result, it is not possible to recommend one specific technique. Our one recommendation is to move the needle through the lesion in a "fanlike pattern" (**Fig. 4**). The trajectory of the needle can be altered using either the "up/down" endoscope dial or the elevator. It is likely that after thrusting the needle deeply into a mass, the path fills with blood on withdrawal of the needle. If one passes the needle back and forth in the same trajectory, one suctions blood into the needle rather than diagnostic cells. In addition, if one feels both soft and firm areas within a pancreatic mass, one should confine the needle movement to the firm areas while avoiding the soft ones, which are usually necrotic. It may be difficult to change the trajectory of the needle in masses located in the uncinate process, which highlights the need for the most flexible needle.

SHOULD I USE SUCTION?

The role of suction during fine-needle sampling is controversial. Suction is thought to increase the cellular yield but may increase the "bloodiness" of the sample, which dilutes diagnostic cells and hinders adequate cytologic analysis.[39] In their study of

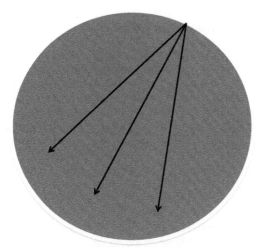

Fig. 4. The authors' recommended technique for EUS-FNA. Move the needle through the lesion in a "fanlike pattern."

100 consecutive patients, Mair and colleagues[41] sampled superficial mass lesions in various body sites with and without syringe suction. The latter technique was termed "fine-needle capillary" (FNC) sampling. The 2 sampling techniques were compared using 5 objective parameters: (1) amount of diagnostic cellular material present, (2) retention of appropriate architecture and cellular arrangement, (3) degree of cellular degeneration, (4) cellular trauma, and (5) volume of obscuring background blood and clots. There was no statistically significant difference between the 2 sampling techniques for any of the parameters studied. In a study of 11 patients, Yue and Zheng[42] found FNC samples caused less trauma and yielded less blood, yet had the same diagnostic yield when compared with FNA. Adequate samples can be obtained in many cases without suction, and when suction is applied, it appears that increasing the suction worsens the specimen quality. In a study using 2 LNs dissected at autopsy, Bhutani and colleagues[43] found that both specimen quality and cellularity were better when lesser degrees of suction were applied with a syringe (10 mL vs 20 mL or 30 mL). If in-room analysis of the FNA sample obtained without suction shows inadequate cellularity, it may be helpful to apply 5 to 10 mL of suction for a few seconds immediately before withdrawing the needle from the lesion. One should also take into consideration the nature of the lesion. Soft lesions (LNs, necrotic and cystic/solid masses) tend to be bloody and avoiding suction is recommended. Very firm lesions tend to be less cellular and suction may be required to obtain adequate cellularity for diagnosis.

Clotting may lead to artifactual grouping of cells. Clotting of blood within the needle can be a particular problem with the smaller-gauge needles. There are 2 ways to overcome this issue. One is to microdissect the clot and tissue fragment with a surgical blade or a separate needle tip and place the fragments in formalin for cell-block preparation. One must be careful because this can cause significant crush effect and render the cells uninterpretable. Another option is to use heparin in the needle.[44] The purpose of heparinizing the needle is to lubricate the lumen of the needle so that tissue material does not stick and to prevent blood from clotting. Care should be taken to avoid using too much heparin, as it can create artifacts, dilute the specimen, and alter cell features. The best way to avoid using too much heparin is to flush the needle with air after filling it with heparin.

DO I NEED AN ON-SITE CYTOPATHOLOGIST?

On-site cytopathology interpretation may not be available in many centers. Up to 32% of FNA interpretation may be "nondiagnostic" because of multiple factors, including scant cellularity and/or "crush artifact" from poor slide preparation.[35] On-site interpretation of FNA specimens has proven to be beneficial for rapid clinical diagnosis.[35,45] Published data suggest that the presence of a cytopathologist during EUS-FNA is cost-effective and useful. Chang and colleagues[46] reported that in the presence of an on-site cytologist during EUS-FNA, adequate specimens were obtained in 100% of patients. In contrast, in the same study, the absence of an on-site cytologist resulted in 29% of patients requiring a second procedure to obtain an adequate specimen. This led to a change in policy at their center, requiring that all EUS-FNA procedures be performed in the presence of an on-site cytologist. Erickson and colleagues[40] also reported that, in addition to prolonging procedure time and potentially increasing the procedural risk from multiple needle passes, the diagnostic yield of EUS-FNA dropped by 10% to 15% when a cytopathologist was not present on-site. In a series of 67 patients[47] with metastatic lung cancer, EUS-FNA with on-site cytopathology interpretation reported a diagnostic accuracy of 92%, thereby avoiding the need for surgery in 68% of patients. Klapman and colleagues[48] also demonstrated that the presence of an on-site cytopathologist improved the diagnostic yield of EUS-FNA. In their study, they reviewed EUS-FNA results from 2 university hospitals. At Center I, 108 patients underwent EUS-FNA in the presence of an on-site cytopathologist. At Center II, 87 patients underwent EUS-FNA in the absence of cytopathologist. All procedures at both hospitals were performed by the same endosonographer. At Center I, a definite diagnosis of positive or negative for malignancy was reported in 78% compared with 52% for Center II ($P = .001$), and the proportion of patients with an unsatisfactory specimen was 9% compared with 20% in Center II ($P = .035$).

These results are not limited to EUS-FNA alone. In a large review of 5688 patients by Nasuti and colleagues,[35] all FNA procedures performed by ultrasound, CT, bronchoscopy, fluoroscopy, and EUS over a period of 5 years were included. The proportion of nondiagnostic specimens was 0.98%, which compared with the published rate of nondiagnostic FNA (20%) when onsite cytologic evaluation was not present. The investigators also reported a significant cost benefit of $404,525 per year by decreasing the number of repeat FNA procedures owing to nondiagnostic specimens.

Alsohaibani and colleagues[49] in their retrospective study in 2009 suggested that on-site cytotechnologist interpretation of adequacy of tissue sampling significantly improves the diagnostic yield of EUS-FNA and this appears to be independent of the total number of needle passes undertaken for tissue sampling. The patients were divided into 2 groups. In group I, slides were prepared by an endoscopy nurse (n = 47) and in group II, slides were prepared by an on-site cytotechnologist (n = 55). Pancreatic masses were the most common target site in both groups. The total number of needle passes was 105 in group I (mean 2.14 passes per patient; range 1 to 5) and 158 in group II (mean 2.63 passes per patient; range 1 to 4). The difference in the number of needle passes was not statistically significant between groups. The final diagnosis was definite in 53% in group I compared with 77% in group II ($P = .01$). The percentage of inconclusive diagnoses was 47% in group I and 23% in group II ($P = .001$). These data suggest that if an on-site cytopathologist cannot be provided, a trained cytopathology technician (or specially train yourself or an EUS nurse) should be present to provide an assessment of "specimen adequacy," as this will positively affect the diagnostic yield of EUS-FNA.

HOW SHOULD THE SPECIMENS BE STAINED?

A smear is the standard method of preparing slides of EUS-FNA specimens. Two types of smears can be prepared from the FNA specimen: air dried or alcohol fixed. Air-dried smears are stained rapidly with Diff-Quik and used for immediate cytologic evaluation. Alcohol fixation preserves nuclear features and is stained by papanicolau or hematoxylin and eosin (H&E) stains. For lesions that may require special staining, however, cell-block preparation is recommended. For cell block, the FNA specimen is placed into liquid media and sent to the laboratory where it is spun into a pellet, formalin fixed, paraffin embedded, and sectioned for standard H&E staining.[50] Liquid-based cytology (Thin prep: Cytyc Inc., Marlborough, MA, USA, and SurePath: TriPath Inc., Burlington, NC, USA) is an automated process designed to minimize the technical problems associated with manual preparation. This method provides high cell preservation and uniform monolayer dispersion of cells into a confined area of the slide.[51,52] Disadvantages of this method include increased cost and inability to provide immediate cytologic assessment to the endosonographer unless the specimen is split into 2 parts, one for Diff-Quik and the other for liquid prep. This preparation may also lead to loss of background mucin, which is problematic, as this is an important diagnostic clue for mucin-producing pancreatic tumors. De Luna and colleagues[53] compared conventional preparations with liquid-based preparation. EUS specimens were split for conventional and liquid-based preparations. Although conventional smears in this study had significantly better diagnostic index, the study provided a proof of principle for this application of cytology. Given the small number of studies of liquid-based EUS-FNA samples, more data are required before this method is more widely adopted.[54] A recently published study by LeBlanc and colleagues[55] showed that the smear method is more sensitive and accurate than ThinPrep in detecting malignancy in pancreatic and LN EUS-FNA samples. They conducted a study of 130 patients who underwent EUS-FNA of 139 sites (50 pancreas, 89 LN). Malignancy was confirmed in 47 pancreas samples (94%) and 48 LN samples (54%). The mean ± SD number of passes made for the smear method was 2.6 ± 1.3. For pancreatic cancer, the sensitivity, specificity, PPV, NPV, and accuracy of the ThinPrep versus the smear method was 62% versus 98%, 100% versus 100%, 100% versus 100%, 14% versus 75%, and 64% versus 98%, respectively.

A new technology called contrast harmonic echo (CHE) has been developed for endoscopic ultrasound. It may improve accuracy in diagnosis of solid pancreatic masses, particularly when trying to differentiate an inflammatory from a neoplastic mass. It may also help guide EUS-FNA. A hyper-enhancing pattern could indicate an inflammatory process and a hypo-enhancing and inhomogeneous mass can strengthen the suspicion of pancreatic adenocarcinoma.[56] The combination of optimal targeting of a lesion (perhaps using CHE) and optimal staining methods has great promise in optimizing the diagnostic accuracy of EUS-FNA.

In cases in which initial cytology is indeterminate, combining routine cytology with fluorescence in situ hybridization (FISH) and K-ras/p53 analysis may improve the diagnostic yield. Reicher and colleagues[57] retrospectively analyzed 50 EUS-FNAs of pancreatic masses in 46 patients. Thirteen initial cytologic samples (26%) were benign, 23 malignant (46%), and 14 atypical (28%). They performed FISH for p16, p53, LPL, c-Myc, MALT1, topoisomerase 2/human epidermal growth factor receptor 2, as well as K-ras/p53 mutational analysis. On final diagnosis, 11 (79%) of atypical FNAs were malignant, and 3 (21%) were benign. FISH was negative in all benign and all atypical samples with final benign diagnosis. FISH plus K-ras analysis correctly identified 60% of atypical FNAs with a final malignant diagnosis. The combination of routine cytology with FISH and K-ras analysis yielded 87.9% sensitivity, 93.8% specificity, 96.7% PPV, 78.9% NPV, and 89.8% accuracy. Kubiliun and colleagues[58] suggested that in patients with suspected pancreatic cancer, FISH analysis can detect additional cases missed by cytology without compromising specificity. FISH analysis to detect polysomy of chromosomes 3, 7, and 17 and deletion of 9p21can be considered when cytology is negative for malignancy in patients with a known pancreatic mass.

HOW DO I MANAGE A NONDIAGNOSTIC FNA?

It is often difficult to diagnose pancreatic cancer in the background of chronic pancreatitis.[59,60] Even in experienced hands, this may be the most common reason for a false-negative EUS-FNA. Also, if the lesion is in the uncinate process or neck of the pancreas, it may be difficult to visualize the lesion and/or obtain tissue. At present, there is no universally accepted protocol on how to manage patients who present with a clinical history and/or imaging suggestive of pancreatic malignancy, but have negative cytology by EUS-FNA. The 3 most viable options are (1) clinical observation with repeat imaging ± FNA in 2 to 4 months (invariably stressful on the patient and

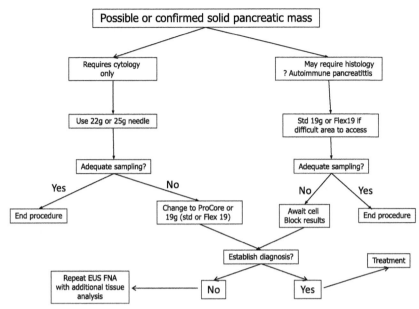

Fig. 5. Diagnosis and treatment algorithm for solid pancreatic mass.

family), (2) surgical exploration, or (3) CT-guided biopsy. CT-guided biopsy is less favorable because of the risk of seeding the needle track and causing a worse outcome even in patients who are not surgical candidates.[61] If suspicion of malignancy is very high, the patient is a good operative candidate, and the lesion appears to be resectable, then the best option is often surgery. As the degree of suspicion for malignancy decreases, the health of the patient decreases, and the resectability becomes more marginal, then repeat imaging and tissue sampling is probably the best course of action. If suspicion is very high but the patient or surgeon is reluctant to move forward with open or laparoscopic exploration, then repeat EUS-FNA has been shown to be another viable option. In this setting, Eloubeidi and colleagues[62] reported repeat EUS-FNA to have an accuracy of 84% in a series of 24 patients. DeWitt and colleagues[63] reported that repeat examination had a clinical impact in 63% of patients and Nicaud and colleagues[64] had an overall accuracy of 61% of patients with repeat EUS-FNA. The literature supports reattempting EUS-FNA, and this is an appealing strategy because of the safety profile for EUS-FNA. On the second EUS-FNA, it may be advisable to combine routine cytology with FISH and K-ras/p53 analysis to improve diagnostic yield.[57,58]

SUMMARY

In this article, we have tried to address some of the challenges of EUS-FNA for solid pancreatic masses. There is no clear optimal-gauge needle in all scenarios, but the take-home points are that smaller-gauge needles have similar cytology yields as large-gauge needles but have the added advantage of greater flexibility for difficult-to-reach areas, such as the uncinate process. In the future, technology may allow greater flexibility in larger-bore needles and then the advantage may sway toward this option, especially if analysis of core samples becomes important in determining optimal treatment.

There is consensus opinion that on-site cytopathology with real-time interpretation of samples is best for optimal patient care. If this cannot be provided, 5 to 7 passes for pancreatic masses and 3 to 4 passes for peripancreatic LNs will provide the maximal yield. If a cytopathologist is not available on-site, however, then one should insist on having an experienced cytopathology technician or to specifically train an EUS nurse to prepare and determine cellular adequacy for each sample.

Suction is not needed for soft lesions and LNs. Gentle suction can be accomplished by withdrawing the stylet as the needle is moved through the lesion. If initial samples without suction are not obtaining adequate cellularity, then suction can be applied with subsequent passes.

Air-dried specimens stained with Diff-Quik is the standard for optimal real-time interpretation. Excess sample should be placed in liquid media and sent for cell block. For indeterminate samples, one can add FISH and K-ras/p53 analysis to improve accuracy.

In cases in which the initial EUS-FNA is negative for malignancy, if suspicion remains high, surgical exploration or repeat EUS-FNA is advised. If suspicion is moderate to low, then repeat imaging ± FNA in 2 to 4 months is a good option.

Indications and a clinical algorithm are shown in **Fig. 5**.

REFERENCES

1. Rösch T, Lorenz R, Braig C, et al. [Endoscopic ultrasound in small pancreatic tumors]. Z Gastroenterol 1991;29:110–5 [in German].
2. Varadarajulu S, Eloubeidi MA. The role of endoscopic ultrasonography in the evaluation of pancreatico-biliary cancer. Gastrointest Endosc Clin N Am 2005; 15:497–511.
3. Chang KJ. State of the art lecture: endoscopic ultrasound (EUS) and FNA in pancreatico-biliary tumors. Endoscopy 2006;38(Suppl 1):S56–60.
4. Buscail L, Faure P, Bournet B, et al. Interventional endoscopic ultrasound in pancreatic diseases. Pancreatology 2006;6:7–16.
5. Săftoiu A, Vilmann P. Role of endoscopic ultrasound in the diagnosis and staging of pancreatic cancer. J Clin Ultrasound 2009;37:1–17.
6. Klapman JB, Chang KJ, Lee JG, et al. Negative predictive value of endoscopic ultrasound in a large series of patients with a clinical suspicion of pancreatic cancer. Am J Gastroenterol 2005;100:2658–61.
7. Rösch T, Lightdale CJ, Botet JF, et al. Localization of pancreatic endocrine tumors by endoscopic ultrasonography. N Engl J Med 1992;326:1721–6.
8. Schumacher B, Lübke HJ, Frieling T, et al. Prospective study on the detection of insulinomas by endoscopic ultrasonography. Endoscopy 1996;28:273–6.
9. Bhutani MS, Gress FG, Giovannini M, et al. The No Endosonographic Detection of Tumor (NEST) Study: a case series of pancreatic cancers missed on endoscopic ultrasonography. Endoscopy 2004;36:385–9.
10. Hunt GC, Faigel DO. Assessment of EUS for diagnosing, staging, and determining resectability of pancreatic cancer: a review. Gastrointest Endosc 2002; 55:232–7.
11. Wiersema MJ. Accuracy of endoscopic ultrasound in diagnosing and staging pancreatic carcinoma. Pancreatology 2001;1:625–32.
12. Papanikolaou IS, Adler A, Neumann U, et al. Endoscopic ultrasound in pancreatic disease—its influence on surgical decision-making. An update 2008. Pancreatology 2009;9:55–65.

13. Giovannini M, Seitz JF, Monges G, et al. Fine-needle aspiration cytology guided by endoscopic ultrasonography: results in 141 patients. Endoscopy 1995;27:171–7.
14. Wiersema MJ, Vilmann P, Giovannini M, et al. Endosonography-guided fine-needle aspiration biopsy: diagnostic accuracy and complication assessment. Gastroenterology 1997;112:1087–95.
15. Chang KJ, Nguyen P, Erickson RA, et al. The clinical utility of endoscopic ultrasound-guided fine-needle aspiration in the diagnosis and staging of pancreatic carcinoma. Gastrointest Endosc 1997;45:387–93.
16. Bhutani MS, Hawes RH, Baron PL, et al. Endoscopic ultrasound guided fine needle aspiration of malignant pancreatic lesions. Endoscopy 1997;29:854–8.
17. Lai R, Stanley MW, Bardales R, et al. Endoscopic ultrasound-guided pancreatic duct aspiration: diagnostic yield and safety. Endoscopy 2002;34:715–20.
18. Levy MJ, Jondal ML, Clain J, et al. Preliminary experience with an EUS-guided trucut biopsy needle compared with EUS-guided FNA. Gastrointest Endosc 2003;57:101–6.
19. Larghi A, Verna EC, Stavropoulos SN, et al. EUS-guided trucut needle biopsies in patients with solid pancreatic masses: a prospective study. Gastrointest Endosc 2004;59:185–90.
20. Pinto MM, Avila NA, Criscuolo EM. Fine needle aspiration of pancreas, a five-year experience. Acta Cytol 1988;32:39–42.
21. Johnson DE, Pendurthi TK, Balshem AM, et al. Implications of fine-needle aspiration in patients with resectable pancreatic cancer. Am Surg 1997;63:675–9.
22. Voss M, Hammel P, Molas G, et al. Value of endoscopic ultrasound guided fine needle aspiration biopsy in the diagnosis of solid pancreatic masses. Gut 2000;46:244–9.
23. O'Toole D, Palazzo L, Arotçarena R, et al. Assessment of complications of EUS-guided fine-needle aspiration. Gastrointest Endosc 2001;53:470–4.
24. Mertz H, Gautam S. The learning curve for EUS-guided FNA of pancreatic cancer. Gastrointest Endosc 2004;59:33–7.
25. Itoi T, Itokawa F, Sofuni A, et al. Puncture of solid pancreatic tumors guided by endoscopic ultrasonography: a pilot study series comparing trucut and 19-gauge and 22-gauge aspiration needle. Endoscopy 2005;37:362–6.
26. Eloubeidi MA, Jhala D, Chhieng DC, et al. Yield of endoscopic ultrasound-guided fine-needle aspiration biopsy in patients with suspected pancreatic carcinoma. Cancer 2003;99:285–92.
27. VanSonnenberg E, Goodacre BW, Wittich GR, et al. Image-guided 25-guage needle biopsy for thoracic lesions: diagnostic feasibility and safety. Radiology 2003; 227:414–8.
28. Sakamoto H, Kitan M, Komaki T, et al. Prospective comparative study of the EUS guided 25-gauge FNA needle with the 19-gauge Trucut needle and 22-gauge FNA needle in patients with solid pancreatic masses. Gastroenterol Hepatol 2009;24:384–90.
29. Fabbri C, Polifemo AM, Luigiano C, et al. Endoscopic ultrasound-guided fine needle aspiration with 22- and 25-gauge needles in solid pancreatic masses: a prospective comparative study with randomisation of needle sequence. Dig Liver Dis 2011;43(8):647–52.
30. Imazu H, Uchiyama Y, Kakutani H, et al. A prospective comparison of EUS-guided FNA using 25-gauge and 22-gauge needles. Gastroenterol Res Pract 2009;2009: 546390.
31. Siddiqui UD, Rossi F, Rosenthal LS, et al. EUS-guided FNA of solid pancreatic masses: a prospective, randomized trial comparing 22-gauge and 25-gauge needles. Gastrointest Endosc 2009;70(6):1098–100.

32. Siddiqui AA, Lyles T, Avula H, et al. Endoscopic ultrasound-guided fine needle aspiration of pancreatic masses in a veteran population: comparison of results with 22- and 25-gauge needles. Pancreas 2010;39(5):685–6.

33. Song TJ, Kim JH, Lee SS, et al. The prospective randomized, controlled trial of endoscopic ultrasound-guided fine-needle aspiration using 22G and 19G aspiration needles for solid pancreatic or peripancreatic masses. Am J Gastroenterol 2010;105(8):1739–45.

34. Pellise Urquiza M, Fernandez-Esparrach G, Sole M, et al. Endoscopic ultrasound-guided fine needle aspiration: predictive factors of accurate diagnosis and cost-minimization analysis of on-site pathologist. Gastroenterol Hepatol 2007;30: 319–24.

35. Nasuti JF, Gupta PK, Baloch ZW. Diagnostic value and cost-effectiveness of on-site evaluation of fine-needle aspiration specimens: review of 5,688 cases. Diagn Cytopathol 2002;27:1–4.

36. Layfield LJ, Bentz JS, Gopez EV. Immediate on-site interpretation of fine-needle aspiration smears: a cost and compensation analysis. Cancer 2001; 93:319–22.

37. Diacon AH, Schuurmans MM, Theron J, et al. Utility of rapid on-site evaluation of transbronchial needle aspirates. Respiration 2005;72:182–8.

38. LeBlanc JK, Ciaccia D, Al-Assi MT, et al. Optimal number of EUS-guided fine needle passes needed to obtain a correct diagnosis. Gastrointest Endosc 2004;59: 475–81.

39. Wallace MB, Kennedy T, Durkalski V, et al. Randomized controlled trial of EUS-guided fine needle aspiration techniques for the detection of malignant lymphadenopathy. Gastrointest Endosc 2000;54:441–7.

40. Erickson RA, Sayage-Rabie L, Beissner RS. Factors predicting the number of EUS-guided fine-needle passes for diagnosis of pancreatic malignancies. Gastrointest Endosc 2000;51:184–90.

41. Mair S, Dunbar F, Becker PJ, et al. Fine needle cytology—is aspiration suction necessary? A study of 100 masses in various sites. Acta Cytol 1989;33:809–13.

42. Yue XH, Zheng SF. Cytologic diagnosis by transthoracic fine needle sampling without aspiration. Acta Cytol 1989;33:805–8.

43. Bhutani MS, Suryaprasad S, Moezzi J, et al. Improved technique for performing endoscopic ultrasound guided fine needle aspiration of lymph nodes. Endoscopy 1999;31:550–3.

44. Kasugai H, Tatsuta YR, Okano Y, et al. Value of heparinized fine needle aspiration biopsy in liver malignancy. Am J Roentgenol 1985;144:243–4.

45. Campisi P, Accinelli G, De Angelis C, et al. [On-site evaluation and triage for endoscopic ultrasound-guided fine needle aspiration cytology. The Turin experience]. Minerva Med 2007;98:395–400 [in Italian].

46. Chang KJ, Katz KD, Durbin TE, et al. Endoscopic ultrasound guided fine-needle aspiration. Gastrointest Endosc 1994;40:694–9.

47. Tournoy KG, Praet MM, Van Maele G, et al. Esophageal endoscopic ultrasound with fine-needle aspiration with an on-site cytopathologist: high accuracy for the diagnosis of mediastinal lymphadenopathy. Chest 2005;128:3004–9.

48. Klapman JB, Logrono R, Dye CE, et al. Clinical impact of on-site cytopathology interpretation on endoscopic ultrasound-guided fine needle aspiration. Am J Gastroenterol 2003;98:1289–94.

49. Alsohaibani F, Girgis S, Sandha GS. Does onsite cytotechnology evaluation improve the accuracy of endoscopic ultrasound-guided fine-needle aspiration biopsy? Can J Gastroenterol 2009;23(1):26–30.

50. Koss LG. Diagnostic cytology and its histopathologic basis, vol. 2. 3rd edition. Philadelphia: JB Lippincott; 1979.
51. Lee KR, Papillo JL, St John R, et al. Evaluation of the ThinPrep processor for fine needle aspiration specimens. Acta Cytol 1996;40:895–9.
52. Michael CW, McConnel J, Pecott J, et al. Comparison of ThinPrep and TriPath prep liquid based preparations in nongynecological specimens: a pilot study. Diagn Cytopathol 2001;25:177–84.
53. de Luna R, Eloubeidi MA, Sheffield MV, et al. Comparison of ThinPrep and conventional preparations in pancreatic fine needle aspiration biopsy. Diagn Cytopathol 2004;30:71–6.
54. Rossi ED, Larghi A, Verna EC, et al. Endoscopic ultrasound-guided fine-needle aspiration with liquid-based cytologic preparation in the diagnosis of primary pancreatic lymphoma. Pancreas 2010;39(8):1299–302.
55. LeBlanc JK, Emerson RE, Dewitt J, et al. A prospective study comparing rapid assessment of smears and ThinPrep for endoscopic ultrasound-guided fine-needle aspirates. Endoscopy 2010;42(5):389–94.
56. Fusaroli P, Spada A, Mancino MG, et al. Contrast harmonic echo-endoscopic ultrasound improves accuracy in diagnosis of solid pancreatic masses. Clin Gastroenterol Hepatol 2010;8(7):629–34.
57. Reicher S, Boyar FZ, Albitar M, et al. Fluorescence in situ hybridization and K-ras analyses improve diagnostic yield of endoscopic ultrasound-guided fine-needle aspiration of solid pancreatic masses. Pancreas 2011;40(7):1057–62.
58. Kubiliun N, Ribeiro A, Fan YS, et al. EUS-FNA with rescue fluorescence in situ hybridization for the diagnosis of pancreatic carcinoma in patients with inconclusive on-site cytopathology results. Gastrointest Endosc 2011;74(3):541–7.
59. Varadarajulu S, Tamhane A, Eloubeidi MA. Yield of EUS-guided FNA of pancreatic masses in the presence or the absence of chronic pancreatitis. Gastrointest Endosc 2005;62:728–36.
60. Fritscher-Ravens A, Brand L, Knofel WT, et al. Comparison of endoscopic ultrasound-guided fine needle aspiration for focal pancreatic lesions in patients with normal parenchyma and chronic pancreatitis. Am J Gastroenterol 2002;97: 2768–75.
61. Micames C, Jowell PS, White R, et al. Lower frequency of peritoneal carcinomatosis in patients with pancreatic cancer diagnosed by EUS-guided FNA vs. percutaneous FNA. Gastrointest Endosc 2003;58(5):690–5.
62. Eloubeidi MA, Varadarajulu S, Desai S, et al. Value of repeat endoscopic ultrasound-guided fine needle aspiration for suspected pancreatic cancer. J Gastroenterol Hepatol 2008;23(4):567–70.
63. DeWitt J, McGreevy K, Sherman S, et al. Utility of a repeated EUS at a tertiary-referral center. Gastrointest Endosc 2008;67(4):610–9.
64. Nicaud M, Hou W, Collins D, et al. The utility of repeat endoscopic ultrasound-guided fine needle aspiration for suspected pancreatic cancer. Gastroenterol Res Pract 2010;2010:268290.

Endoscopic Ultrasonography-Guided Fine-Needle Aspiration of Pancreatic Cystic Lesions: A Practical Approach to Diagnosis and Management

Jason B. Samarasena, MD[a], Yousuke Nakai, MD, PhD[a,b], Kenneth J. Chang, MD[a],*

KEYWORDS

• Fine-needle aspiration • Pancreatic cystic lesions
• Cyst analysis • Endoscopic ultrasonography • Tumor markers

INTRODUCTION

Pancreatic cysts are common in the general population. The reported incidence of cysts varies widely in the literature, ranging from 0.7% to 24.3%.[1–3] The incidence estimated from cross-sectional imaging is lower than that estimated from autopsy studies. The incidence of truly asymptomatic cysts in the general population is estimated to be around 2.6% and increases with advancing age.[2] In the last 2 decades the proportion of pancreatic resections performed for cystic lesions has grown substantially. As pancreatic cysts can be either benign or neoplastic, with variable malignant potential based on their subtype, there has been a substantial effort to establish an accurate preoperative diagnosis using minimally invasive techniques.

[a] Division of Gastroenterology and Hepatology, H.H. Chao Comprehensive Digestive Disease Center, University of California, Irvine, 101 The City Drive, Orange, CA 92868, USA; [b] Department of Gastroenterology, Graduate School of Medicine, The University of Tokyo, 7-3-1 Hongo, Bunkyo-ku, Tokyo 113-8655, Japan
* Corresponding author.
E-mail address: kchang@uci.edu

Gastrointest Endoscopy Clin N Am 22 (2012) 169–185
doi:10.1016/j.giec.2012.04.007
1052-5157/12/$ – see front matter © 2012 Elsevier Inc. All rights reserved.
giendo.theclinics.com

Endoscopic ultrasonography has been a valuable tool in this effort, given its ability to provide not only high-resolution imaging of these cysts but also the ability to safely aspirate cyst fluid for detailed analysis.

TYPES OF PANCREATIC CYSTIC LESIONS

Pancreatic cysts can be classified as either neoplastic or nonneoplastic. Nonneoplastic cysts include pseudocysts, retention cysts, lymphoepithelial cysts, duplication cysts, and infectious cysts. Neoplastic pancreatic cysts comprise a heterogeneous group of lesions that are histopathologically different and demonstrate a diverse natural history. These cysts can be broadly classified as mucinous and nonmucinous cysts. Nonmucinous neoplastic cysts include serous cystadenoma (SCA) and solid pseudopapillary neoplasm (SPN). Mucinous cysts are premalignant lesions, and include mucinous cystic neoplasm (MCN) and intraductal papillary mucinous neoplasm (IPMN). IPMN can be further divided into a main-duct subtype and a branched-duct subtype, depending on the relationship with the main pancreatic duct. The main-duct subtype is considered to carry a higher risk of malignancy than the side-branch subtype.[4] Morphologic variations of IPMNs have also been recognized, with 4 distinct subtypes distinguished based on the histomorphologic features of papillae and the immunohistochemical features of mucin glycoproteins. Recent consensus studies have labeled these IPMN types as gastric, intestinal, pancreaticobiliary, and oncocytic, and suggest that each type may demonstrate a distinct clinical course.[5]

DIAGNOSTIC MODALITIES TO EVALUATE PANCREATIC CYSTS

Differentiating among these cysts is challenging, and a variety of modalities including cross-sectional imaging, endoscopic imaging, cytology, and cyst fluid analysis have been found to be useful. The 2 noninvasive imaging modalities used most frequently to evaluate pancreatic cysts are computed tomography (CT) and magnetic resonance imaging (MRI). CT is a good test for cystic lesions of the pancreas because of its widespread availability and ability to detect cysts, and it is often the modality with which cystic lesions are initially suspected or diagnosed. Pancreas protocol CT scanning has become a preferred modality to evaluate the pancreas given its ease, relatively low expense, and accuracy with cyst detection. Pancreas protocol uses an intravenous contrast bolus timed for both arterial and venous phases, typically with water as the oral contrast, to minimize artifacts arising from denser contrast media. MRI has the advantage over CT of not involving ionizing radiation, and MR cholangiopancreatography (MRCP) has the added benefit of being able to examine the relationship of the lesion and the pancreatic duct in a noninvasive manner. T2-weighted images acquired on MRI (both MRCP and cross-sectional MRI) are excellent for serial follow-up of cyst size. Both CT and MRI, however, have limited ability in differentiating between mucinous and nonmucinous cystic lesions of the pancreas.[6,7]

Endoscopic retrograde cholangiopancreatography (ERCP), although more invasive than MRCP, is very useful in defining the communication of the cyst with the main pancreatic duct and provides another method for tissue acquisition. However, diagnostic ERCP, with its associated risk of pancreatitis, has largely been replaced by MRCP and endoscopic ultrasonography (EUS).

EUS has many attributes that make the procedure an ideal tool for evaluation of cystic lesions in the pancreas. EUS is a low-risk procedure that produces high-resolution imaging of the pancreas (both parenchyma and ducts) and surrounding structures. More importantly, it affords the ability to sample cyst contents for analysis.

The diagnostic accuracy of EUS morphology alone is widely variable. In a large prospective multicenter trial using morphologic criteria to distinguish mucinous cysts (macrocystic septations or adjacent mass) from nonmucinous cystic lesions (unilocular, honeycombed, or thickened wall), the sensitivity and specificity were low, at 56% and 45%, respectively, which resulted in a poor accuracy of 51%.[8] Furthermore, a study by Ahmad and colleagues[9] evaluated the degree of agreement among endosonographers for EUS diagnosis of neoplastic versus nonneoplastic pancreatic cystic lesions and the specific type of lesion. There was only fair agreement between endosonographers for the diagnosis of neoplastic versus nonneoplastic lesions ($\kappa = 0.24$). Agreement of individual types of lesions was moderately good for serous cystadenoma ($\kappa = 0.46$) but only fair for the remainder of lesions. As a result, the investigators concluded that there is little more than chance interobserver agreement among experienced endosonographers for the diagnosis of neoplastic versus nonneoplastic and specific type of pancreatic cystic lesions. The reason for this low diagnostic accuracy, despite excellent visualization by EUS, probably lies in the considerable overlap of morphologic features among the different kinds of cystic structures.

INDICATIONS FOR EUS-GUIDED FINE-NEEDLE ASPIRATION

The imaging modalities discussed are very sensitive for detecting pancreatic cystic neoplasms. However, once a pancreatic cystic lesion is identified, the key clinical issue becomes diagnosis of the cyst type, at the least categorizing the cyst as benign, premalignant, or malignant, to guide subsequent management decisions. Imaging information alone is often not sufficient to accurately characterize the lesions. In cases of diagnostic uncertainty, EUS-guided fine-needle aspiration (EUS-FNA) can be valuable because of its ability to evaluate viscosity, cytology, chemistry, tumor markers, and molecular arrangement in the cyst fluid. As such, the American Society of Gastrointestinal Endoscopy support the use of EUS-FNA for pancreatic cyst diagnosis.[10] However, before performing EUS-FNA, the question must be asked as to how management would be affected by the information obtained. For example, in the case of a macrocystic lesion in the head of the pancreas, given the operative morbidity with a resection of a pancreatic head cyst, confirmation that the cyst is mucinous before surgery is advisable. Alternatively, if the patient is symptomatic and is a good surgical candidate, resection without EUS-FNA may be the appropriate next step. Similarly, if a lesion is a benign-appearing unilocular cyst, or the lesion has characteristic morphology for SCA or demonstrates overt malignant features, the incremental value of FNA to confirm the clinical impression may be limited.

Cyst size is often the most important determinant of success for cyst aspiration and acquisition of adequate fluid for analysis. Walsh and colleagues[11] conducted a study to determine whether cyst size or cyst location predicted success of cyst fluid collection and analysis. It was concluded that successful aspiration of cysts was independent of cyst location in the pancreas and that the larger the cyst, the larger number of diagnostic variables (cytology, carcinoembryonic antigen [CEA], amylase) were able to be obtained. The investigators stated that a minimum cyst size of 1.5 cm was needed to successfully result in at least 1 variable with an 84% success rate. The authors agree with this threshold of 1.5 cm, and endorse FNA of pancreatic cysts 1.5 cm or larger.

VISCOSITY

In an early study by Lewandrowski and colleagues,[12] pancreatic cyst fluid was obtained by surgical exploration, and relative viscosity (RV) was measured using a viscometer. Water was used as a standard, and had an RV equal to 1. Cyst fluid from serous cystadenomas and pseudocysts had mean RV values of 1.24 and 1.25, respectively. By contrast, mean RV values of mucinous cysts were significantly higher, ranging from 1.2 to 30. In this study it was calculated that an RV of less than 1.63 seemed helpful for distinguishing mucinous from nonmucinous cystic lesions, with an 89% sensitivity and 100% specificity. Similar findings were found in a more recent study by Linder and colleagues,[13] who concluded that viscosity greater than 1.6 predicted mucinous cystic adenoma/adenocarcinoma.

In a study by Leung and colleagues,[14] a novel surrogate marker of cyst viscosity was used, described as the "string sign." This test, which was performed by the endosonographer, was determined by placing a drop of fluid between the thumb and index finger and measuring the maximum length of stretch before disruption of the mucous string. Benign lesions in the study had a median string length of 0 mm compared with a significantly longer string length of 3.5 mm in potentially malignant/malignant cysts (P<.0001). The investigators concluded that a long string sign was associated with premalignant or malignant lesions.[14] The string sign is a simple manual technique that can quickly and easily be performed at the time of EUS-FNA and may complement existing tests. The authors use the string sign routinely, and believe that a positive string sign is highly predictive of a mucinous lesion.

CYTOLOGY

Pancreatic cystic neoplasms have epithelial cells that either are columnar and stain for mucin (in mucinous neoplasms) or are cuboidal and stain for glycogen (in SCA). These cell types are easily distinguishable by cytology and when positive results are yielded, cytology is one of the most accurate methods of cyst diagnosis. However, obtaining sufficient cells for diagnostic cytology is often difficult because of the limited volume and low cellularity of aspirated cyst fluid, with sensitivity generally less than 50%.[8,15,16] In a large multicenter study from the United States, for diagnosis of a MCN based on cytology the sensitivity was 35%, specificity 83%, and accuracy 59%, which was similar to the overall accuracy of EUS morphology.[8] By contrast, in a single-center study[17] whereby all the cytopathologic examinations were performed by the same pathologist, FNA provided a correct diagnosis in 65 of 67 cases. In this study, 77% of the FNA contained enough material for definitive diagnosis. Sensitivity, specificity, positive predictive value (PPV), and negative predictive value (NPV) was 97%, 100%, 100%, and 95%, respectively.[17] A pooled analysis including the aforementioned studies and 5 others that evaluated cytologic examination calculated sensitivities of diagnosing mucinous neoplasm, malignancy, and SCA at 45%, 48%, and 38%, respectively.[16]

A recent study by Rogart and colleagues[18] showed that EUS-FNA with cyst-wall puncture increased the cytologic yield by 37% compared with simple FNA with fluid analysis alone. The investigators in this study used a 22-gauge FNA needle and sent fluid for CEA and amylase if at least 1 mL was obtained for each. Any additional fluid beyond 2 mL was sent for cytology. Without removing the needle, FNA of the cyst wall was then performed by puncturing the far wall of the cyst and moving the needle back and forth through the wall to sample the wall epithelium. For 32 cysts in the study, despite inadequate fluid obtained for CEA or fluid cytology, cyst-wall puncture was performed and a positive diagnosis was still obtained in 15 of 32 cysts (47%). These results are very encouraging, and this technique warrants further study.

CHEMISTRY

Amylase and lipase levels can be elevated in any cystic lesion having a communication with the pancreatic ductal system, such as pseudocysts, IPMN, and also some

MCN.[16,19] As a result, elevated amylase levels are often not helpful clinically in differentiating mucinous from nonmucinous cysts. A low amylase level, however, can be helpful because pseudocysts rarely demonstrate low amylase level in cyst fluid. In a pooled analysis by Van der Waaij and colleagues[16] evaluating amylase concentration in a total of 155 cysts, an amylase level of less than 250 U/L indicated SCA, mucinous cystadenoma, or mucinous cystadenocarcinoma, with sensitivity of 44%, specificity of 98%, PPV 98%, NPV 53%, and accuracy 65%, thus virtually excluding pseudocyst.

A recent single-center study by Park and colleagues[19] found that amylase may also be helpful in differentiating benign from malignant mucinous cysts. The study included 126 patients, and evaluated CEA and amylase in differentiating (1) mucinous from nonmucinous cystic lesions, (2) benign mucinous from malignant mucinous cystic lesions, and (3) pseudocysts from nonpseudocysts. The median amylase level for benign mucinous cysts was 5090 IU/L, compared with 60 IU/L for malignant mucinous cysts and 94 IU/L for malignant cystic neuroendocrine tumors ($P = .0008$). The investigators speculated that malignant transformation may be associated with uncontrolled cellular growth that occludes any microscopic ductal connections. These results should be accepted with caution given the limitations of the study, including that this was a retrospective analysis in a single-center tertiary-care center with likely referral and selection bias. Also, use of amylase to differentiate benign and malignant mucinous neoplasms was not appreciated in the pooled analysis by Van der Waaij and colleagues.[16]

TUMOR MARKERS

Since Hammel and colleagues[20] first demonstrated that tumor markers were present in high concentrations in the cyst fluid from MCNs, multiple subsequent studies have evaluated the use of tumors markers to predict mucinous and malignant cystic pancreatic lesions. A large Unites States multicenter study conducted by Brugge and colleagues[8] evaluated CEA, carbohydrate antigen (CA) 72-4, CA 125, CA 19-9, and CA 15-3. In this study CEA was found to be the most accurate marker in differentiating mucinous from nonmucinous cysts. The median cyst CEA concentration for mucinous cysts was 500 mg/mL and that for nonmucinous cysts 21 ng/mL. A cutoff value of 192 ng/mL provided the greatest accuracy (79%) for differentiating between mucinous and nonmucinous cysts, with moderate sensitivity (73%) and specificity (84%).[8] Other investigators have found similar results. Khalid and colleagues[21] reported on fluid CEA on 76 cysts, and the cutoff value of 192 ng/mL yielded a sensitivity of 64% and specificity of 83% for detecting mucinous cysts. Park and colleagues[19] demonstrated in 104 patients that a CEA cutoff level of 200 ng/mL had a sensitivity of 60%, specificity of 93%, and diagnostic accuracy of 58% for mucinous cysts. In the pooled analysis by Van der Waaij and colleagues,[16] a CEA level greater than 800 ng/mL showed a 79% accuracy for distinguishing mucinous adenoma/adenocarcinoma from a serous cystadenoma or pseudocyst, with 48% sensitivity and 98% specificity. Another large study by Snozek and colleagues[22] analyzed tumor marker levels in 442 patients with pancreatic cysts, in which an optimal CEA cutoff of 30 ng/mL resulted in 79% sensitivity, 73% specificity, and 84% PPV for detection of a mucinous cyst. A low CEA level has also been shown to be useful in predicting serous cystadenoma and pseudocyst. In an early study, Hammel and colleagues[20] showed that a CEA level below 4 ng/mL predicted an SCA with a sensitivity of 100% and specificity of 93%. In the pooled analysis by Van der Waaij and colleagues,[16] a CEA level below 5 ng/mL predicted SCA or PC with a specificity of 95%, sensitivity of 50% and accuracy of 67%.

As one can appreciate, there is a wide variation in the literature regarding the optimal CEA level at which to predict a mucinous cystic lesion, which is largely due to the significant overlap in CEA levels between mucinous and nonmucinous cysts. Other factors may include laboratory variation (see Technical Considerations section), differences in study design, and differences in study population. Nonetheless, studies have consistently shown that increasing the CEA value raises specificity for a mucinous lesion but at the cost of falling sensitivity for detection. At the authors' institution, for clinical decision making, a cutoff of greater than 192 ng/mL is used to differentiate mucinous from nonmucinous cysts.

Several other tumor markers have been evaluated for differentiating mucinous from nonmucinous cysts but have not performed as well as CEA. For example, in the pooled analysis by Van der Waaij and colleagues[16] a cutoff CA 19-9 value of less than 37 U/mL predicted SCA or pseudocyst with a sensitivity of 19%, specificity 98%, and accuracy 46%. In the United States multicenter study already discussed, a CA 72-4 value greater than 7 ng/mL demonstrated a sensitivity of 80% and specificity of 61% for differentiating mucinous and nonmucinous lesions.[8]

MOLECULAR ANALYSIS OF CYST FLUID

Molecular testing of cyst fluid has increased over the past few years, largely due to the availability of a commercially available test (PathFinderTG; RedPath Integrated Pathology, Pittsburgh, PA, USA). Similar to pancreatic ductal adenocarcinoma, molecular alterations in neoplastic mucinous cysts have demonstrated multistep genetic changes involving KRAS mutation, p53, loss of p16, and SMAD4.[23–26] Detection of these underlying molecular changes using cyst fluid DNA from exfoliated epithelial cells has become a major research focus. Early studies showed that increased levels of DNA, the presence of the KRAS mutation or 2 or more loci of allelic imbalance was each associated more significantly with a mucinous neoplasm, whereas a high amplitude of mutations and allelic loss was predictive of malignancy.[27]

The largest multicenter prospective study (PANDA study) evaluating the molecular analysis of cyst fluid included 113 cysts with histologic follow-up based on surgical resection or cytologic findings from EUS-FNA. The goals of this study were to evaluate molecular characteristics of cyst fluid that differentiated mucinous from nonmucinous cysts as well as premalignant from malignant cysts. The investigators found that among the parameters of DNA level, presence of KRAS mutation, and 2 or more loci of allelic loss, presence of KRAS mutation showed the highest specificity for mucinous cysts at 96% but sensitivity was low, at 45%. It was therefore concluded that in the presence of the KRAS mutation, the cyst very likely represents a mucinous cyst. When the presence of KRAS mutation was combined with CEA, the sensitivity of CEA (cutoff level 148 ng/mL) was improved from 67% to 84% while specificity remained at 67%. In the absence of a KRAS mutation, the cyst fluid CEA remains significantly associated with mucinous cysts, although with a less optimal sensitivity (69%) and specificity (68%). For premalignant versus malignant cysts, the most accurate test diagnosing a malignant cyst was an allelic-loss amplitude of greater than 80%, achieving sensitivity of 70% and specificity of 85%.[21]

Other studies have shown more mixed results with molecular analysis. Sawhney and colleagues[28] conducted a retrospective study of 100 pancreatic cysts (with 17 mucinous neoplasms) that evaluated both CEA and molecular analysis in predicting a mucinous lesion. In this study, there was poor agreement between CEA and molecular analysis for the classification of mucinous pancreatic cysts ($\kappa = 0.2$). A CEA level higher than 192 ng/mL had a higher sensitivity of 82% for mucinous cysts, compared with 77% with molecular analysis. However, the combination of CEA and molecular analysis yielded a 100% sensitivity and specificity, indicating that these data may be complementary. The small sample size was the major limitation of this study. A recent retrospective study by Klochan, Dewitt and colleagues[29] on 270 patients with pancreatic cystic lesions evaluated CEA, KRAS mutation, and DNA analysis for the diagnosis of mucinous cysts. CEA performed better than DNA analysis with sensitivity of 54.5% and specificity 80% compared with 45.5% and 80%, respectively. Using a combination of CEA, KRAS mutation, and DNA analysis, sensitivity increased to 75% but specificity decreased to 66.7%.

One of the major benefits of molecular analysis is that only 0.2 mL of cyst fluid is needed. Given that increasingly small cysts are being detected with fluid aspirate volumes often inadequate for CEA analysis or cytology, there may be a role for molecular analysis to provide information in these cases. In cysts with adequate aspirate volumes for CEA and cytology, the value-added benefit of molecular analysis may not be sufficient enough at this time to justify its high cost.

CYSTOSCOPY USING SPYGLASS

Endoscopy of pancreatic lesions has been reported via peroral pancreatoscopy (POPS) through the ampulla. The yield of POPS is limited to lesions in the main pancreatic duct (PD), but most pancreatic cystic lesions or dilated ducts are not necessarily associated with the main PD. Recently, EUS-guided cystoscopy using the Spyglass system (Boston Scientific, Natick, MA, USA) has been reported. Antillon and colleagues[30] first reported a case of a suspected pseudocyst undergoing diagnostic cystoscopy using the Spyglass system. In their report, the Spyglass access and a 10F delivery catheter were introduced into the cyst after puncture of the cyst under EUS guidance and fistula dilation. The spyglass view of the debris inside the cyst and the biopsy specimen using Spybite confirmed the diagnosis of pseudocyst, and cystogastrostomy was then performed. This case report was not a through-the-needle procedure, but did demonstrate the feasibility of Spyglass for pancreatic cystic lesions.

EUS-guided cystoscopy with biopsy through an FNA needle has since been reported in 2 cases with pancreatic cystic lesions.[31] Cystoscopy was performed using the Spyglass through a 19-gauge needle, and showed smooth mucosa without papillary projections. The cyst wall was then biopsied with small biopsy forceps used for ERCP (220 × 0.8 mm; PolyScope; Lumenis Surgical, Yokneam, Israel) through the needle under EUS guidance. Biopsy specimens showed mucin-like cylindrical epithelium without cellular atypia in both cases, suggesting mucinous cystadenoma. In one case, a late complication of severe acute pancreatitis developed 1 month after the procedure. A prospective trial is currently under way, with preliminary data in 21 patients suggesting specific cystoscopy findings that may predict mucinous cysts.[32]

NEEDLE-BASED CONFOCAL LASER–INDUCED ENDOMICROSCOPY

The utility of confocal laser–induced endomicroscopy (CLE) has been reported in many diseases of the gastrointestinal tract including Barrett esophagus and colon polyps. Recently, a prototype miniaturized CLE probe that can be passed through an FNA needle was developed (Mauna Kea Technologies, France; diameter 350 μm; lateral resolution 3.5 μm; field of view, 300 × 300 μm). This needle-based CLE (nCLE) enables an "optical" biopsy of intra-abdominal organs. An optical-biopsy approach is more useful in deep organs where conventional biopsies are difficult, and the pancreas is one such organ than can benefit from such an optical biopsy. The feasibility of nCLE was first reported in a porcine model by Becker and colleagues.[33] After puncture of the organ using a 22-gauge FNA needle, the nCLE probe was advanced into the organ with moderate compression. Various intra-abdominal structures and organs (lymph nodes, diaphragm, ovaries, liver, spleen, and pancreas) were imaged after intravenous injection of fluorescein. The authors' group[34] also reported the feasibility of nCLE through a 19-gauge FNA needle for intra-abdominal organs in a porcine model. In this study the nCLE imaging of the pancreas, liver, spleen, gallbladder, and lymph nodes correlated well with histologic findings. These studies have demonstrated the feasibility of nCLE in abdominal organs in a porcine model.

The first human clinical trial of nCLE in the pancreas was reported by Konda and colleagues.[35] In this study, nCLE of 16 cysts and 3 masses were performed, using a new prototype probe compatible with a 19-guage FNA needle (Mauna Kea Technologies; diameter 850 μm, lateral resolution 3.5 μm, field of view 320 μm). The imaging of nCLE was obtained in 17 cases, but in 1 case the probe could not be advanced into the needle tip. The nCLE imaging after injection of fluorescein was assessed as good or very good in 10 cases. In 3 cases villous structures were identified, consistent with the papillary formations seen on histopathologic specimens of IPMN lesions. With regard to complications, there were 2 patients with postprocedural pancreatitis that resolved with conservative treatment. This study demonstrated the clinical feasibility of nCLE in cystic lesions of the pancreas. A more recent multicenter study published in abstract form aimed to define nCLE interpretation criteria for pancreatic cystic lesions and to determine whether pancreatic cystic neoplasms (PCN) could be identified using nCLE. In this study, 8 centers performed nCLE in patients with pancreatic cystic lesions with video captured with the nCLE probe via a 19-gauge needle during EUS. Sixty-five video cases were reviewed. The presence of epithelial villous structures based on nCLE was associated with PCN ($P = .004$), providing sensitivity of 59% and specificity of 100%. The diagnostic yield of nCLE (41.9%) was higher than either CEA level above 192 ng/mL (28.6%) or cytology results (29.6%). Identification of pancreatic parenchymal structures with presumed histologic correlates to acinar tissue, adipose tissue, and pancreaticobiliary ductal lining did not provide significant differentiation between PCN and other lesions.[36]

COMBINATION OF CYSTOSCOPY AND nCLE

A prospective study of pancreatic cystic lesions using the combination of Spyglass and nCLE through a 19-gauge FNA needle (DETECT study) is now under way at the authors' center (**Figs. 1–3**).[32] With direct visualization of the cyst wall using Spyglass, the macroscopic characteristics of the cyst wall can be evaluated. In addition, with nCLE one can obtain optical biopsy of the cyst wall. These 2 new technologies are complementary to each other and, in combination with cyst fluid analysis, show promise in helping differentiate pancreatic cystic lesions. However, further study of these techniques with comparative histopathology is needed.

TECHNICAL CONSIDERATIONS

EUS-FNA is performed with a linear echoendoscope from either the duodenum or the stomach. Pancreatic cystic lesions are seen as anechoic or hypoechoic (dark) lesions within the pancreatic parenchyma on EUS. FNA should be performed with a 19-gauge or 22-gauge needle containing an occluding stylet. With the echoendoscope transducer in close proximity to the cystic lesion, the needle is guided through the wall of cyst into the lumen of the cyst, ideally in one passage. The cyst fluid should be aspirated until the cyst collapses, to prevent infectious complications.[37] High-viscosity fluid may require a considerable amount of time for evacuation of the cyst contents,

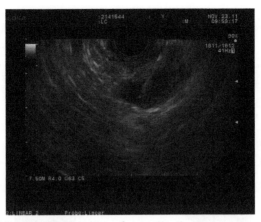

Fig. 1. EUS-guided fine-needle aspiration of a pancreatic cyst.

and this is often a clue that the cyst is mucinous. Focal nodules, thick septations, and adjacent masses should be targeted for aspiration and cytologic examination. The prevailing opinion is to administer an antibiotic such as a fluoroquinolone during and for 3 to 5 days after EUS-FNA of a pancreatic cystic lesion to prevent infection.[10]

Measurement of CEA in cyst fluid has not been approved by the US Food and Drug Administration, and therefore represents an off-label application in this setting. Furthermore, no commercially available CEA assays have been formally validated

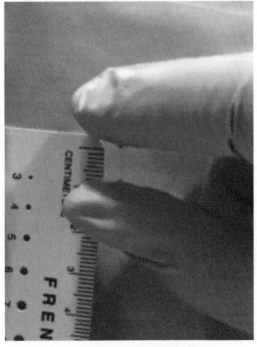

Fig. 2. A positive string sign from cyst fluid aspiration in **Fig. 1.**

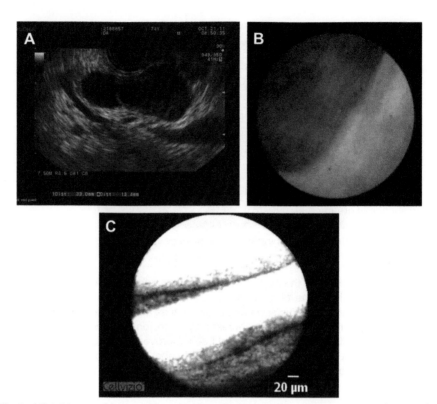

Fig. 3. (A) A 74-year-old man with an incidentally found 33.0 × 13.4-mm septated cyst in the body of the pancreas. EUS-FNA showed viscous fluid. (B) Cystoscopy of the same cyst showing smooth wall with septum and normal vessels. (C) nCLE of the cyst wall showing finger-like projections consistent with IPMN.

for any of the cyst fluid analyses encountered in clinical practice. Published cyst fluid data and cutoff values must therefore be viewed with caution, because important validation parameters such as linearity, precision, accuracy, and stability have not been reported. In addition, the handling of cyst fluid submitted for CEA analysis is not standardized, with some laboratories receiving fluid undiluted, whereas others are diluted or placed in fixative. Approximately 0.5 to 1 mL of fluid is needed for CEA analysis. If samples are too scant, too viscous for a pipette, or inhomogeneous because of mucin clumps in watery fluid, the cyst fluid can be diluted with saline and or/vortexed to achieve homogeneity. The dilution factor must be accounted for in the final CEA value reported, and often it is best to let the laboratory handle the fresh, undiluted fluid.[38] At their institution the authors are performing a study to evaluate the accuracy of CEA after 1 or more dilutions of the fresh sample, and results thus far have been consistently accurate over a wide range of CEA values.[39]

COMPLICATIONS

The overall complication rate of EUS-FNA of pancreatic cysts is low. Lee and colleagues[37] reviewed all complications related to EUS-FNA of pancreatic cysts at their institution in 603 patients, in whom 651 pancreatic cysts were evaluated. Complications were identified in 13 of 603 patients (2.2%). All complications were immediate or early and there were no late complications, deaths, or patients requiring surgery. Six patients developed pancreatitis (1%), 1 of whom had severe pancreatitis with necrosis. Four patients developed nonspecific abdominal pain, 1 patient developed fever and leukocytosis, 1 patient had retroperitoneal bleeding, and 1 patient had bradycardia. Other complications reported in the literature include hemorrhage within the cyst (<1%) and infection (<1%).[10]

THE AUTHORS' DIAGNOSTIC APPROACH TO CYST-FLUID ANALYSIS

The first question we ask when contemplating cyst aspiration is: will fluid analysis change management of the patient? If it is decided that fluid analysis can potentially change management, cyst aspiration is performed. At our institution, following antibiotic administration, cyst fluid is aspirated with a 22-gauge FNA needle using 10-mL syringe suction. If greater than 0.5 mL of fluid is aspirated, a tiny drop of fluid is placed onto the endoscopist's gloved thumb and the string sign is evaluated. If the string sign is greater than 4 mm, the cyst is classified as a mucinous cyst and is managed as such, even in the setting of a low CEA level and negative cytology. If the string sign is negative, CEA values are interpreted, as mucinous cysts may have low viscosity. At least 1 mL of fluid is required for CEA analysis at our institution and if the fluid volume available is less than 1 mL, the cyst fluid is diluted to constitute 1 mL of total fluid with the dilution factor recorded.[39] If cyst fluid CEA is greater than 192 ng/mL, the cyst is considered a mucinous cyst. If additional fluid beyond 1 mL is available, the fluid is sent for cytology and amylase. If cytologic analysis shows columnar cells staining for mucin, the cyst is classified as a mucinous cyst. If less than 0.5 mL of fluid is obtained, a string sign is evaluated, and if this is positive the cyst is considered to be mucinous. In situations where the string sign is negative and insufficient fluid is present for CEA and cytology evaluation, molecular analysis of the fluid is considered (**Fig. 4**).

MANAGEMENT OF NEOPLASTIC PANCREATIC CYSTS

Strategies for management of PCN include surveillance, surgical resection and, in select cases, cyst ablation. Clinical decision making regarding resection versus surveillance is based largely on cyst imaging and fluid analysis, with cost-effectiveness studies supporting this approach.[40,41] Other considerations when assessing which strategy to follow involve nonimaging findings such as symptoms attributable to the cyst, rapid growth, and young age such that lifelong surveillance will be prohibitively burdensome for the patient.

Based on imaging and cyst fluid analysis, there are several characteristics that indicate a high risk for malignancy, and as such the recommended management of these cysts is surgical resection. The Sendai International Consensus Guidelines published by the International Association of Pancreatology identified several risk factors as relative indications for resection of IPMN. These factors include cysts with a main-duct component, cyst size greater than 3 cm, cysts with a solid mural component, positive cytology for malignancy, and the presence of symptoms attributable to the cyst such as abdominal pain, weight loss, and pancreatitis (**Fig. 5**). The rationale for these guidelines lies in the differing risk of malignancy in IPMN lesions. The percentage of main-duct IPMN found with invasive malignancy at diagnosis ranges from 23% to 57%.[42] Estimates of malignancy in side-branch IPMN is lower, ranging from 0% to 31%.[42] However, mural nodules and size greater than 3 cm have been shown to be predictors of malignancy in side-branch IPMN.[43] Despite the risk of malignancy in MCN being similar to that in side-branch IPMN (6%–36%), guidelines recommend resection of

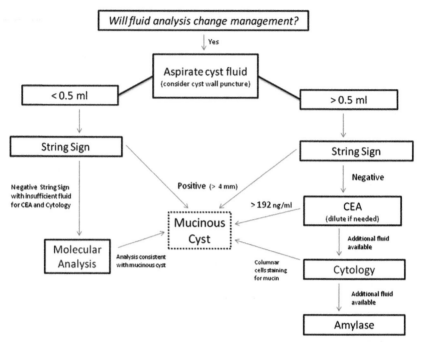

Fig. 4. Fluid-analysis algorithm for diagnosing mucinous cystic lesions of the pancreas.

all MCN lesions. The rationale for this recommendation relates to MCNs typically affecting middle-aged women, with many of these lesions having the potential to progress to cystadenocarcinoma over the remaining lifetime. Furthermore, the operation for MCN, usually a distal pancreatectomy, has a low morbidity and practically no

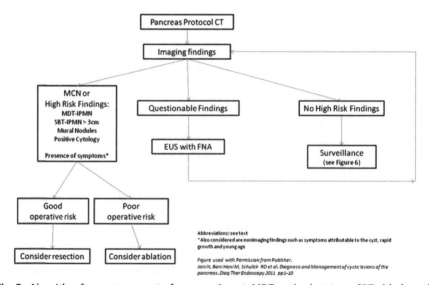

Fig. 5. Algorithm for management of pancreatic cyst. MDT, main-duct type; SBT, side-branch type.

mortality.[42] When possible, it is important to differentiate MCN and IPMN either before resection or with final histology. MCN and IPMN have important clinical differences. MCNs are generally solitary and do not recur after complete resection. On the other hand, branch-duct IPMN can by multifocal in up to 30% of patients and there is at least a 10% recurrence rate.[44] Thus, although no follow-up is needed after resection of MCN, young patients with IPMN may need follow-up.[42] SCA lesions have a very low risk for malignancy of less than 3%, and therefore do not warrant surveillance or resection unless they are the cause of symptoms.[45]

Although surgical resection is curative for many cystic lesions of the pancreas, it does carry a significant perioperative morbidity rate of 30% to 60% and a mortality rate ranging from less than 1% to 2%.[46–48] As a result, for patients who are poor operative candidates, a novel technique of cyst ablation with alcohol may be considered. Although limited data from few centers exist currently on cyst ablation, this technique holds significant promise in the future for the management of pancreatic cysts. The reader is referred to the article by John DeWitt on cyst ablation elsewhere in this issue for information on efficacy, technique, and patient selection.

In the absence of high-risk imaging or fluid-analysis features, a surveillance strategy should be used (**Fig. 6**). At the authors' institution, for cysts less than 1 cm in size, follow-up imaging with CT or MRI is performed at 1 year. For cysts between 1 and 2 cm in size, MRI, CT, or EUS is performed in 6 to 12 months. For cysts between 2 and 3 cm in size, MRI, CT, or EUS is performed in 3 to 6 months. If cysts are stable in size after 3 successive imaging studies, lengthening the interval of future surveillance studies is considered. If MR or CT studies demonstrate concerning changes such as rapid growth, possible high-risk features, or interval development of new symptoms, the authors typically perform EUS-FNA and then consider resection.

The optimal management of PCN remains challenging. The approaches discussed for resection and surveillance have been shaped based on the Sendai guidelines. However, it should be noted that no randomized prospective trials have been performed for pancreatic cystic disease, and guidelines rely predominantly on data from retrospective surgical studies that are subject to their own biases. The Sendai guidelines also did not take into account issues relating to operative mortality, patient age, functional status, or patient preference. Consequently, using Markov modeling, Weinberg and colleagues developed evidence-based nomograms to help guide clinical decision making. Using these models, the decision to resect or survey is based on age, comorbidities, and cyst size as well as whether the patient values quality or

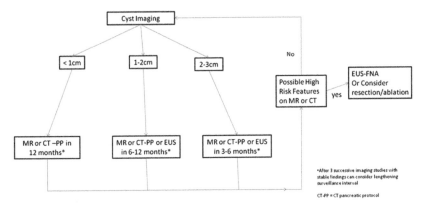

Fig. 6. Algorithm for surveillance of pancreatic cyst.

quantity of life more. This study revealed that those patients valuing primarily survival, irrespective of quality of life, would benefit most from resection of lesions larger than 2 cm, which is a deviation from the Sendai guidelines. However, for patients valuing quality of life over longevity, a 3-cm threshold for resection would be more appropriate. This study further emphasizes that providers and their patients must together carefully weigh the risks and benefits of resection and surveillance on a case-by-case basis.

SUMMARY

The diagnosis and management of pancreatic cystic lesions remains a challenging area in gastroenterology. Differentiating benign from premalignant or premalignant from malignant cysts is complicated by the large overlap in morphologic, chemical, and clinical characteristics between these lesions. At present a multimodal approach is required to maximize diagnostic accuracy, with EUS-FNA at the center of this workup. The use of cyst-fluid molecular markers currently does not add sufficient additional information to justify its use in routine practice, but holds a great deal of promise for the future. In vivo imaging with cystoscopy and endomicroscopy are currently in their infancy, but with refinement may add significant value to the EUS-FNA examination. After the diagnostic hurdles are overcome, management of these lesions can still be a challenge, given that surgical resection carries significant morbidity. However, with the advent of cyst ablation and other options for therapy on the horizon, the future of the diagnosis and management of pancreatic cystic lesions appears bright.

REFERENCES

1. Spinelli KS, Fromwiller TE, Daniel RA, et al. Cystic pancreatic neoplasms: observe or operate. Ann Surg 2004;239(5):651–7 [discussion: 657–9].
2. Laffan TA, Horton KM, Klein AP, et al. Prevalence of unsuspected pancreatic cysts on MDCT. AJR Am J Roentgenol 2008;191(3):802–7.
3. Kimura W, Nagai H, Kuroda A, et al. Analysis of small cystic lesions of the pancreas. Int J Pancreatol 1995;18(3):197–206.
4. Khalid A, Brugge W. ACG practice guidelines for the diagnosis and management of neoplastic pancreatic cysts. Am J Gastroenterol 2007;102(10):2339–49.
5. Furukawa T, Hatori T, Fujita I, et al. Prognostic relevance of morphological types of intraductal papillary mucinous neoplasms of the pancreas. Gut 2011;60(4): 509–16.
6. Curry CA, Eng J, Horton KM, et al. CT of primary cystic pancreatic neoplasms: can CT be used for patient triage and treatment? AJR Am J Roentgenol 2000; 175(1):99–103.
7. Kawamoto S, Lawler LP, Horton KM, et al. MDCT of intraductal papillary mucinous neoplasm of the pancreas: evaluation of features predictive of invasive carcinoma. AJR Am J Roentgenol 2006;186(3):687–95.
8. Brugge WR, Lewandrowski K, Lee-Lewandrowski E, et al. Diagnosis of pancreatic cystic neoplasms: a report of the cooperative pancreatic cyst study. Gastroenterology 2004;126(5):1330–6.
9. Ahmad NA, Kochman ML, Brensinger C, et al. Interobserver agreement among endosonographers for the diagnosis of neoplastic versus non-neoplastic pancreatic cystic lesions. Gastrointest Endosc 2003;58(1):59–64.
10. Jacobson BC, Baron TH, Adler DG, et al. ASGE guideline: the role of endoscopy in the diagnosis and the management of cystic lesions and inflammatory fluid collections of the pancreas. Gastrointest Endosc 2005;61(3):363–70.

11. Walsh RM, Zuccaro G, Dumot JA, et al. Predicting success of endoscopic aspiration for suspected pancreatic cystic neoplasms. JOP 2008;9(5):612–7.
12. Lewandrowski KB, Southern JF, Pins MR, et al. Cyst fluid analysis in the differential diagnosis of pancreatic cysts. A comparison of pseudocysts, serous cystadenomas, mucinous cystic neoplasms, and mucinous cystadenocarcinoma. Ann Surg 1993;217(1):41–7.
13. Linder JD, Geenen JE, Catalano MF. Cyst fluid analysis obtained by EUS-guided FNA in the evaluation of discrete cystic neoplasms of the pancreas: a prospective single-center experience. Gastrointest Endosc 2006;64(5):697–702.
14. Leung KK, Ross WA, Evans D, et al. Pancreatic cystic neoplasm: the role of cyst morphology, cyst fluid analysis, and expectant management. Ann Surg Oncol 2009;16(10):2818–24.
15. Walsh RM, Henderson JM, Vogt DP, et al. Prospective preoperative determination of mucinous pancreatic cystic neoplasms. Surgery 2002;132(4):628–33 [discussion: 633–4].
16. van der Waaij LA, van Dullemen HM, Porte RJ. Cyst fluid analysis in the differential diagnosis of pancreatic cystic lesions: a pooled analysis. Gastrointest Endosc 2005;62(3):383–9.
17. Frossard JL, Amouyal P, Amouyal G, et al. Performance of endosonography-guided fine needle aspiration and biopsy in the diagnosis of pancreatic cystic lesions. Am J Gastroenterol 2003;98(7):1516–24.
18. Rogart JN, Loren DE, Singu BS, et al. Cyst wall puncture and aspiration during EUS-guided fine needle aspiration may increase the diagnostic yield of mucinous cysts of the pancreas. J Clin Gastroenterol 2011;45(2):164–9.
19. Park WG, Mascarenhas R, Palaez-Luna M, et al. Diagnostic performance of cyst fluid carcinoembryonic antigen and amylase in histologically confirmed pancreatic cysts. Pancreas 2011;40(1):42–5.
20. Hammel P, Voitot H, Vilgrain V, et al. Diagnostic value of CA 72-4 and carcinoembryonic antigen determination in the fluid of pancreatic cystic lesions. Eur J Gastroenterol Hepatol 1998;10(4):345–8.
21. Khalid A, Zahid M, Finkelstein SD, et al. Pancreatic cyst fluid DNA analysis in evaluating pancreatic cysts: a report of the PANDA study. Gastrointest Endosc 2009;69(6):1095–102.
22. Snozek CL, Mascarenhas RC, O'Kane DJ. Use of cyst fluid CEA, CA19-9, and amylase for evaluation of pancreatic lesions. Clin Biochem 2009;42(15):1585–8.
23. Izeradjene K, Combs C, Best M, et al. Kras (G12D) and Smad4/Dpc4 haploinsufficiency cooperate to induce mucinous cystic neoplasms and invasive adenocarcinoma of the pancreas. Cancer Cell 2007;11(3):229–43.
24. Biankin AV, Biankin SA, Kench JG, et al. Aberrant p16(INK4A) and DPC4/Smad4 expression in intraductal papillary mucinous tumours of the pancreas is associated with invasive ductal adenocarcinoma. Gut 2002;50(6):861–8.
25. Jimenez RE, Warshaw AL, Z'Graggen K, et al. Sequential accumulation of K-ras mutations and p53 overexpression in the progression of pancreatic mucinous cystic neoplasms to malignancy. Ann Surg 1999;230(4):501–9 [discussion: 509–11].
26. Sasaki S, Yamamoto H, Kaneto H, et al. Differential roles of alterations of p53, p16, and SMAD4 expression in the progression of intraductal papillary-mucinous tumors of the pancreas. Oncol Rep 2003;10(1):21–5.
27. Khalid A, McGrath KM, Zahid M, et al. The role of pancreatic cyst fluid molecular analysis in predicting cyst pathology. Clin Gastroenterol Hepatol 2005;3(10): 967–73.

28. Sawhney MS, Devarajan S, O'Farrel P, et al. Comparison of carcinoembryonic antigen and molecular analysis in pancreatic cyst fluid. Gastrointest Endosc 2009;69(6):1106–10.
29. Klochan C, Dewitt J, Schmidt C, et al. Performance Characteristics of Molecular (DNA) Analysis of Pancreatic Cyst Fluid. Am J Gastroenterol 2011; 106:S584–611.
30. Antillon MR, Tiwari P, Bartalos CR, et al. Taking SpyGlass outside the GI tract lumen in conjunction with EUS to assist in the diagnosis of a pancreatic cystic lesion (with video). Gastrointest Endosc 2009;69(3 Pt 1):591–3.
31. Aparicio JR, Martinez J, Niveiro M, et al. Direct intracystic biopsy and pancreatic cystoscopy through a 19-gauge needle EUS (with videos). Gastrointest Endosc 2010;72(6):1285–8.
32. Nakai Y, Iwashita T, Park DH, et al. Diagnosis of pancreatic cysts: Endoscopic ultrasound Through-the-needle confocal laser-induced Endomicroscopy and Cystoscopy Trial (DETECT Study). Abstract submitted to Digestive Disease Week 2012, 2011.
33. Becker V, Wallace MB, Fockens P, et al. Needle-based confocal endomicroscopy for in vivo histology of intra-abdominal organs: first results in a porcine model (with videos). Gastrointest Endosc 2010;71(7):1260–6.
34. Shinoura S, Iwashita T, Chang KJ. EUS-guided needle-based confocal laser induced endomicroscopy (nCLE): a correlation study of "through the needle" imaging with normal histology in a porcine model. Gastrointest Endosc 2011; 73:AB325–6.
35. Konda VJ, Aslanian HR, Wallace MB, et al. First assessment of needle-based confocal laser endomicroscopy during EUS-FNA procedures of the pancreas (with videos). Gastrointest Endosc 2011;74(5):1049–60.
36. Konda V. An international, multi-center trial on needle-based confocal laser endomicroscopy (nCLE): results from the in vivo NCLE study in the pancreas with endosonography of cystic tumors (INSPECT) Abstract submitted to digestive disease 2012, 2012.
37. Lee LS, Saltzman JR, Bounds BC, et al. EUS-guided fine needle aspiration of pancreatic cysts: a retrospective analysis of complications and their predictors. Clin Gastroenterol Hepatol 2005;3(3):231–6.
38. Pitman MB, Lewandrowski K, Shen J, et al. Pancreatic cysts: preoperative diagnosis and clinical management. Cancer Cytopathol 2010;118(1):1–13.
39. Hamerski C, Iwashita T, Lee JG, et al. Low volume pancreatic cyst fluid acquired by endoscopic ultrasound (EUS) guided FNA: is it okay to dilute it for CEA measurement? Abstract submitted to Digestive Disease Week 2012, 2011.
40. Das A, Ngamruengphong S, Nagendra S, et al. Asymptomatic pancreatic cystic neoplasm: a cost-effectiveness analysis of different strategies of management. Gastrointest Endosc 2009;70(4):690–9, e6.
41. Lim SJ, Alasadi R, Wayne JD, et al. Preoperative evaluation of pancreatic cystic lesions: cost-benefit analysis and proposed management algorithm. Surgery 2005;138(4):672–9 [discussion: 679–80].
42. Tanaka M, Chari S, Adsay V, et al. International consensus guidelines for management of intraductal papillary mucinous neoplasms and mucinous cystic neoplasms of the pancreas. Pancreatology 2006;6(1-2):17–32.
43. Sugiyama M, Izumisato Y, Abe N, et al. Predictive factors for malignancy in intraductal papillary-mucinous tumours of the pancreas. Br J Surg 2003;90(10): 1244–9.

44. Chari ST, Yadav D, Smyrk TC, et al. Study of recurrence after surgical resection of intraductal papillary mucinous neoplasm of the pancreas. Gastroenterology 2002;123(5):1500–7.
45. Strobel O, Z'Graggen K, Schmitz-Winnenthal FH, et al. Risk of malignancy in serous cystic neoplasms of the pancreas. Digestion 2003;68(1):24–33.
46. Lillemoe KD, Kaushal S, Cameron JL, et al. Distal pancreatectomy: indications and outcomes in 235 patients. Ann Surg 1999;229(5):693–8 [discussion: 698–700].
47. DeOliveira ML, Winter JM, Schafer M, et al. Assessment of complications after pancreatic surgery: a novel grading system applied to 633 patients undergoing pancreaticoduodenectomy. Ann Surg 2006;244(6):931–7 [discussion: 937–9].
48. Vin Y, Sima CS, Getrajdman GI, et al. Management and outcomes of postpancreatectomy fistula, leak, and abscess: results of 908 patients resected at a single institution between 2000 and 2005. J Am Coll Surg 2008;207(4):490–8.

Endoscopic Ultrasonography-Guided Diagnosis of Subepithelial Tumors

Amer A. Alkhatib, MD, Douglas O. Faigel, MD, AGAF*

KEYWORDS

- Endoscopic ultrasonography • Subepithelial tumors
- Submucosal lesions • Gastrointestinal stromal tumor
- Leiomyoma • Lipoma • Fine-needle aspiration

INTRODUCTION

It is estimated that more than 4.5 million endoscopic procedures are performed on Medicare patients yearly.[1] Bumps and lumps in the lumen of the gastrointestinal tract are frequently encountered, and are referred to as subepithelial lesions/masses or subepithelial lesions (**Fig. 1**). These lesions represent a diagnostic dilemma for the endoscopist because of difficulties in delineating the origin of the lesion (extramural vs intramural), with an overall accuracy of 89% (sensitivity 98%, specificity 64%) and challenges in obtaining adequate tissue.[2]

Subepithelial masses encompass a large, heterogeneous group of lesions. Such masses are classified into intramural, when the lesion originates from within the layers of the gastrointestinal wall, and extramural, when the lesion originates from outside the gastrointestinal wall. These lesions can be benign and require no additional evaluation, whereas others are premalignant and may need close follow-up and still others are malignant, thus requiring medical and/or surgical interventions.[3,4] The prevalence of subepithelial lesions in the gastrointestinal tract is currently unknown. Postmortem studies found mesenchymal tumors (eg, gastrointestinal stromal tumor [GIST], leiomyoma) in the esophagus in 5% of cases and in the stomach in 50% of cases, with minute gastric GIST in 2.9% to 35% of cases.[5,6] Gastric subepithelial tumors are encountered in approximately 1 in every 300 endoscopies.[4]

The authors have no conflicts of interests related to this subject.

Division of Gastroenterology and Hepatology, Mayo Clinic, 13400 East Shea Boulevard, Scottsdale, AZ 85259, USA

* Corresponding author.

E-mail address: faigel.douglas@mayo.edu

Gastrointest Endoscopy Clin N Am 22 (2012) 187–205
doi:10.1016/j.giec.2012.04.006
1052-5157/12/$ – see front matter © 2012 Elsevier Inc. All rights reserved.

giendo.theclinics.com

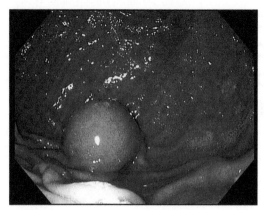

Fig. 1. A gastric subepithelial lesion found during a routine upper endoscopic examination.

CLINICAL PRESENTATION

The majority of subepithelial lesions are asymptomatic.[7] Sixty percent are encountered in the stomach, followed by the esophagus (30%) and duodenum (10%).[6,8] Occasionally the lesions may present with gastrointestinal hemorrhage, obstruction, and dysphagia. If the lesion is close to the ampulla, it may cause jaundice or pancreatitis.[7] However, the majority are encountered incidentally during endoscopy being done for other reasons.

EXAMPLES OF SUBEPITHELIAL LESIONS
Gastrointestinal Stromal Tumor

GISTs (see **Fig. 1**; **Fig. 2**) are considered a subset of mesenchymal tumors.[9] A GIST is the most common mesenchymal neoplasm of the gastrointestinal tract.[9] In the past,

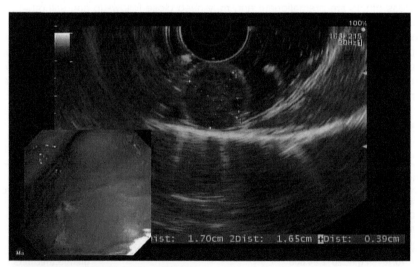

Fig. 2. Endoscopic ultrasonogram of a GIST.

GISTs were confused with leiomyomas of the gastrointestinal tract. However, GISTs are phenotypically and genetically different from leiomyomas.[9,10] GISTs usually express CD34, which is a hematopoietic progenitor cell antigen.[10] Studies found that the marker was not specific for GIST, being expressed in fibroblastic and endothelial cell tumors. This finding led to the pursuance of more specific markers for GISTs. In 1998, CD117, which is the product of the c-kit proto-oncogene, was found in around 85% to 95% of GISTs.[11–13] CD117 is known to be expressed by interstitial cells of Cajal of the gastrointestinal tract, the pacemaker cells associated with the Auerbach plexus. It is debatable whether GISTs originate from interstitial cells of Cajal of the gastrointestinal tract or from multipotential mesenchymal stem cells.[9,14] Other mesenchymal tumors that are positive for CD117 include clear-cell sarcoma, metastatic melanoma, and malignant fibrous histiocytoma.[11] DOG-1 (discovered on GIST) is a recently described immunohistochemical marker for GISTs, useful for differentiating GISTs from these other entities and when CD117 is negative.[15]

The pathogenesis of a GIST is largely atributable to gain-of-function mutations in the tyrosine kinases cKIT and platelet-derived growth factor receptor α (PDGFRA) genes. More than 85% have identifiable mutations in cKIT, whereas the remainder usually have mutations in PDGFRA.[16] The presence of these mutations forms the basis of treatment with the tyrosine kinase inhibitors imatinib mesylate and sunitib.[17]GISTs mainly affect the stomach (around 60%) and small intestine (around 30%), and rarely affect the colon (around 5%), esophagus (2%–4%), and appendix (<2%).[13,18] Extragastrointestinal GISTs have been reported.[19–21] The incidence of GISTs is estimated at around 10 to 20 per 1 million people.[9] Around 90% of cases are diagnosed in patients older than 40 years, with a median age of 63 years.[9,13] Most patients are symptomatic at presentation (70%–90%).[9,22] Presentations include abdominal pain, gastrointestinal bleeding, nausea/vomiting, weight loss, early satiety, and gastrointestinal obstruction.[22] It is estimated that 50% of GISTs are high-risk for malignant behavior.[23] Risk factors for aggressive behavior include size greater than 5 cm, mitotic index greater than 5 mitoses per 50 high-power fields, and location in the intestine.[17] Treatment is generally surgical resection for localized tumors and imatinib mesylate for advanced disease.[9]

Leiomyoma

Leiomyoma is a benign tumor of the smooth muscle. Most leiomyomas are intraluminal or intramural tumors, and are often asymptomatic until they have reached a large size. The clinical presentation depends on the size, location, and direction of tumor growth, and includes bleeding, intestinal obstruction, dysphagia, and perforation into the peritoneal cavity.[24,25] Endoscopically, leiomyomas can present as pedunculated intramural or intraluminal polyps, or as a smooth subepithelial mass indistinguishable from a GIST.[24] Endoscopic ultrasonography (EUS) shows a hypoechoic lesion arising from the second (muscularis mucosae) or fourth layer (muscularis propria). In contrast to GIST, leiomyomas stain positive for smooth muscle actin (SMA) and desmin, and negative for CD34 and CD117.[26] Asymptomatic cases do not require intervention.

Carcinoid Tumors

Carcinoid tumors originate from neuroendocrine cells. Although they commonly occur in the ileum, at endoscopy they are usually discovered in the rectum, stomach, or duodenum.[27] EUS examination of gastrointestinal carcinoids shows a hypoechoic and homogeneous oval to round tumor with clear margin and smooth contour, arising from the third layer (submucosa).[28] Gastric carcinoid is classified into 3 types: type 1, linked with autoimmune chronic atrophic gastritis type A; type 2, associated with the

Zollinger-Ellison syndrome and MEN1; and type 3, sporadic gastric carcinoid tumors unaccompanied by hypergastrinemia. Type 3 is considered the most aggressive type, with 60% of cases being associated with metastases at the time of diagnosis[29,30] Endoscopic mucosal resection (EMR) is recommended for type 1 and type 2 carcinoids, associated with hypergastrinemia and the presence of 3 to 5 tumors, none of them greater 1 cm in diameter. Duodenal (**Fig. 3**)[29] and rectal carcinoids may be endoscopically resected if they are less than 1 cm in size.

Lipoma

Lipomas are most commonly encountered in the right side of the colon but occur anywhere in the gastrointestinal tract.[31] Endoscopically lipomas show pillow and tent signs, both specific but not very sensitive features.[2] Primary gastrointestinal liposarcomas are extremely rare tumors.[31] Lipomas are usually asymptomatic but rarely can cause gastrointestinal hemorrhage, intussusception, and bowel obstruction.[32] On EUS, a lipoma appears as a homogeneous hyperechoic (bright) mass localized in the submucosal (third) layer.[32]

Schwannoma

Schwannomas are tumors of the nerve sheath.[33] Gastrointestinal schwannomas present more frequently in females (male to female ratio 1:1.6) at an average age of 58 years.[33] Schwannomas stain positive for S-100 and glial fibrillary acidic protein (GFAP), and negative for c-kit, CD34, and SMA.[33,34] Usually they have a favorable outcome.[34,35] Schwannomas can present with vague abdominal pain, vomiting, weight loss, dysphagia, obstruction, and gastrointestinal hemorrhage.[35] In a series of gastrointestinal schwannoma, most of the cases arose in the stomach (around 70%), around 15% in the colon and rectum, and the rest in the esophagus, whereas none originated in the small intestine.[35] Multiple schwannomas should raise the suspicion of von Recklinghausen disease.[36] On EUS, a schwannoma appears as a hypoechoic lesion that originates from the third or fourth layer and has an appearance similar to a GIST or leiomyoma.

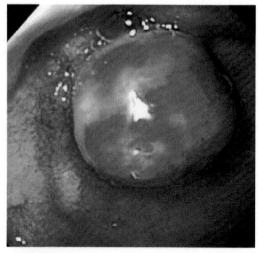

Fig. 3. Duodenal carcinoid tumor.

Pancreatic Rest

Pancreatic rest, or pancreatic heterotopia or aberrant pancreas, refers to pancreatic tissue that is found outside the pancreas without anatomic or vascular connection with the pancreas itself.[37] The overall surgical incidence is estimated as 1 case per 500 cases of upper abdominal exploration. In autopsy studies, the incidence is estimated 0.55% to 13.7%. Most of the cases are asymptomatic. When symptomatic, patients may present with mucosal ulcer and hemorrhage, intussusception, intestinal obstruction, and bile duct obstruction.[37] Endoscopically, pancreatic heterotopia can present as an umbilicated subepithelial lesion of the gastric antrum (>90%) or a duodenal mass, ulcer, or duodenal obstruction.[37] As of 2004 there were fewer than 30 well-documented cases of adenocarcinoma arising from heterotopic pancreas.[38] On EUS, most of the lesions originate from the second, third, and/or fourth layers. Ninety-five percent of the lesions have a heterogeneous echotexture, and are mainly hypoechoic or of mixed echogenicity. In 65% the borders are indistinct, and 35% exhibit anechoic cystic or a tubular structure within the lesion.[39]

Duplication Cyst

Foregut duplication cysts are uncommon congenital anomalies. Duplication cysts are usually asymptomatic in adults. Nevertheless, abdominal pain, dyspnea, dysphagia, or coughing have been reported with these cysts. Malignant transformation in foregut duplication cysts is extremely rare.[40] On EUS they appear as anechoic, homogeneous lesions with regular margins arising from the third layer or extrinsic to the gut wall. It is important to bear in mind that a hypoechoic, and not necessarily anechoic, echo pattern should not exclude the diagnosis of a duplication cyst.[40] In the past, it was believed that fine-needle aspiration (FNA) was necessary to establish the diagnosis of foregut duplication cyst. Nevertheless, because of several reported cases of infection from FNA of mediastinal duplication cysts, despite the use of prophylactic antibiotics, it is recommended that FNA be avoided for cysts with typical EUS appearance of duplication cyst in the mediastinum.[40]

Glomus Tumor

Glomus tumors are typically found in the skin and the subcutaneous tissue. These tumors originate from modified smooth muscle cells that behave like perivascular glomus bodies.[41] Gastrointestinal glomus tumors are mostly encountered in the antrum.[41,42] Close to half of these tumors present as a submucosal ulcerated mass,[42] and originate mostly from the fourth layer. Nevertheless, a glomus tumor can originate from the third layer and on rare occasion extends to the second layer. Glomus tumors are either hypoechogenic or hyperechogenic. Internal hyperechoic spots, corresponding to the calcifications found on histologic examination, can be seen in more than half of the cases.[42] Doppler EUS can be helpful, as it shows a prominent vascular signal corresponding to the hypervascular nature of the tumor.[42] Glomus tumors are usually benign; however, cases of malignant transformation have been reported. Hence surgical resection is usually recommended.[41,42]

Metastasis

More than 50% of metastases to the stomach may present as subepithelial lesions. Metastases to the stomach tend to involve the upper and middle third of the stomach. Endoscopic biopsy may be diagnostic in up to 90% of cases. Metastasis to the stomach most commonly originates from the lung, esophagus, breast, and malignant melanoma.[43] The EUS appearance of the tumors can show a hypoechoic or heterogeneous mass.[7]

Table 1 summarizes the characteristic clinical and endosonographic features of subepithelial lesions.

INVESTIGATIONS

Radiographic imaging as well as standard endoscopy cannot reliably differentiate the nature of subepithelial lesions.[44,45] On the other hand, EUS has revolutionized our approach to investigating subepithelial lesions. EUS has many advantages over standard endoscopy, including delineation of the origin of the mass (intramural vs extramural), depth and the extent of the tumor, presence of lymphadenopathy, and vascularity of the lesion. Using FNA, EUS has paved the way to obtain cytologic biopsy and thus has improved the diagnostic yield. EUS is considered the first choice for evaluation of subepithelial gastrointestinal lesions in the upper and the lower gastrointestinal tract.[44,46–49]

Endoscopic Ultrasonography and Subepithelial Lesions

To understand the role of EUS in evaluating subepithelial lesions, one should be familiar with the histologic layers of the gastrointestinal wall and their sonographic counterparts. The layers of the gastrointestinal wall are the epithelium, lamina propria, submucosa, muscularis propria, and serosa (adventitia).[7] At usual EUS frequencies (5–12 MHz) these are displayed in a 5-layer pattern numbered from the lumen out: first and second (mucosa including the muscularis mucosa), third (submucosa), fourth (muscularis propria), and fifth (serosa or adventitia).

Like any other ultrasound examination, the interpretation of the EUS images is operator dependent. Overall agreement for subepithelial lesions evaluation using EUS appears to be good ($\kappa = 0.63$). Nonetheless, the interobserver agreement varies according to the lesion type whereby κ is highest (>0.8) for cystic lesions and extrinsic compressions, and good for lipomas ($\kappa = 0.65$), fair for leiomyoma and vascular lesions ($\kappa = 0.53$ and 0.54, respectively), and poor for other subepithelial lesions ($\kappa = 0.34$). There is also a significant relationship between operators' years of experience and their ability to reach accurate diagnoses using EUS.[50]

Whenever EUS is performed to examine a subepithelial lesion, the operator should try to address the following points:

1. Location of the lesion (esophagus, stomach, small intestine, colon)
2. The general endoscopic appearance (presence of ulcerated mass, umbilicated mass, yellowish appearance, and so forth)
3. Whether the mass is intramural versus extramural
4. Layer of origin
5. Echogenicity of the mass by comparing the mass to the spleen or 3rd and 4th layer of the gastrointestinal wall
6. Define internal structures, for example presence of calcifications, tubular structures, cystic changes, and so forth
7. Size
8. Extent of the mass
9. Presence of vessels around or within the lesion
10. Relationship to surrounding structures
11. Presence of lymphadenopathy.

Addressing these points can help to narrow the differential diagnosis. Determining the location of the lesion in the gastrointestinal tract can be very helpful. For example, finding a fourth-layer subepithelial lesion in the esophagus makes it less likely to be a GIST, whereas finding the same lesion in the stomach makes it more likely to be a GIST.[34] On other hand, finding a subepithelial lesion in the colon raises the suspicion for lipomas and lymphangiomas, and to a lesser extent endometriosis and leiomyoma.[49]

Conducting EUS should not deter the operator from paying attention to the gross endoscopic appearance of the lesion, as it may provide pivotal information. For example, finding an ulcerated GIST increases the likelihood that the lesion is malignant,[51] finding an umbilicated lesion in the antrum raises the suspicion of pancreatic heterotopia,[52] and finding yellowish subepithelial lesion in the rectum supports the diagnosis of rectal carcinoid.[53,54] Finding a lesion with a positive pillow sign (probing leaves an indentation) or a tent sign (pulling with a biopsy forceps raises the mucosa off the lesion) are highly suggestive of a lipoma.[2,55]

One of the strengths of EUS is its ability to differentiate between intramural and extramural lesions or external compressions.[47] EUS is superior to other studies (computed tomography, barium studies, endoscopic studies with biopsies) in delineating the origin of the mass, hence EUS should be the first choice to investigate any subepithelial lesion.[3] Studies have shown that around 14% to 42% of the lesions suspected to be subepithelial lesions during a routine endoscopic examination turned out to be extramural lesions or compressions during EUS examinations.[6,56] Structures that are commonly found to be compressing the gastrointestinal wall during EUS are usually benign. In one study that included 238 patients who underwent EUS to investigate subepithelial lesions, 55 lesions were found to represent extramural structures. More than half of these cases (58%) were impressed upon by neighboring organs such as the spleen, splenic vessels, gallbladder, liver, and pancreas. Twelve cases were related to benign lesions (hepatic cysts, hepatic hemangiomas, splenic cyst, and pancreatic cyst). Ten percent of extramural cases were thought to represent transient impression. Nine percent of the cases represented malignant lesions (pancreas, liver, and spleen).[56] Hence extramural lesions may be malignant, though as such are encountered infrequently.

The EUS operator should try to identify the layer of origin for any subepithelial lesion because this can help significantly to narrow the diagnosis. Lesions originating from the submucosal layer are usually lipomas, fibromas, carcinoid tumors, granular cell tumors, pancreatic rests, and duplication cysts. Lesions arising from the muscularis propria usually represent gastrointestinal stromal tumors, leiomyomas, and schwannomas.[6,7]

Echogenicity is an important feature to describe when investigating subepithelial lesions. Anechoic lesions may represent cysts, varices, lymphangiomas, or cavernous hemangiomas. A hypoechoic lesion can represent gastrointestinal mesenchymal tumor (GIST, leiomyoma, schwannoma), granular cell tumor, neuroendocrine tumor, inflammatory fibroid polyp, metastasis, subepithelial cancer, lymphoma, amyloid, focal inflammation, and endometriosis. Hyperechoic lesions usually represent lipomas or fibrolipomas. Mixed echogenicity (bright and dark areas) can be seen, and may represent heterotopic pancreas, malignant mesenchymal tumor, fibrovascular polyp, spontaneous esophageal hematoma, or wall abscess.[6,57]

Measuring the size of the lesion is important because it may help to narrow the diagnosis and may provide prognostic value in certain situations. For example, in a patient with a GIST, size of less than 1 cm is less likely than size of 5 cm to be malignant.[57,58]

The extent of the mass has implications for treatment and prognosis. If the subepithelial lesion is seen to extend to the fourth layer or beyond, it makes the chance of removing the lesion endoscopically risky because of the high risk of perforation.[59] In

Table 1
Characteristics of subepithelial mass lesions at endoscopy and endoscopic ultrasonography (EUS)

Subepithelial Lesion	Endoscopic Appearance	EUS Layer	EUS Appearance
Benign			
GIST, benign	No specific characteristics, lack ulcerations	4th (rarely 2nd or 3rd)	Hypoechoic, majority <3–5 cm, smooth margins, round, homogeneous, rarely malignant GIST were reported with size <3 cm
Leiomyoma	No specific characteristics	2nd, 3rd, or 4th	Hypoechoic, well circumscribed
Lipoma	Yellow hue, pillow sign (high specificity, low sensitivity), tent sign, usually isolated	3rd	Intensely hyperechoic, homogeneous, smooth margins, may be polypoid
Varices	Bluish tinge, tortuous, easily compressible	3rd	Anechoic, serpiginous, Doppler positive
Neural origin: schwannoma, neuroma, neurofibroma	No specific characteristics	3rd or 4th	Hypoechoic
Granular cell tumor	No specific characteristics, majority small (<4 cm) and solitary	2nd or 3rd	Hypoechoic, heterogeneous echotexture
Inflammatory fibroid polyp	Smooth, usually solitary, sessile polyp with ulceration of the overlying mucosa, 2–5 cm	3rd or 4th	Hypo- to hyperechoic, indistinct margin, homogeneous appearance
Duplication cyst	Smooth and regular appearance, slightly translucent, compressible	Any or extramural	Anechoic, 3–5-layer wall, round or oval, absent Doppler signal
Lymphangioma	Cystlike bulging mass, easily compressed, more common in intestine	3rd	Anechoic with internal septa

Pancreatic rest	90% have umbilicated surface corresponding to a draining duct, >90% located in the antrum	2nd, 3rd, or 4th	Hypoechoic or mixed echogenicity (heterogeneous = acinous tissue, anechoic = ductal structures), indistinct margin; anechoic cystic or tubular structures within the lesions can be seen in one-third of cases
Brunner gland hyperplasia	Duodenal bulb, usually single	2nd and 3rd	Hyperechoic, anechoic area due to duct, smooth margin
Malignant (potential)			
GIST, malignant	Presence of ulcerations	4th (rarely 2nd or 3rd)	Hypoechoic, >3 cm, irregular extraluminal margins, cystic spaces, heterogeneous, lymph node changes, echogenic foci
Carcinoid	No specific characteristics, may be yellowish in appearance, gastric carcinoids often multiple; types 1 and 2 are usually benign and type 3 is usually malignant; rectal and duodenal usually solitary	2nd or 3rd	Mildly hypoechoic or isoechoic, homogeneous, oval or round, smooth margin
Lymphoma	No specific characteristics	2nd, 3rd, or 4th	Hypoechoic
Metastasis	No specific characteristics	Any or all	Hypoechoic, heterogeneous mass
Glomus tumor	No specific characteristics, mostly seen in the antrum	3rd << 4th	Hypo- or hyperechogenicity; more than half have internal hyperechoic spots that correspond to calcifications; Doppler EUS shows a prominent vascular signal consistent with the hypervascular nature of the tumor

Data from Refs.[2,7,39,55,103–109]

addition, if the lesion is seen to extend to invade surrounding organs, this raises the concern of an invasive malignancy.

Determining vascularity and presence of surrounding vessels is also important, especially before attempting to obtain a biopsy or remove a lesion. For example, gastric varices can be easily misdiagnosed as a gastric mass. EUS can safely and reliably identify gastric varices and vessels with tumors, improving safety.[60,61]

Identifying the presence of lymphadenopathy and performing EUS-guided FNA of suspicious lymph nodes can be helpful in the locoregional staging of malignant lesions, with implications for the management of these lesions.[62,63]

Cytologic and Histopathological Diagnosis

With this range of diagnostic potentials, reaching a definite diagnosis of subepithelial tumor/lesion can be challenging. In many cases EUS is not capable of providing a definitive diagnosis of the subepithelial lesion, requiring tissue sampling for a histologic diagnosis.[64] EUS may guide the choice of technique for tissue sampling, or obtain a cytologic specimen through EUS-guided FNA.

Methods to Obtain Cytologic and Histopathologic Samples

There are several endoscopic methods to obtain biopsy, including biopsy forceps, Trucut needle biopsy, EUS-guided FNA, endoscopic submucosal resection (ESMR), and a variety of unroofing and resection techniques.[7,65,66] Using standard cold forceps biopsy is not helpful in most cases. To obtain deep biopsy the tunnel biopsy technique, stacked jumbo forceps, and bite-on-bite forceps have been described. The diagnostic yield for third-layer lesions using stacked jumbo forceps biopsy is low, estimated at between 14% and 42%, compared with almost 90% for endoscopic mucosal resection.[59,65,66] The yield of bite-on-bite forceps is related to the site and not the size.[65] The highest yield is in the esophagus, where the yield can reach up to 58%.[65]

A Trucut biopsy (Quick-Core; Wilson-Cook Medical Inc, Winston-Salem, NC, USA) can be used with linear echoendoscopes. This device uses a 19-gauge needle with an 18-mm tissue tray with a built-in spring-loaded mechanism allowing a core of tissue to be obtained for histologic diagnosis.[7] The Trucut biopsy is considered a safe procedure when used by experienced operators in appropriate locations. The device functions well in the esophagus, rectum, and most of the stomach. However, use of the Trucut biopsy in the antrum, fundus, and duodenum is cumbersome and technically difficult, with lower yields for an adequate specimen because echoendoscope angulations produce sluggish advancement of the cutting sheath.[7,67–69] The use of the device beyond the duodenal apex is not recommended.[69] It was initially postulated that the Trucut has the advantage of decreasing the number of passes needed. Nevertheless, conflicting results exist regarding whether Trucut biopsy really decreases the number of biopsy passes required to establish cytologic/pathologic diagnosis.[67–69] Trucut needle biopsy has the higher accuracy than FNA biopsy when sampling subepithelial lesions and lymphoma (88%–100% vs 29%–66%).[67,69] A new biopsy needle, the ProCore needle (Wilson-Cook Medical Inc), is now available in 22-gauge and 19-gauge sizes. It was designed to increase diagnostic yield and obtain a histologic core, but whether it improves the sampling of subepithelial lesions is as yet unknown.

ESMR adapts a variety of endoscopic mucosal resection techniques to removing lesions from the submucosa (third layer). ESMR involves raising the lesion away from the fourth layer, the muscularis propria, either by injection of saline solution (strip biopsy) or suction of the lesion into a cap fitted to the endoscope (aspiration lumpectomy), followed by electrosurgical snare resection.[7,64,70,71] Subepithelial lesions that are confined to layers 1 to 3 and up to 20 mm in size are amenable to safe resection.[7,64,72] ESMR is helpful in establishing a histologic diagnosis and in providing definitive therapy for smaller lesions.[73–75] The main complication of ESMR is bleeding in 4% to 13% of cases.[59,70,76,77] Bleeding is usually managed endoscopically.[76,78] Perforation after EMR has been reported in up to 5% of the cases,[78] but may be less common after ESMR.

Endoscopic tissue sampling and resection of fourth-layer lesions such as GISTs is more challenging. The location of the tumor deep to the submucosa makes it less accessible to biopsy, and resecting the muscularis propria from which they arise runs the risk of perforation. A variety of techniques to unroof the lesion followed by biopsy or resection has been described. One method is to perform endoscopic submucosal dissection using an insulated tipped knife to dissect and enucleate the tumor, followed by closure with clips.[79–82] These techniques are technically challenging and run the risk of perforation in up to 28% of cases. Other techniques to unroof the tumor include aggressive bite-on-bite forceps biopsies with on-site pathologic guidance to ensure an adequate sample, and using a standard electrocautery snare to unroof the mass. Endoscopic band ligation without endoscopic resection has been described for GISTs smaller than 2 cm. Tumors completely slough within several weeks.

EUS-guided FNA is frequently applied to submucosal lesions, particularly those arising from the fourth layer (muscularis propria). Whereas earlier studies reported relatively poor accuracy,[83] more recent studies have reported high diagnostic yields reaching 75% to 100%.[84–89] The sensitivity of EUS FNA for GISTs has been estimated at 84% to 89%.[86,90] Higher yield of EUS FNA of subepithelial lesions may be obtained from larger lesions, from a gastric location, and in the presence of on-site cytopathology.[91] The overall rate of EUS FNA–specific morbidity is low, estimated to be 0% to 2%.[92] Complications after FNA of subepithelial masses are very rare, and mostly consists of postprocedural abdominal pain.[92] Antibiotic prophylaxis should be considered in cases of cystic lesions.[98]

Immunohistochemistry is an important tool in the diagnostic arsenal when evaluating subepithelial lesions, and can be performed on FNA material. For example, GISTs are usually positive for CD117 or c-kit.[85,92] In addition to CD117, other commonly used markers are CD34, SMA, S-100, desmin, and vimentin. Ki67 (MIB-1) is considered a marker of proliferation and can be assessed in resected GISTs and EUS FNA specimens. Nonetheless, it is not clear whether it improves the ability to predict GIST behavior.[7,93,94] Up to 14% of GISTs are cKIT negative, but are positive for PDGFRA gene mutation. These lesions may be diagnosed through mutational analyses of c-kit and PDGFRA genes or staining for DOG-1.[95–97]

Management of Subepithelial Lesions

Management of subepithelial lesions depends on the etiology, location, size, symptoms, and patients' characteristics such as age, comorbidities, and need and frequency of follow-up examinations. Asymptomatic benign lesions do not require follow-up or intervention. Such lesions include most pancreas rests, leiomyomas, schwannomas, lipomas, duplication cysts, hemangiomas, and inflammatory fibroid polyps. Lesions with malignant or invasive risk should be resected or undergo endoscopic or EUS surveillance. These lesions include carcinoids, granular cell tumors, and GISTs. Endoscopic resection is indicated for all carcinoids of less than 1 cm in size as well as most type 1 and type 2 gastric carcinoids. Most granular cell tumors may be resected endoscopically, as can small GISTs arising from the third layer (submucosa or muscularis mucosae).[98]

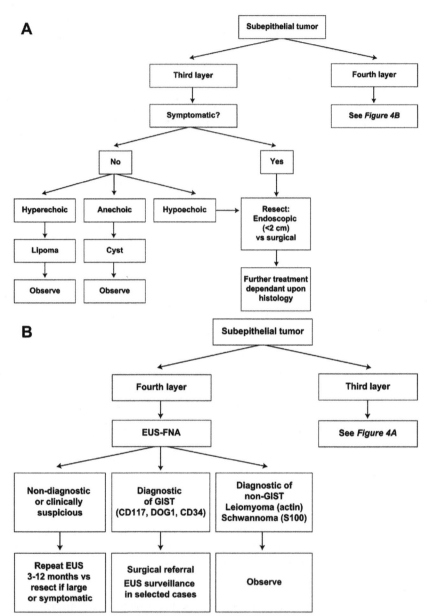

Fig. 4. (*A*) Management algorithm for subepithelial lesions. EUS is performed to determine layer of origin, echogenicity, and size. Symptomatic third-layer lesions should be resected either endoscopically (<2 cm) or surgically. Asymptomatic hyperechoic lesions are lipomas and asymptomatic anechoic lesions are cysts; these do not require intervention. Hypoechoic lesions may be resected endoscopically. Further treatment depends on the final histology. (*B*) Management algorithm for subepithelial lesions. Fourth-layer lesions are sampled with EUS-guided FNA. Tumors diagnostic of GIST by immunohistochemistry should undergo evaluation by surgery and oncology. Small (<2 cm) gastric tumors may considered for EUS surveillance. Tumors diagnostic of a non-GIST such as a leiomyoma or schwannoma generally do not require any intervention. Nondiagnostic results should prompt repeat EUS FNA within 1 year if there is a clinical suspicion of GIST; otherwise large or symptomatic tumors should be resected.

Controversy exists as to the management of small incidentally found GISTs, especially gastric lesions less than 2 cm in size. These tumors appear to have a low risk of malignant behavior and may be considered for EUS surveillance without resection.[99] Factors to be considered in selecting patients for surveillance include patient's age, comorbidities, and life expectancy. Although the optimal timing and number of surveillance examinations and duration are unknown, a recent survey reported 70% would survey annually.[100] Any change in size should prompt surgical resection (**Fig. 4**).[101,102]

SUMMARY

Subepithelial masses in the gastrointestinal tract are a frequently encountered endoscopic finding. These masses encompass a heterogeneous group of lesions that range from benign to malignant. EUS is highly useful in the evaluation of these lesions, and guides subsequent tissue sampling and therapy if needed. Management of these lesions depends on many factors and should be considered case by case.

REFERENCES

1. Sonnenberg A, Amorosi SL, Lacey MJ, et al. Patterns of endoscopy in the United States: analysis of data from the Centers for Medicare and Medicaid Services and the National Endoscopic Database. Gastrointest Endosc 2008; 67(3):489–96.
2. Hwang JH, Saunders MD, Rulyak SJ, et al. A prospective study comparing endoscopy and EUS in the evaluation of GI subepithelial masses. Gastrointest Endosc 2005;62(2):202–8.
3. Brand B, Oesterhelweg L, Binmoeller KF, et al. Impact of endoscopic ultrasound for evaluation of submucosal lesions in gastrointestinal tract. Dig Liver Dis 2002; 34(4):290–7.
4. Papanikolaou IS, Triantafyllou K, Kourikou A, et al. Endoscopic ultrasonography for gastric submucosal lesions. World J Gastrointest Endosc 2011;3(5):86–94.
5. Muenst S, Thies S, Went P, et al. Frequency, phenotype, and genotype of minute gastrointestinal stromal tumors in the stomach: an autopsy study. Hum Pathol 2011;42(12):1849–54.
6. Jenssen C, Dietrich CF. Endoscopic ultrasound in subepithelial tumors of the gastrointestinal tract. In: Dietrich CF, editor. Endoscopic ultrasound: an introductory manual and atlas. New York: Thieme; 2006. p. 121–54.
7. Humphris JL, Jones DB. Subepithelial mass lesions in the upper gastrointestinal tract. J Gastroenterol Hepatol 2008;23(4):556–66.
8. Polkowski M. Endoscopic ultrasound and endoscopic ultrasound-guided fine-needle biopsy for the diagnosis of malignant submucosal tumors. Endoscopy 2005;37(7):635–45.
9. Stamatakos M, Douzinas E, Stefanaki C, et al. Gastrointestinal stromal tumor. World J Surg Oncol 2009;7:61.
10. Miettinen M, Virolainen M, Maarit Sarlomo R. Gastrointestinal stromal tumors—value of CD34 antigen in their identification and separation from true leiomyomas and schwannomas. Am J Surg Pathol 1995;19(2):207–16.
11. Sarlomo-Rikala M, Kovatich AJ, Barusevicius A, et al. CD117: a sensitive marker for gastrointestinal stromal tumors that is more specific than CD34. Mod Pathol 1998;11(8):728–34.
12. Corless CL, Schroeder A, Griffith D, et al. PDGFRA mutations in gastrointestinal stromal tumors: frequency, spectrum and in vitro sensitivity to imatinib. J Clin Oncol 2005;23(23):5357–64.

13. Kim KM, Kang DW, Moon WS, et al. Gastrointestinal stromal tumors in Koreans: its incidence and the clinical, pathologic and immunohistochemical findings. J Korean Med Sci 2005;20(6):977–84.
14. Dei Tos AP, Laurino L, Bearzi I, et al. Gastrointestinal stromal tumors: the histology report. Dig Liver Dis 2011;43(Suppl 4):S304–9.
15. Miettinen M, Wang ZF, Lasota J. DOG1 antibody in the differential diagnosis of gastrointestinal stromal tumors: a study of 1840 cases. Am J Surg Pathol 2009; 33(9):1401–8.
16. Hirota S, Ohashi A, Nishida T, et al. Gain-of-function mutations of platelet-derived growth factor receptor alpha gene in gastrointestinal stromal tumors. Gastroenterology 2003;125(3):660–7.
17. Demetri GD, von Mehren M, Antonescu CR, et al. NCCN Task Force report: update on the management of patients with gastrointestinal stromal tumors. J Natl Compr Canc Netw 2010;8(Suppl 2):S1–41 [quiz: S42–4].
18. Tryggvason G, Kristmundsson T, Orvar K, et al. Clinical study on gastrointestinal stromal tumors (GIST) in Iceland, 1990-2003. Dig Dis Sci 2007;52(9):2249–53.
19. Petrou A, Alexandrou P, Papalambros A, et al. A malignant gastrointestinal stromal tumor of the gallbladder immunoreactive for PDGFRA and negative for CD 117 Antigen (c-KIT). HPB Surgery 2011;2011:327192.
20. Cecka F, Jon B, Ferko A, et al. Long-term survival of a patient after resection of a gastrointestinal stromal tumor arising from the pancreas. Hepatobiliary Pancreat Dis Int 2011;10(3):330–2.
21. Long KB, Butrynski JE, Blank SD, et al. Primary extragastrointestinal stromal tumor of the pleura: report of a unique case with genetic confirmation. Am J Surg Pathol 2010;34(6):907–12.
22. Alvarado-Cabrero I, Vazquez G, Sierra Santiesteban FI, et al. Clinicopathologic study of 275 cases of gastrointestinal stromal tumors: the experience at 3 large medical centers in Mexico. Ann Diagn Pathol 2007;11(1):39–45.
23. Goettsch WG, Bos SD, Breekveldt-Postma N, et al. Incidence of gastrointestinal stromal tumours is underestimated: results of a nation-wide study. Eur J Cancer 2005;41(18):2868–72.
24. De Palma GD, Rega M, Masone S, et al. Lower gastrointestinal bleeding secondary to a rectal leiomyoma. World J Gastroenterol 2009;15(14):1769–70.
25. Mutrie CJ, Donahue DM, Wain JC, et al. Esophageal leiomyoma: a 40-year experience. Ann Thorac Surg 2005;79(4):1122–5.
26. Miettinen M, Sarlomo-Rikala M, Sobin LH. Mesenchymal tumors of muscularis mucosae of colon and rectum are benign leiomyomas that should be separated from gastrointestinal stromal tumors–a clinicopathologic and immunohistochemical study of eighty-eight cases. Mod Pathol 2001;14(10):950–6.
27. Stamatakos M, Kontzoglou K, Sargedi C, et al. Gastrointestinal carcinoid tumors: diagnosis and treatment. Chirurgia 2010;105(6):759–66.
28. Yoshikane H, Tsukamoto Y, Niwa Y, et al. Carcinoid tumors of the gastrointestinal tract: evaluation with endoscopic ultrasonography. Gastrointest Endosc 1993; 39(3):375–83.
29. Ichikawa J, Tanabe S, Koizumi W, et al. Endoscopic mucosal resection in the management of gastric carcinoid tumors. Endoscopy 2003;35(3):203–6.
30. Rindi G, Bordi C, Rappel S, et al. Gastric carcinoids and neuroendocrine carcinomas: pathogenesis, pathology, and behavior. World J Surg 1996;20(2):168–72.
31. Plesec TP. Gastrointestinal mesenchymal neoplasms other than gastrointestinal stromal tumors: focusing on their molecular aspects. Pathol Res Int 2011;2011: 952569.

32. Yu HG, Ding YM, Tan S, et al. A safe and efficient strategy for endoscopic resection of large, gastrointestinal lipoma. Surg Endoscopy 2007;21(2):265–9.
33. Daimaru Y, Kido H, Hashimoto H, et al. Benign schwannoma of the gastrointestinal tract: a clinicopathologic and immunohistochemical study. Hum Pathol 1988;19(3):257–64.
34. Kwon MS, Lee SS, Ahn GH. Schwannomas of the gastrointestinal tract: clinicopathological features of 12 cases including a case of esophageal tumor compared with those of gastrointestinal stromal tumors and leiomyomas of the gastrointestinal tract. Pathol Res Pract 2002;198(9):605–13.
35. Hou YY, Tan YS, Xu JF, et al. Schwannoma of the gastrointestinal tract: a clinicopathological, immunohistochemical and ultrastructural study of 33 cases. Histopathology 2006;48(5):536–45.
36. Quiroga S, Alvarez-Castells A, Pallisa E, et al. Duodenal schwannoma causing gastrointestinal bleeding: helical CT findings. Abdom Imaging 1997;22(2):154–5.
37. Pang LC. Pancreatic heterotopia: a reappraisal and clinicopathologic analysis of 32 cases. South Med J 1988;81(10):1264–75.
38. Emerson L, Layfield LJ, Rohr LR, et al. Adenocarcinoma arising in association with gastric heterotopic pancreas: a case report and review of the literature. J Surg Oncol 2004;87(1):53–7.
39. Chen SH, Huang WH, Feng CL, et al. Clinical analysis of ectopic pancreas with endoscopic ultrasonography: an experience in a medical center. J Gastrointest Surg 2008;12(5):877–81.
40. Diehl DL, Cheruvattath R, Facktor MA, et al. Infection after endoscopic ultrasound-guided aspiration of mediastinal cysts. Interact Cardiovasc Thorac Surg 2010;10(2):338–40.
41. Miettinen M, Paal E, Lasota J, et al. Gastrointestinal glomus tumors: a clinicopathologic, immunohistochemical, and molecular genetic study of 32 cases. Am J Surg Pathol 2002;26(3):301–11.
42. Chou KC, Yang CW, Yen HH. Rare gastric glomus tumor causing upper gastrointestinal bleeding, with review of the endoscopic ultrasound features. Endoscopy 2010;42(Suppl 2):E58–9.
43. Oda I, Kondo H, Yamao T, et al. Metastatic tumors to the stomach: analysis of 54 patients diagnosed at endoscopy and 347 autopsy cases. Endoscopy 2001; 33(6):507–10.
44. Boyce GA, Sivak MV Jr, Rosch T, et al. Evaluation of submucosal upper gastrointestinal tract lesions by endoscopic ultrasound. Gastrointest Endosc 1991; 37(4):449–54.
45. Rosch T, Kapfer B, Will U, et al. Accuracy of endoscopic ultrasonography in upper gastrointestinal submucosal lesions: a prospective multicenter study. Scand J Gastroenterol 2002;37(7):856–62.
46. Yasuda K, Cho E, Nakajima M, et al. Diagnosis of submucosal lesions of the upper gastrointestinal tract by endoscopic ultrasonography. Gastrointest Endosc 1990;36(Suppl 2):S17–20.
47. Shen EF, Arnott ID, Plevris J, et al. Endoscopic ultrasonography in the diagnosis and management of suspected upper gastrointestinal submucosal tumours. Br J Surg 2002;89(2):231–5.
48. Yasuda K, Nakajima M, Yoshida S, et al. The diagnosis of submucosal tumors of the stomach by endoscopic ultrasonography. Gastrointest Endosc 1989;35(1):10–5.
49. Kameyama H, Niwa Y, Arisawa T, et al. Endoscopic ultrasonography in the diagnosis of submucosal lesions of the large intestine. Gastrointest Endosc 1997; 46(5):406–11.

50. Gress F, Schmitt C, Savides T, et al. Interobserver agreement for EUS in the evaluation and diagnosis of submucosal masses. Gastrointest Endosc 2001;53(1): 71–6.
51. Jeon SW, Park YD, Chung YJ, et al. Gastrointestinal stromal tumors of the stomach: endosonographic differentiation in relation to histological risk. J Gastroenterol Hepatol 2007;22(12):2069–75.
52. Bromberg SH, Camilo Neto C, Borges AF, et al. Pancreatic heterotopias: clinicopathological analysis of 18 patients. Rev Col Bras Cir 2010;37(6):413–9 [in Portuguese].
53. Burke M, Shepherd N, Mann CV. Carcinoid tumours of the rectum and anus. Br J Surg 1987;74(5):358–61.
54. Hamada H, Shikuwa S, Wen CY, et al. Pedunculated rectal carcinoid removed by endoscopic mucosal resection: a case report. World J Gastroenterol 2003; 9(12):2870–2.
55. De Beer RA, Shinya H. Colonic lipomas. An endoscopic analysis. Gastrointest Endosc 1975;22(2):90–1.
56. Chen TK, Wu CH, Lee CL, et al. Endoscopic ultrasonography to study the causes of extragastric compression mimicking gastric submucosal tumor. J Formos Med Assoc 2001;100(11):758–61.
57. Miettinen M, El-Rifai W, H L Sobin L, et al. Evaluation of malignancy and prognosis of gastrointestinal stromal tumors: a review. Hum Pathol 2002;33(5): 478–83.
58. Burkill GJ, Badran M, Al-Muderis O, et al. Malignant gastrointestinal stromal tumor: distribution, imaging features, and pattern of metastatic spread. Radiology 2003;226(2):527–32.
59. Hunt GC, Smith PP, Faigel DO. Yield of tissue sampling for submucosal lesions evaluated by EUS. Gastrointest Endosc 2003;57(1):68–72.
60. Chien CH, Chien RN, Yen CL, et al. The role of endoscopic ultrasonography examination for evaluation and surveillance of gastric subepithelial masses. Chang Gung Med J 2010;33(1):73–81.
61. Romero-Castro R, Pellicer-Bautista F, Giovannini M, et al. Endoscopic ultrasound (EUS)-guided coil embolization therapy in gastric varices. Endoscopy 2010;42(Suppl 2):E35–6.
62. Takizawa K, Matsuda T, Kozu T, et al. Lymph node staging in esophageal squamous cell carcinoma: a comparative study of endoscopic ultrasonography versus computed tomography. J Gastroenterol Hepatol 2009;24(10):1687–91.
63. Botet JF, Lightdale CJ, Zauber AG, et al. Preoperative staging of esophageal cancer: comparison of endoscopic US and dynamic CT. Radiology 1991; 181(2):419–25.
64. Karaca C, Turner BG, Cizginer S, et al. Accuracy of EUS in the evaluation of small gastric subepithelial lesions. Gastrointest Endosc 2010;71(4):722–7.
65. Ji JS, Lee BI, Choi KY, et al. Diagnostic yield of tissue sampling using a bite-on-bite technique for incidental subepithelial lesions. Korean J Intern Med 2009; 24(2):101–5.
66. Cantor MJ, Davila RE, Faigel DO. Yield of tissue sampling for subepithelial lesions evaluated by EUS: a comparison between forceps biopsies and endoscopic submucosal resection. Gastrointest Endosc 2006;64(1):29–34.
67. Saftoiu A, Vilmann P, Guldhammer Skov B, et al. Endoscopic ultrasound (EUS)-guided Trucut biopsy adds significant information to EUS-guided fine-needle aspiration in selected patients: a prospective study. Scand J Gastroenterol 2007;42(1):117–25.

68. Levy MJ, Jondal ML, Clain J, et al. Preliminary experience with an EUS-guided Trucut biopsy needle compared with EUS-guided FNA. Gastrointest Endosc 2003;57(1):101–6.
69. Levy MJ, Wiersema MJ. EUS-guided Trucut biopsy. Gastrointest Endosc 2005; 62(3):417–26.
70. Kajiyama T, Hajiro K, Sakai M, et al. Endoscopic resection of gastrointestinal submucosal lesions: a comparison between strip biopsy and aspiration lumpectomy. Gastrointest Endosc 1996;44(4):404–10.
71. Tanabe S, Koizumi W, Kokutou M, et al. Usefulness of endoscopic aspiration mucosectomy as compared with strip biopsy for the treatment of gastric mucosal cancer. Gastrointest Endosc 1999;50(6):819–22.
72. Faigel DO, Gopal D, Weeks DA, et al. Cap-assisted endoscopic submucosal resection of a pancreatic rest. Gastrointest Endosc 2001;54(6):782–4.
73. Barr H, Kendall C, Hutchings J, et al. Rapid endoscopic identification and destruction of degenerating Barrett's mucosal neoplasia. Surgeon 2011;9(3): 119–23.
74. Tanabe S, Koizumi W, Mitomi H, et al. Clinical outcome of endoscopic aspiration mucosectomy for early stage gastric cancer. Gastrointest Endosc 2002;56(5): 708–13.
75. Tanabe S, Koizumi W, Mitomi H, et al. Usefulness of EMR with an oblique aspiration mucosectomy device compared with strip biopsy in patients with superficial esophageal cancer. Gastrointest Endosc 2004;59(4):558–63.
76. Martinez-Ares D, Lorenzo MJ, Souto-Ruzo J, et al. Endoscopic resection of gastrointestinal submucosal tumors assisted by endoscopic ultrasonography. Surg Endosc 2005;19(6):854–8.
77. Kojima T, Takahashi H, Parra-Blanco A, et al. Diagnosis of submucosal tumor of the upper GI tract by endoscopic resection. Gastrointest Endosc 1999;50(4):516–22.
78. Ahmadi A, Draganov P. Endoscopic mucosal resection in the upper gastrointestinal tract. World J Gastroenterol 2008;14(13):1984–9.
79. Lee IL, Lin PY, Tung SY, et al. Endoscopic submucosal dissection for the treatment of intraluminal gastric subepithelial tumors originating from the muscularis propria layer. Endoscopy 2006;38(10):1024–8.
80. Jeong ID, Jung SW, Bang SJ, et al. Endoscopic enucleation for gastric subepithelial tumors originating in the muscularis propria layer. Surg Endosc 2011; 25(2):468–74.
81. Park YS, Park SW, Kim TI, et al. Endoscopic enucleation of upper-GI submucosal tumors by using an insulated-tip electrosurgical knife. Gastrointest Endosc 2004;59(3):409–15.
82. Bai J, Wang Y, Guo H, et al. Endoscopic resection of small gastrointestinal stromal tumors. Dig Dis Sci 2010;55(7):1950–4.
83. Williams DB, Sahai AV, Aabakken L, et al. Endoscopic ultrasound guided fine needle aspiration biopsy: a large single centre experience. Gut 1999;44(5): 720–6.
84. Hoda KM, Rodriguez SA, Faigel DO. EUS-guided sampling of suspected GI stromal tumors. Gastrointest Endosc 2009;69(7):1218–23.
85. Akahoshi K, Sumida Y, Matsui N, et al. Preoperative diagnosis of gastrointestinal stromal tumor by endoscopic ultrasound-guided fine needle aspiration. World J Gastroenterol 2007;13(14):2077–82.
86. Vander Noot MR 3rd, Eloubeidi MA, Chen VK, et al. Diagnosis of gastrointestinal tract lesions by endoscopic ultrasound-guided fine-needle aspiration biopsy. Cancer 2004;102(3):157–63.

87. Philipper M, Hollerbach S, Gabbert HE, et al. Prospective comparison of endoscopic ultrasound-guided fine-needle aspiration and surgical histology in upper gastrointestinal submucosal tumors. Endoscopy 2010;42(4):300–5.
88. Chatzipantelis P, Salla C, Karoumpalis I, et al. Endoscopic ultrasound-guided fine needle aspiration biopsy in the diagnosis of gastrointestinal stromal tumors of the stomach. A study of 17 cases. J Gastrointest Liver Dis 2008;17(1):15–20.
89. Sasaki Y, Niwa Y, Hirooka Y, et al. The use of endoscopic ultrasound-guided fine-needle aspiration for investigation of submucosal and extrinsic masses of the colon and rectum. Endoscopy 2005;37(2):154–60.
90. Sepe PS, Moparty B, Pitman MB, et al. EUS-guided FNA for the diagnosis of GI stromal cell tumors: sensitivity and cytologic yield. Gastrointest Endosc 2009; 70(2):254–61.
91. Watson RR, Binmoeller KF, Hamerski CM, et al. Yield and performance characteristics of endoscopic ultrasound-guided fine needle aspiration for diagnosing upper GI tract stromal tumors. Dig Dis Sci 2011;56(6):1757–62.
92. Hirota S, Isozaki K, Moriyama Y, et al. Gain-of-function mutations of c-kit in human gastrointestinal stromal tumors. Science 1998;279(5350):577–80.
93. Toquet C, Le Neel JC, Guillou L, et al. Elevated (> or = 10%) MIB-1 proliferative index correlates with poor outcome in gastric stromal tumor patients: a study of 35 cases. Dig Dis Sci 2002;47(10):2247–53.
94. Terada T. Gastrointestinal stromal tumor of the digestive organs: a histopathologic study of 31 cases in a single Japanese institute. Int J Clin Exp Pathol 2009;3(2):162–8.
95. Hirota S, Isozaki K. Pathology of gastrointestinal stromal tumors. Pathol Int 2006; 56(1):1–9.
96. Heinrich MC, Corless CL, Duensing A, et al. PDGFRA activating mutations in gastrointestinal stromal tumors. Science 2003;299(5607):708–10.
97. Wong NA. Gastrointestinal stromal tumours–an update for histopathologists. Histopathology 2011;59:807–21.
98. American Gastroenterological Association Institute medical position statement on the management of gastric subepithelial masses. Gastroenterology 2006; 130(7):2215–6.
99. Al-Haddad M, Dewitt J. EUS-guided sampling of suspected GI mesenchymal tumors: cells, cores, or a combination? Gastrointest Endosc 2009;69(7):1224–7.
100. Ha CY, Shah R, Chen J, et al. Diagnosis and management of GI stromal tumors by EUS-FNA: a survey of opinions and practices of endosonographers. Gastrointest Endosc 2009;69(6):1039–44, e1.
101. Tanaka J, Oshima T, Hori K, et al. Small gastrointestinal stromal tumor of the stomach showing rapid growth and early metastasis to the liver. Dig Endosc 2010;22(4):354–6.
102. Okada K, Maruyama K, Nagase H, et al. [A case of gastrointestinal stromal tumor of the stomach with rapid growth in a short term]. Gan To Kagaku Ryoho 2008;35(12):2080–2 [in Japanese].
103. Eckardt AJ, Wassef W. Diagnosis of subepithelial tumors in the GI tract. Endoscopy, EUS, and histology: bronze, silver, and gold standard? Gastrointest Endosc 2005;62(2):209–12.
104. Chak A. EUS in submucosal tumors. Gastrointest Endosc 2002;56(Suppl 4):S43–8.
105. Fujimoto Y, Nakanishi Y, Yoshimura K, et al. Clinicopathologic study of primary malignant gastrointestinal stromal tumor of the stomach, with special reference to prognostic factors: analysis of results in 140 surgically resected patients. Gastric Cancer 2003;6(1):39–48.

106. Palazzo L, Landi B, Cellier C, et al. Endosonographic features predictive of benign and malignant gastrointestinal stromal cell tumours. Gut 2000;46(1): 88–92.
107. Chak A, Canto MI, Rosch T, et al. Endosonographic differentiation of benign and malignant stromal cell tumors. Gastrointest Endosc 1997;45(6):468–73.
108. Tsai TL, Changchien CS, Hu TH, et al. Differentiation of benign and malignant gastric stromal tumors using endoscopic ultrasonography. Chang Gung Med J 2001;24(3):167–73.
109. Orellana F, Onetto C, Balbontin P, et al. Gastric glomus tumor: report of one case and review. Endoscopy 2011;43(Suppl 2):E71–2.

Endoscopic Ultrasonography/Fine-Needle Aspiration and Endobronchial Ultrasonography/Fine-Needle Aspiration for Lung Cancer Staging

Ali Lankarani, MD, Michael B. Wallace, MD, MP*

KEYWORDS

- Lung cancer • Mediastinal adenopathy
- Nonsmall cell lung cancer • Endoscopic ultrasonography
- Transthoracic needle aspirate • Transbronchial needle aspirate
- Fine-needle aspiration • Endobronchial ultrasonography

INTRODUCTION

This review covers recent developments in techniques for staging patients with lung cancer, focusing on the different modalities available for staging mediastinal adenopathy and highlighting the advantages and disadvantages of each method. The controversies regarding the sequence of tests required for nodal staging in the mediastinum are reviewed and evidence is provided for current best practice. The role of endoscopic ultrasonography (EUS) and the gastroenterologist in mediastinal nodal staging is explored. An algorithm is proposed that incorporates EUS as one of the staging modalities for patients with non–small cell lung cancer (NSCLC).

EPIDEMIOLOGY

Lung cancer is the second most common cancer and the most common cause of cancer-related death in both men and women in the United States and in the world.

Disclosures: Dr Wallace receives research funding from the National Cancer Institute, Olympus, Red Path Integrated Pathology, Fujinon, Mauna Kea Technologies, The Bankhead Coley Research Program, and The Boston Scientific Foundation.
Department of Gastroenterology, Mayo Clinic, 4500 San Pablo Road South, Jacksonville, FL 32224, USA
* Corresponding author.
E-mail address: wallace.michael@mayo.edu

Gastrointest Endoscopy Clin N Am 22 (2012) 207–219
doi:10.1016/j.giec.2012.04.005
1052-5157/12/$ – see front matter © 2012 Elsevier Inc. All rights reserved.

Most new cases of lung cancer (up to 80%) are NSCLC. Incidence and mortality for men have decreased in the past decade in the United States and in those countries in which smoking cessation efforts have been successful[1]; however, internationally, especially in Asia, this disease is becoming epidemic.[2]

DIAGNOSIS AND STAGING

In cases in which small cell lung cancer is suspected, tissue diagnosis should be made by the easiest available method. Radiologic imaging is usually sufficient to distinguish limited from extensive disease.[3]

In contrast, in patients who are suspected to have NSCLC, diagnosis and staging should occur concurrently. It is critical to stage the disease accurately, because the choice of therapy is dictated by the stage of the disease. Patients with mediastinal nodal metastases (ie, N2 or N3) are not likely to benefit from surgical resection.[4] In some patients with limited ipsilateral lymph node involvement, surgery can still be advised. Incomplete or inaccurate staging can result in patients undergoing futile thoracotomies. Mediastinal metastases are missed in 7% to 17% of all patients NSCLC who undergo lung resection.[5,6]

Lung cancer is staged by TNM classification. The current TNM staging system for NSCLC was last revised in 1997.[7,8] The distribution and mapping of lymph nodes in the mediastinum was initially described by Mountain and colleagues,[9] and its various revisions are used to describe the N factor in TNM staging. The American Thoracic Society regional lymph node station criteria are frequently used to divide the mediastinal lymph node stations (**Fig. 1**).

Noninvasive, minimally invasive, and invasive staging methods have been used for staging lung cancer.

Cross-sectional imaging studies of the chest, along with imaging of the liver and adrenal glands, are the first steps of assessment in patients with suspected NSCLC who may undergo treatment.[10] Computed tomography (CT) and positron emission tomography (PET) scans, especially with their excellent safety profiles, are among the first noninvasive modalities that are used. They are widely available; however, their limited sensitivity and specificity undermine their usefulness.

The pooled sensitivity and specificity of CT for identifying mediastinal lymph node metastasis are 51% and 85%, respectively. PET has a sensitivity and specificity of 74% and 85%, respectively, for identifying mediastinal lymph node metastasis.[10] Patients with negative CT for mediastinal adenopathy can have up to 35% prevalence of malignant mediastinal lymph nodes.[11] Therefore, tissue sampling is often required.

Bronchoscopy is often necessary in every patient to confirm the diagnosis and to evaluate for synchronous occult contralateral lesions. Bronchoscopy is falsely negative in up to 30% of cases even if brushings, washings, and transbronchial biopsies are performed.[12] To stage the cancer, confirm the diagnosis, and assess for respectability, patients usually need to undergo other investigations.

The American College of Chest Physicians (ACCP) guidelines for lung cancer staging recommend that patients with abnormal lymph nodes on CT or PET, or centrally located tumors without mediastinal adenopathy, should undergo invasive staging for tissue diagnosis and confirmation.[13] Mediastinal tissue can be obtained by needle techniques or surgical biopsies.

NEEDLE TECHNIQUES

Needle techniques are generally less invasive, less expensive, and less associated with complications compared with surgical methods. Deep sedation is usually not

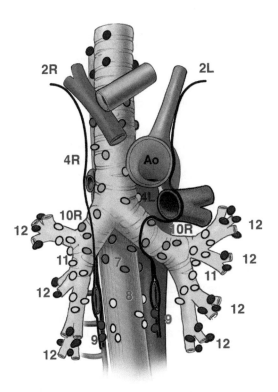

Fig. 1. Mediastinal lymph node stations based on the American Thoracic Society regional lymph node station criteria.

necessary for needle techniques. The following techniques have been used for needle sampling of the mediastinal area.

Transthoracic Needle Aspirate

CT or fluoroscopy-guided transthoracic needle aspirate (TTNA) is mainly used for the sampling of a lung mass that is not reachable during bronchoscopy. In addition, large mediastinal lymph nodes can be sampled via this method.[13,14] The major adverse event associated with TTNA is pneumothorax, which can happen in up to 10% of cases.[13]

Transbronchial Needle Aspirate

Conventional transbronchial needle aspirate (TBNA) can be performed through indirect or blind guidance of a needle by using information derived from CT on the location of lymph nodes, transbronchially during bronchoscopy., TBNA was originally described in 1949 using a rigid bronchoscope. It gained more popularity after the introduction of flexible endoscopes and the Wang needle in the mid-1980s.[15] TBNA is an underused procedure; only 12% of North American bronchoscopists routinely use TBNA, and 29% of all bronchoscopists use it occasionally.[16,17] The blind nature of the procedure along with the limitations of CT, especially its inability to identify smaller nodes, are the main factors contributing to the underuse of TBNA.[18] Pneumothorax can happen in 0.4% to 5% of TBNA cases.[19]

Endobronchial Ultrasonography with TBNA

The accuracy of TBNA can be improved by addition of endobronchial ultrasonography (EBUS).[20] Two types of EBUS system are available: radial catheter probe and convex probe EBUS (CP-EBUS). Radial catheter probe EBUS does not allow real-time needle biopsy; however, with the introduction of CP-EBUS, real-time ultrasound-guided transesophageal mediastinal lymph node biopsies became possible.[21–23]

EBUS can identify lymph nodes in the anterior and superior mediastinum (stations 1, 2, 4, and anterior nodes of station 7; see **Fig. 1**), as well as intrapulmonary and hilar nodes (stations 10, 11, and 12).[24] EBUS-TBNA is reported to have a sensitivity of 85% to 100%, a specificity of 100% and an accuracy of more than 96% in distinguishing benign from malignant mediastinal lymph nodes in patients with lung cancer.[25–28] EBUS-TBNA is considered to be a safe procedure, with a reported 0.05% risk for major complications in systematic reviews. Pneumothorax and respiratory failure requiring ventilation are the major complications of EBUS-TBNA.[29]

EUS–Fine-Needle Aspiration

A radial or linear scope can be used during the mediastinal staging of lung cancer. The radial scope is generally used for staging purposes, after which a linear echoendoscope is used for targeted EUS–fine-needle aspiration (FNA). Alternatively, the entire examination can be performed with a linear echoendoscope. Because echo characteristics alone have limited accuracy, EUS staging of lung cancer almost always requires FNA of lymph nodes.[30]

EUS can identify lymph nodes in the posterior and inferior mediastinum. Stations 8, 9, and posterior nodes at station 7 are accessible during EUS. When enlarged, station 5 nodes can also be accessible.[31–34]

Unlike the trachea, the esophagus is flexible. Considerable excursions in the lateral direction of the esophagus are possible so that structures, which on a CT scan look relatively remote from the esophagus, can often be seen and biopsied during EUS examinations. In the superior mediastinum, the trachea is to the right of the esophagus, which often makes it possible to reach area 2L and 4L lymph nodes.[35] 4R nodes are usually not accessible with EUS unless enlarged.[36]

The feasibility of EUS-FNA of the aortopulmonary window lymph nodes (station 5) has been believed to be a major advantage of EUS. Evaluation of this station has traditionally required a paramedian mediastinotomy (Chamberlain procedure). EUS-FNA is recommended as the first-line method for assessment of stage 5 nodes by the American Society for Gastrointestinal Endoscopy.[37]

Another advantage of EUS is that it can detect metastatic disease to subdiaphragmatic sites such as left adrenal, celiac lymph nodes, and liver. The importance of EUS in the evaluation of the celiac lymph nodes has been emphasized by several investigators.[38,39]

Major limitations of EUS arise because EUS-FNA is performed through the esophagus and ultrasonic rays do not penetrate air-filled structures, thus regions immediately anterior to the trachea are a blind spot for EUS-FNA.[34] In general, EUS is most appropriate for evaluation of the posterior inferior mediastinum, whereas EBUS is better for the lymph nodes in the anterior superior mediastinum.

With regard to the detection of malignant mediastinal lymph nodes in NSCLC, EUS-FNA has an overall sensitivity of 84%, and an overall false-negative (FN) rate of 19% (range, 0%–61%). The overall specificity is 99.5% and the overall false-positive rate is 0.4%.[32,34–36,38–44] With a positive predictive value (PPV) greater than 99% and a negative predictive value (NPV) of 81%, EUS-FNA is proved to be a great tool for mediastinal lymph node staging in patients who have lung cancer.[13]

Complications from EUS-FNA in a recent meta-analysis of 18 studies with a total of 1201 patients were reported to be 0.8% (only 10 cases).[11]

Multiple publications have evaluated the role of EUS in the staging of patients with NSCLC. In a study involving 107 Dutch patients, 16% of thoracotomies could have been avoided by using EUS in addition to mediastinoscopy.[45] In another study, the role of preoperative EUS in addition to standard staging for detection of malignant lymph nodes was examined. It was shown that the addition of EUS can reduce the need of resective surgery in patients who have lung cancer with advanced disease.[46] In a retrospective study, EUS-guided FNA was performed on 35 patients with biopsy-proven negative mediastinoscopies. Thirteen patients were found to have malignant N2 or N3 lymph nodes.[33]

In a cost-analysis model using Monte-Carlo techniques,[45] the investigators postulated that if EUS-FNA had been performed initially (rather than mediastinoscopy) an average cost saving of $11,033 per patient would have resulted.

COMBINED EUS-FNA AND EBUS-TBNA

EBUS-TBNA assesses and samples the same nodal stations as cervical mediastinoscopy.[37] However, the FN rate of EBUS-TBNA is 24%, whereas mediastinoscopy has an FN rate of approximately 10%.[13] This rate has been partly attributed to the fact that EBUS-TBNA cannot access the posterior and inferior mediastinum, or stage 5 lymph nodes.

EUS has the highest yield in the posterior inferior mediastinum. The addition of EUS-FNA to EBUS-TBNA provides a safe way to sample the posterior inferior mediastinal lymph nodes. EUS and EBUS complement each other and provide access to most of the mediastinal lymph nodes in patients with NSCLC. In 1 study, it was shown that if mediastinoscopy had been performed only when results from EUS plus EBUS were negative, this surgical procedure would have been avoided in 28% of patients.[20] Similarly, encouraging results using a combined approach have been reported by other investigators.[27,35,47]

Herth and colleagues[48] recently reported a sensitivity of 96% and NPV of 96% in 150 consecutive patients with suspected lung cancer and enlarged mediastinal lymph node (>1 cm) on CT who underwent combined endoscopic-endobronchial ultrasound-guided FNA using a single bronchoscope.

Two prospective studies looked at the feasibility, performance characteristics, and safety of combined EUS-EBUS for staging in patients with NSCLC.

Szlubowski and colleagues[49] prospectively evaluated 120 patients with NSCLC with a radiologically normal mediastinum. PPV and NPV of combined EUS-EBUS was found to be 91%. Wallace and colleagues[20] reported an NPV of 97% using a combined EUS-EBUS staging protocol in a prospective study that evaluated 138 patients with NSCLC. No complications were reported related to the combined EUS-EBUS procedure in any of these studies.

SURGICAL TECHNIQUES

Traditionally, surgical techniques are considered the gold standard method for obtaining mediastinal lymph node biopsy samples (NPV, 89%; PPV, 100%).[13] Mediastinoscopy is an underused procedure and its yield varies considerably based on the training and the experience of the surgeon.[50]

In a US study of 11,668 patients who underwent thoracotomy for lung cancer, only 27% of these patients had preoperative mediastinoscopy. Lymphoid tissue samples were obtained in only 47% of these patients.[51] Another study from the Netherlands showed that only 40% of the surgeons adhere to the examination of the 5 nodal stations that routinely should be examined during mediastinoscopy.[52] Nevertheless, mediastinoscopy, if performed by experienced surgeons, will continue to have a role in the invasive staging of NSCLC.

Surgical techniques normally require deep sedation and general anesthesia after endotracheal intubation, and tend to be more expensive compared with the needle techniques.[13,53,54] The risk of morbidity and serious complications, including stroke and aortic injury, is higher in surgical techniques.[13,55,56] The following surgical techniques have been used for sampling of the mediastinal area.

Cervical Mediastinoscopy

Cervical mediastinoscopy can be used for lymph node sampling or complete excision of nodal stations 1, 2, 3, 4, and anterior nodes of 7.[13,57] This procedure can be performed as an outpatient surgical procedure. It has a morbidity of 1% to 2% and a mortality of 0.05% to 0.08%.[13,58] Cervical mediastinoscopy has limited access to the inferior and posterior mediastinum as well as to the aortopulmonary window (station 5).

Extended Cervical Mediastinoscopy

Extended cervical mediastinoscopy is mainly useful when evaluation of the stage 5 nodes is needed in cases of carcinoma of the left lung.[59–61] The drawback of this surgical procedure is the higher incidence of complications, including aortic artery injuries.[13,58,62]

Anterior Mediastinoscopy

Anterior mediastinoscopy is more commonly used to obtain samples from the station 5 nodes.[60,61] A complication rate of 6.8%, including pneumothorax, bleeding, nerve injury, and transient ischemia, has been associated with this surgical procedure.[9,63]

Video-Assisted Thoracoscopy

When video-assisted thoracoscopy (VATS) is used for staging of mediastinal adenopathy, one of the patient's lungs commonly needs to be collapsed after general anesthesia; therefore, the procedure typically evaluates either the right or the left mediastinum. Nodal stations 5 and 6 can be accessed when the left mediastinum is studied.

Right paratracheal nodes (stations 2 and 4), subcarinal nodes (station 7), and inferior mediastinal nodes (stations 8 and 9) can be accessed during VATS. The morbidity of VATS is approximately 2%.[13]

CURRENT BEST PRACTICE

One of 4 patients with resectable lung cancer based on the cross-sectional imaging studies has mediastinal metastases that has not been detected.[10] The ACCP guidelines recommend invasive staging for patients with or without mediastinal lymph node enlargement on CT, regardless of the PET scan findings. If needle techniques are used (such as EUS-FNA, TBNA, EBUS-TBNA, or TTNA) a nonmalignant result should be further confirmed by mediastinoscopy if the suspicion for mediastinal node metastasis is high.[13]

Historically, surgical mediastinoscopy served as a gold standard for mediastinal adenopathy to sample or excise lymph nodes.[64] Combined EUS and EBUS, also known as complete medical mediastinoscopy, has been proposed as an alternative modality to evaluate the entire mediastinum without a need for a surgical procedure.[27,28]

Combined EUS and EBUS can access mediastinal stations beyond the scope of mediastinoscopy.[65] These complimentary techniques are proposed as a further gold standard for diagnosis of mediastinal adenopathy.[49]

Use of less invasive techniques before mediastinoscopy has been advocated to be implemented in staging mediastinal adenopathy in patients with NSCLC. A staging algorithm that takes advantage of such modalities can be considered the current best practice. Based on the currently available data, EUS and EBUS can serve as a replacement for mediastinoscopy in many patients; however, the order in which they need to be performed is not clear.

ROLE OF THE GASTROENTEROLOGIST AND EUS

Numerous recent publications have shown the role of EUS-FNA as a valuable adjunct to the diagnosis and staging of patients with lung cancer. EUS-FNA combined with EBUS-TBNA allows a complete minimally invasive mediastinal staging at a lesser cost and can help avoid thoracotomies.

Despite the overwhelming evidence supporting the role of EUS in mediastinal staging, EUS-FNA is often not incorporated into staging of the patients with NSCLC. This observation has been made both in the United States[66] and in Australia.[67] In a US survey, more than 60% of oncologists believed that EUS would not improve staging of NSCLC and even when EUS was available, less than 20% of them would use EUS for staging of lung cancer.[68]

Multiple factors have been attributed to the lack of incorporation of EUS-FNA into diagnostic protocols. EUS-FNA requires a linear array echoendoscope, a compatible needle system, cytopathology support, and a trained endosonographer. EUS is traditionally performed by gastroenterologists and EBUS-TBNA by thoracic specialists. Only a few centers offer EUS and EBUS for lung cancer staging as a single combined procedure.[45,69] In most cases, EUS and EBUS are performed by different practitioners, and the patients cannot undergo both of these tests at 1 session.

Performing the EUS and EBUS as a single combined procedure prevents the patient from undergoing sedation on 2 different occasions and saves the patient a second procedure day. It also maximizes the resource use and decreases the cost. However, arranging for 2 skilled endoscopists together can at times be logistically difficult. It also requires an endoscopy unit equipped with 2 sets of endoscopic instruments that can be used during each portion of the procedure. It is not clear whether EUS and EBUS for lung cancer should be performed by 1 practitioner trained in both techniques, or whether they should be performed by a multispecialty team.

LUNG CANCER STAGING CLINICAL ALGORITHM

Here, we propose a staging algorithm that uses combined EUS-FNA and EBUS-TBNA as a minimally invasive technique for sampling mediastinal adenopathy. Because of the high accuracy of the combined EUS-FNA and EBUS-TBNA and its excellent safety profile, we recommend combined EUS-EBUS as the first-line test for staging in patients with NSCLC. If no metastasis was found on the sampling the of the mediastinal nodes, patients with low suspicion for mediastinal metastasis can undergo thoracotomy. Patients with mediastinal adenopathy on CT, positive node on PET scan, or

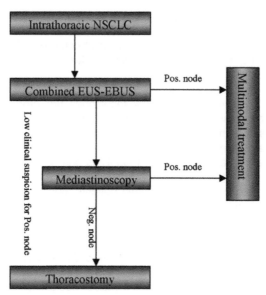

Fig. 2. Staging algorithm for patients with suspected NSCLC when combined EUS-EBUS is available. Pos., positive; Neg., negative.

centrally located primary tumor have a higher chance of mediastinal node metastasis. We recommend that these patients undergo mediastinoscopy before thoracotomy (**Fig. 2**).

When a combined procedure is not available, we recommend a targeted approach based on the location of the node or site of the primary lung tumor (**Fig. 3**).[65]

In patients in whom the imaging study shows enlarged lymph nodes in the mediastinum, the choice of EUS or EBUS as the first staging test can be made depending on the location of the enlarged lymph node. Patients with enlarged lymph nodes in the posterior inferior mediastinum or subcarinal area are recommended to undergo EUS as the first staging procedure. Those patients with anterior, superior, or paratracheal lymph adenopathy may benefit from EBUS as the first staging test.

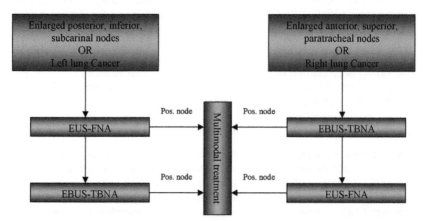

Fig. 3. Targeted approach for patients with suspected NSCLC when combined EUS-EBUS is not available. Pos., positive; Neg., negative.

Patients without mediastinal adenopathy still need sampling of their mediastinal lymph nodes for staging of the NSCLC. The choice of the first test depends on the site of the primary lung tumor. Left lung tumors have a predilection for metastasis to stations 5 and 6 nodes; therefore, we recommend EUS-FNA as the initial procedure for these patients. On the other hand, patients with right lung cancer have a predilection for metastasis to stations 4R and 7. In these patients, EBUS-TBNA is the preferred initial staging procedure.[70–72] Patients who had either EUS or EBUS as their initial staging procedure are required to undergo the other complementary test, if the initial sampling does not show evidence of metastasis.

REFERENCES

1. Alberg AJ, Ford JG, Samet JM. Epidemiology of lung cancer: ACCP evidence-based clinical practice guidelines (2nd edition). Chest 2007;132(Suppl 3):29S–55S.
2. Huxley R, Jamrozik K, LamR TH, et al. Impact of smoking and smoking cessation on lung cancer mortality in the Asia-Pacific region. Am J Epidemiol 2007;165(11): 1280–6.
3. Rivera MP, Mehta AC. Initial diagnosis of lung cancer: ACCP evidence-based clinical practice guidelines (2nd edition). Chest 2007;132(Suppl 3):131S–48S.
4. Robinson LA, Ruckdeschel JC, Wagner H Jr, et al. Treatment of non-small cell lung cancer-stage IIIA: ACCP evidence-based clinical practice guidelines (2nd edition). Chest 2007;132(Suppl 3):243S–65S.
5. Herder GJ, Verboom P, Smit EF, et al. Practice, efficacy and cost of staging suspected non-small cell lung cancer: a retrospective study in two Dutch hospitals. Thorax 2002;57(1):11–4.
6. van Tinteren H, Hoekstra OS, Smit EF, et al. Effectiveness of positron emission tomography in the preoperative assessment of patients with suspected non-small-cell lung cancer: the PLUS multicentre randomised trial. Lancet 2002; 359(9315):1388–93.
7. Goldstraw P, Crowley J, Chansky K, et al. The IASLC Lung Cancer Staging Project: proposals for the revision of the TNM stage groupings in the forthcoming (seventh) edition of the TNM classification of malignant tumours. J Thorac Oncol 2007;2(8):706–14.
8. Silvestri GA. A seismic shift in staging. J Thorac Oncol 2007;2(8):682–3.
9. Toloza EM, Harpole L, McCrory DC. Noninvasive staging of non-small cell lung cancer: a review of the current evidence. Chest 2003;123(Suppl 1):137S–46S.
10. Silvestri GA, Gould MK, Margolis ML, et al. Noninvasive staging of non-small cell lung cancer: ACCP evidenced-based clinical practice guidelines (2nd edition). Chest 2007;132(Suppl 3):178S–201S.
11. Micames CG, McCrory DC, Pavey DA, et al. Endoscopic ultrasound-guided fine-needle aspiration for non-small cell lung cancer staging: a systematic review and metaanalysis. Chest 2007;131(2):539–48.
12. Arroliga AC, Matthay RA. The role of bronchoscopy in lung cancer. Clin Chest Med 1993;14(1):87–98.
13. Detterbeck FC, Jantz MA, Wallace M, et al. Invasive mediastinal staging of lung cancer: ACCP evidence-based clinical practice guidelines (2nd edition). Chest 2007;132(Suppl 3):202S–20S.
14. Protopapas Z, Westcott JL. Transthoracic needle biopsy of mediastinal lymph nodes for staging lung and other cancers. Radiology 1996;199(2):489–96.
15. Wang KP, Brower R, Haponik EF, et al. Flexible transbronchial needle aspiration for staging of bronchogenic carcinoma. Chest 1983;84(5):571–6.

16. Haponik EF, Shure D. Underutilization of transbronchial needle aspiration: experiences of current pulmonary fellows. Chest 1997;112(1):251–3.
17. Dasgupta A, Mehta AC. Transbronchial needle aspiration. An underused diagnostic technique. Clin Chest Med 1999;20(1):39–51.
18. Patelli M, Lazzari Agli L, Poletti V, et al. Role of fiberscopic transbronchial needle aspiration in the staging of N2 disease due to non-small cell lung cancer. Ann Thorac Surg 2002;73(2):407–11.
19. Milman N, Faurschou P, Munch EP, et al. Transbronchial lung biopsy through the fibre optic bronchoscope. Results and complications in 452 examinations. Respir Med 1994;88(10):749–53.
20. Wallace MB, Pascual JM, Raimondo M, et al. Minimally invasive endoscopic staging of suspected lung cancer. JAMA 2008;299(5):540–6.
21. Wiersema MJ, Kochman ML, Chak A, et al. Real-time endoscopic ultrasound-guided fine-needle aspiration of a mediastinal lymph node. Gastrointest Endosc 1993;39(3):429–31.
22. Wiersema MJ, Kochman ML, Cramer HM, et al. Preoperative staging of non-small cell lung cancer: transesophageal US-guided fine-needle aspiration biopsy of mediastinal lymph nodes. Radiology 1994;190(1):239–42.
23. Yasufuku K, Nakajima T, Chiyo M, et al. Endobronchial ultrasonography: current status and future directions. J Thorac Oncol 2007;2(10):970–9.
24. Herth FJ, Eberhardt R, Vilmann P, et al. Real-time endobronchial ultrasound guided transbronchial needle aspiration for sampling mediastinal lymph nodes. Thorax 2006;61(9):795–8.
25. Li SY, Chen XB, He Y, et al. [Real-time endobronchial ultrasound-guided transbronchial needle aspiration: preliminary study on mediastinal and hilar lymph nodes of lung cancer]. Zhonghua Yi Xue Za Zhi 2009;89(24):1672–5 [in Chinese].
26. Yasufuku K, Chiyo M, Koh E, et al. Endobronchial ultrasound guided transbronchial needle aspiration for staging of lung cancer. Lung Cancer 2005;50(3):347–54.
27. Rintoul RC, Skwarski KM, Murchison JT, et al. Endobronchial and endoscopic ultrasound-guided real-time fine-needle aspiration for mediastinal staging. Eur Respir J 2005;25(3):416–21.
28. Vilmann P, Krasnik M, Larsen SS, et al. Transesophageal endoscopic ultrasound-guided fine-needle aspiration (EUS-FNA) and endobronchial ultrasound-guided transbronchial needle aspiration (EBUS-TBNA) biopsy: a combined approach in the evaluation of mediastinal lesions. Endoscopy 2005;37(9):833–9.
29. Varela-Lema L, Fernandez-Villar A, Ruano-Ravina A. Effectiveness and safety of endobronchial ultrasound-transbronchial needle aspiration: a systematic review. Eur Respir J 2009;33(5):1156–64.
30. Gill KR, Ghabril MS, Jamil LH, et al. Endosonographic features predictive of malignancy in mediastinal lymph nodes in patients with lung cancer. Gastrointest Endosc 2010;72(2):265–71.
31. Cerfolio RJ, Bryant AS, Eloubeidi MA. Accessing the aortopulmonary window (#5) and the paraaortic (#6) lymph nodes in patients with non-small cell lung cancer. Ann Thorac Surg 2007;84(3):940–5.
32. Silvestri GA, Hoffman BJ, Bhutani MS, et al. Endoscopic ultrasound with fine-needle aspiration in the diagnosis and staging of lung cancer. Ann Thorac Surg 1996;61(5):1441–5 [discussion: 1445–6].
33. Eloubeidi MA, Tamhane A, Chen VK, et al. Endoscopic ultrasound-guided fine-needle aspiration in patients with non-small cell lung cancer and prior negative mediastinoscopy. Ann Thorac Surg 2005;80(4):1231–9.

34. Wallace MB, Ravenel J, Block MI, et al. Endoscopic ultrasound in lung cancer patients with a normal mediastinum on computed tomography. Ann Thorac Surg 2004;77(5):1763–8.
35. Larsen SS, Vilmann P, Krasnik M, et al. Endoscopic ultrasound guided biopsy versus mediastinoscopy for analysis of paratracheal and subcarinal lymph nodes in lung cancer staging. Lung Cancer 2005;48(1):85–92.
36. Annema JT, Hoekstra OS, Smit EF, et al. Towards a minimally invasive staging strategy in NSCLC: analysis of PET positive mediastinal lesions by EUS-FNA. Lung Cancer 2004;44(1):53–60.
37. Jue TL, Sharaf RN, Appalaneni V, et al. Role of EUS for the evaluation of mediastinal adenopathy. Gastrointest Endosc 2011;74(2):239–45.
38. LeBlanc JK, Devereaux BM, Imperiale TF, et al. Endoscopic ultrasound in non-small cell lung cancer and negative mediastinum on computed tomography. Am J Respir Crit Care Med 2005;171(2):177–82.
39. Kramer H, van Putten JW, Post WJ, et al. Oesophageal endoscopic ultrasound with fine needle aspiration improves and simplifies the staging of lung cancer. Thorax 2004;59(7):596–601.
40. Gress FG, Savides TJ, Sandler A, et al. Endoscopic ultrasonography, fine-needle aspiration biopsy guided by endoscopic ultrasonography, and computed tomography in the preoperative staging of non-small-cell lung cancer: a comparison study. Ann Intern Med 1997;127(8 Pt 1):604–12.
41. Fritscher-Ravens A, Soehendra N, Schirrow L, et al. Role of transesophageal endosonography-guided fine-needle aspiration in the diagnosis of lung cancer. Chest 2000;117(2):339–45.
42. Wallace MB, Silvestri GA, Sahai AV, et al. Endoscopic ultrasound-guided fine needle aspiration for staging patients with carcinoma of the lung. Ann Thorac Surg 2001;72(6):1861–7.
43. Wiersema MJ, Vazquez-Sequeiros E, Wiersema LM. Evaluation of mediastinal lymphadenopathy with endoscopic US-guided fine-needle aspiration biopsy. Radiology 2001;219(1):252–7.
44. Eloubeidi MA, Tamhane A, Chen VK, et al. Endoscopic ultrasound-guided fine needle aspiration of mediastinal lymph node in patients with suspected lung cancer after positron emission tomography and computed tomography scans. Ann Thorac Surg 2005;79(1):263–8.
45. Annema JT, Versteegh MI, Veseliç M, et al. Endoscopic ultrasound-guided fine-needle aspiration in the diagnosis and staging of lung cancer and its impact on surgical staging. J Clin Oncol 2005;23(33):8357–61.
46. Sawhney MS, Bakman Y, Holmstrom AM, et al. Impact of preoperative endoscopic ultrasound on non-small cell lung cancer staging. Chest 2007;132(3):916–21.
47. Herth FJ, Lunn W, Eberhardt R, et al. Transbronchial versus transesophageal ultrasound-guided aspiration of enlarged mediastinal lymph nodes. Am J Respir Crit Care Med 2005;171(10):1164–7.
48. Herth FJ, Krasnik M, Kahn N, et al. Combined endoscopic-endobronchial ultrasound-guided fine-needle aspiration of mediastinal lymph nodes through a single bronchoscope in 150 patients with suspected lung cancer. Chest 2010;138(4):790–4.
49. Szlubowski A, Zieliński M, Soja J, et al. A combined approach of endobronchial and endoscopic ultrasound-guided needle aspiration in the radiologically normal mediastinum in non-small-cell lung cancer staging–a prospective trial. Eur J Cardiothorac Surg 2010;37(5):1175–9.
50. Rusch VW. Mediastinoscopy: an endangered species? J Clin Oncol 2005;23(33):8283–5.

51. Little AG, Rusch VW, Bonner JA, et al. Patterns of surgical care of lung cancer patients. Ann Thorac Surg 2005;80(6):2051–6 [discussion: 2056].
52. Smulders SA, Smeenk FW, Janssen-Heijnen ML, et al. Surgical mediastinal staging in daily practice. Lung Cancer 2005;47(2):243–51.
53. Harewood GC, Wiersema MJ, Edell ES, et al. Cost-minimization analysis of alternative diagnostic approaches in a modeled patient with non-small cell lung cancer and subcarinal lymphadenopathy. Mayo Clin Proc 2002;77(2):155–64.
54. Aabakken L, Silvestri GA, Hawes R, et al. Cost-efficacy of endoscopic ultrasonography with fine-needle aspiration vs. mediastinotomy in patients with lung cancer and suspected mediastinal adenopathy. Endoscopy 1999;31(9):707–11.
55. Call S, Rami-Porta R, Serra-Mitjans M, et al. Extended cervical mediastinoscopy in the staging of bronchogenic carcinoma of the left lung. Eur J Cardiothorac Surg 2008;34(5):1081–4.
56. Urschel JD, Vretenar DF, Dickout WJ, et al. Cerebrovascular accident complicating extended cervical mediastinoscopy. Ann Thorac Surg 1994;57(3):740–1.
57. Leschber G, Holinka G, Linder A. Video-assisted mediastinoscopic lymphadenectomy (VAMLA)–a method for systematic mediastinal lymphnode dissection. Eur J Cardiothorac Surg 2003;24(2):192–5.
58. Lemaire A, Nikolic I, Petersen T, et al. Nine-year single center experience with cervical mediastinoscopy: complications and false negative rate. Ann Thorac Surg 2006;82(4):1185–9 [discussion: 1189–90].
59. Metin M, Citak N, Sayar A, et al. The role of extended cervical mediastinoscopy in staging of non-small cell lung cancer of the left lung and a comparison with integrated positron emission tomography and computed tomography: does integrated positron emission tomography and computed tomography reduce the need for invasive procedures? J Thorac Oncol 2011;6(10):1713–9.
60. Freixinet Gilart J, García PG, de Castro FR, et al. Extended cervical mediastinoscopy in the staging of bronchogenic carcinoma. Ann Thorac Surg 2000;70(5):1641–3.
61. Ginsberg RJ. Extended cervical mediastinoscopy. Chest Surg Clin North Am 1996;6(1):21–30.
62. Lopez L, Varela A, Freixinet J, et al. Extended cervical mediastinoscopy: prospective study of fifty cases. Ann Thorac Surg 1994;57(3):555–7 [discussion: 557–8].
63. Nechala P, Graham AJ, McFadden SD, et al. Retrospective analysis of the clinical performance of anterior mediastinotomy. Ann Thorac Surg 2006;82(6):2004–9.
64. De Leyn P, Lardinois D, Van Schil P, et al. European trends in preoperative and intraoperative nodal staging: ESTS guidelines. J Thorac Oncol 2007;2(4):357–61.
65. Navani N, Spiro SG, Janes SM. Mediastinal staging of NSCLC with endoscopic and endobronchial ultrasound. Nat Rev Clin Oncol 2009;6(5):278–86.
66. Hernandez LV, Geenen JE, Schmalz MJ, et al. The underutilization of EUS-guided FNA in the lymph-node staging of non-small-cell lung cancer: perceptions of chest physicians in Wisconsin. Gastrointest Endosc 2005;62(4):517–20.
67. Walsh PR, Williams DB. Mediastinal adenopathy: finding the answer with endoscopic ultrasound-guided fine-needle aspiration biopsy. Intern Med J 2005;35(7):392–8.
68. Reddy NK, Markowitz AB, Abbruzzese JL, et al. Knowledge of indications and utilization of EUS: a survey of oncologists in the United States. J Clin Gastroenterol 2008;42(8):892–6.

69. Herth FJ, Rabe KF, Gasparini S, et al. Transbronchial and transoesophageal (ultrasound-guided) needle aspirations for the analysis of mediastinal lesions. Eur Respir J 2006;28(6):1264–75.
70. Cerfolio RJ, Bryant AS. Distribution and likelihood of lymph node metastasis based on the lobar location of nonsmall-cell lung cancer. Ann Thorac Surg 2006;81(6):1969–73 [discussion: 1973].
71. Naruke T, Tsuchiya R, Kondo H, et al. Lymph node sampling in lung cancer: how should it be done? Eur J Cardiothorac Surg 1999;16(Suppl 1):S17–24.
72. Kotoulas CS, Foroulis CN, Kostikas K, et al. Involvement of lymphatic metastatic spread in non-small cell lung cancer accordingly to the primary cancer location. Lung Cancer 2004;44(2):183–91.

Endoscopic Ultrasonography-Guided Pancreatic Drainage

Marc Giovannini, MD

KEYWORDS

- Pancreatic pseudocysts • Endoscopic ultrasonography
- Pancreatic drainage

The management of pancreatic pseudocysts (PPCs) has traditionally been surgical. Although highly effective, surgery may be associated with a complication rate of 35% and a mortality of 10%, a situation that has encouraged the development of nonsurgical approaches. Percutaneous puncture and aspiration under computed tomography (CT) or ultrasound guidance has been used, but aspiration alone has been found to be ineffective because of high recurrence rates of up to 71%. Continuous percutaneous drainage with indwelling catheters reduces the relapse rates, but may be associated with a complication rate ranging from 5% to 60%. Complications include fistula formation, infection, and bleeding.

Endoscopic transmural drainage of a PPC is an alternative nonsurgical approach. Since the first reports by Sahel and colleagues[1] and Cremer and colleagues,[2] endoscopic drainage of PPCs has become established. This procedure entails the creation of a fistulous tract between the PPC and the gastric lumen (cystogastrostomy) or duodenal lumen (cystoduodenostomy). Having established endoscopic access to the PPC, a nasocystic catheter or a stent can be placed for continuous drainage. The obvious limitation of endoscopic transmural drainage of a PPC is its relatively blind approach. The risk of perforation is particularly high when endoscopically visible intraluminal bulging is absent. A major risk of endoscopic cystoduodenostomy or cystogastrostomy is hemorrhage (6% of cases).[1,2] The ideal approach for PPC puncture combines endoscopy with real-time endosonography using an interventional echoendoscope. Several investigators have described the use of endoscopic ultrasonography (EUS) longitudinal scanners for guidance of transmural punctures[3–5] and drainage procedures. The same technique could be used to access a dilated pancreatic duct in cases where the duct cannot be drained by conventional endoscopic retrograde cholangiopancreatography (ERCP) because of complete obstruction.

Endoscopic Unit, Paoli-Calmettes Institute, 232 Boulevard St-Marguerite, 13273 Marseille Cedex 9, France
E-mail address: giovanninim@marseille.fnclcc.fr

Gastrointest Endoscopy Clin N Am 22 (2012) 221–230
doi:10.1016/j.giec.2012.04.004
1052-5157/12/$ – see front matter © 2012 Published by Elsevier Inc.

EUS-GUIDED DRAINAGE OF PANCREATIC PSEUDOCYSTS
Indications

PPCs are reported to complicate between 10% and 20% of patients with acute and chronic pancreatitis. Most of these PPCs are asymptomatic and do not require treatment. Spontaneous regression of PPCs is reported to occur in 7% to 60% of patients. The indication for PPC drainage will differ depending on whether the cyst develops in the setting of acute or chronic pancreatitis. For PPCs that complicate acute pancreatitis, drainage is indicated when pancreatitis fails to resolve with conservative measures. PPCs that are not associated with persistent pancreatitis should be kept under observation, as there is a high probability of spontaneous resolution. A 6-week observation period is generally recommended before considering decompression. Spontaneous regression after persistence of more than 6 weeks is considered by some to be unlikely. In fact, this cutoff time of 6 weeks is heavily doubted in the literature nowadays, and large pseudocysts (>4 cm) should be treated.

For PPCs complicating chronic pancreatitis, drainage is indicated to relieve symptoms associated with a space-occupying mass, including neighboring organ compression. Such patients have chronic cysts that remain unchanged over a period of months. Patients typically complain of a dull and constant pain, and may develop symptoms of gastric outlet obstruction or jaundice from bile duct compression.

Multiple or multiloculated PPCs sometimes cannot be adequately treated by an endoscopic approach, and warrant surgical resection. It should be remembered that an endoscopic approach contaminates the cyst and risks infection if the contents of the PPC cannot be completely drained.

Is EUS Necessary?

The main question is: what is the best route for draining a PPC? To obtain a response, Kahaleh and colleagues[6] have reported a prospective comparative study on the two techniques of endoscopic transmural drainage and EUS-guided drainage. A total of 99 consecutive patients underwent endoscopic management of PPC according to a predetermined treatment algorithm as follows. Patients with bulging lesions without obvious portal hypertension underwent endoscopic transmural drainage, and all remaining patients underwent EUS-guided drainage. Patients were followed prospectively, with cross-sectional imaging during visits to the clinic. The investigators compared short-term and long-term results (effectiveness and complications) at 1 and 6 months postprocedure. Forty-six patients (37 men) underwent EUS drainage and 53 patients (39 men) had endoscopic transmural drainage. There were no significant differences between the two groups regarding short-term success (93% vs 94%) or long-term success (84% vs 91%); 68 of the 99 patients completed 6 months of follow-up. Complications occurred in 19% of EUS patients versus 18% of endoscopic patients, and consisted of bleeding in 3, infection of the collection in 8, stent migration into the pseudocyst in 3, and pneumoperitoneum in 5 patients. All complications except one were able to be managed conservatively. No clear differences in efficacy or safety were observed between conventional and EUS-guided cystenterostomy. The choice of technique is likely best predicated by individual patient presentation and local expertise.

From the technical point of view, the EUS-guided approach has two crucial steps. The first is the identification of an optimal point to puncture, without intervening vessels and with a short distance between the cyst and the gut wall. Once this point is identified, the endoscope should be straightened as much as possible in a stable position. The second critical step is that once the puncture has been performed and the guide wire is curled inside the cyst cavity, the wall dilator must be introduced without losing the endoscope position and under ultrasonographic view. Once the dilator has been inserted through the parietal fistula the ultrasonographic view is no longer needed, and the dilation and stent insertion can be made under endoscopic view.

A Web-based survey concerning the technique of pancreatic collection drainage was sent to members of the American Society for Gastrointestinal Endoscopy (ASGE) in the United States and internationally.[7] Of the 3054 endoscopists to whom the survey was sent, 266 (8.7%) replied; 198 performed pseudocyst drainage (103 [52%] ASGE members from the United States and 95 [48%] international members). The median of the total number of drainages per physician was 15 (range 1–364). The transgastric route was the most commonly used drainage route (65%). Transmural entry was performed using a needle-knife in 53% of transmural drainages that were not EUS-guided. The number of stents placed ranged from 1 to 5, and these remained in place for 2 to 30 weeks. A CT scan was used before drainage by 95% of all respondents. EUS imaging was used before drainage by 72 of 103 (70%) United States endoscopists compared with 56 of 95 (59%) international endoscopists ($P = .1$). EUS-guided drainage was used by 56% of United States endoscopists compared with 43% of international endoscopists ($P = .06$). The most common site of transmural entry for drainage of PPCs appears to be the transgastric route. Although CT is the most commonly used predrainage imaging modality, EUS is used before and during transmural drainage of pseudocysts in both the United States and abroad, particularly in academic medical centers. Use of EUS before or during drainage does not appear to differ significantly among endoscopists in the United States and internationally.

More recently, Varadarajulu and colleagues[8] reported a randomized study to compare the rate of technical success between EUS and esophagogastroduodenoscopy (EGD) for transmural drainage of PPCs. Thirty patients were randomized to undergo pseudocyst drainage by EUS (n = 15) or EGD (n = 15) over a 6-month period. Except for the sex, there was no difference in patient or clinical characteristics between the two cohorts. Although all the patients (n = 14) randomized to EUS underwent successful drainage (100%), the procedure was technically successful in only 5 of 15 patients (33%) randomized to an EGD ($P<.001$). All 10 patients who failed drainage by EGD underwent successful drainage of the pseudocyst on a crossover to EUS. There was no significant difference in the rates of treatment success between EUS and EGD after stenting, either by intention-to-treat (ITT) analysis (100% vs 87%; $P = .48$) or as-treated analysis (95.8% vs 80%; $P = .32$). Major procedure-related bleeding was encountered in 2 patients in whom drainage by EGD was attempted; one resulted in death and the other necessitated a blood transfusion. No significant difference was observed between EUS and EGD with regard to complications either by ITT (0% vs 13%; $P = .48$) or as-treated analysis (4% vs 20%; $P = .32$). Technical success was significantly greater for EUS than for EGD, even after adjusting for luminal compression and sex (adjusted exact odds ratio 39.4; $P = .001$). The investigators concluded that when available, EUS should be considered as the first-line treatment modality for endoscopic drainage of a PPC, given its high technical success rate.

A second randomized study was published in 2009[9] and came to a different conclusion, suggesting that EUS-guided PPC drainage is equivalent to EGD, and should be performed in nonbulging PPCs. A total of 60 consecutive patients with PPCs were randomly divided into two groups to undergo either EUS (n = 31) or EGD (n = 29). The technical success rate, complications, and short-term and long-term results were prospectively evaluated.

The rate of technical success of the drainage was higher for EUS (94%, 29/31) than for EGD (72%, 21/29; $P = .039$) in ITT analysis. In cases where EGD failed (n = 8) because the PPCs were nonbulging, a crossover was made to EUS, which was successfully performed in all these patients. Complications occurred in 7% of the EUS group and in 10% of the EGD group ($P = .67$). During short-term follow-up, PPC resolution was achieved in 97% (28/29) in the EUS group and in 91% (19/21) in the EGD group ($P = .565$). Long-term results analyzed on a per-protocol basis showed no significant difference in clinical outcomes between EUD (89%, 33/37) and conventional transmural drainage (86%, 18/21, $P = .696$).[9]

Recently, a large study on EUS-guided PPC drainage showed a low rate of complications.[10] Of 148 patients who underwent EUS, perforation was encountered at the site of transmural stenting in 2 (1.3%, 95% confidence interval [CI] 0.41–4.76) patients with a PPC in the uncinate. Other complications included bleeding in 1 (0.67%, 95% CI 0.16–3.68), stent migration in 1 (0.67%, 95% CI 0.16–3.68), and infection in 4 (2.7%, 95% CI 1.09–6.73) patients. Bleeding occurred in a patient with underlying acquired factor VIII inhibitors, there was stent migration in a patient who underwent drainage via the gastric cardia, and infection occurred in 2 patients with pseudocysts and in 2 with necrosis. Whereas 2 patients who developed postprocedural infection and 1 with stent migration were managed endoscopically, both perforations required surgery. Surgical debridement was performed in 2 patients who developed infection, with a successful outcome in one and death from underlying comorbidity in another.

In addition to its safety and therapeutic success rate, EUS also allows a diagnostic evaluation of the pancreatic cystic lesions. Thus, based on the EUS findings, the management plan is changed in 5% to 9% of patients because EUS identifies other cystic lesions misdiagnosed as pseudocysts.[11–13]

Which Technique and Accessories are Best?

EUS-guided PPC drainage should be performed under propofol anesthesia with endotracheal intubation to avoid regurgitation in the fluoroscopy suite, with the patient in the left lateral or prone position. The patient should receive broad-spectrum antibiotics during and after the procedure to reduce the risk of PPC infection. A CT scan should be performed immediately before the intervention. CT is less invasive than endoscopy and gives information about important anatomic details (eg, varices, arterial pseudoaneurysms, multiple cysts or extended necrosis, ascites, large or atypically located gall bladder, pleural effusion).

The individual steps are (**Fig. 1**):

1. Locate the cyst and the contact zone between the gastric or duodenal wall and the cyst wall.
2. Doppler assessment of the stomach or duodenal wall is performed for interposed vessels. Doppler ultrasonography is now mandatory before cyst drainage.
3. Having determined the optimal site for puncture, the PPC is punctured using a 19-gauge fine-needle aspiration needle or the new Access 19-gauge needle (Cook Medical, Bloomington, IN, USA), which prevents damage to the Teflon part of the 0.0035-in guide wire. A sample of the cyst contents is aspirated and submitted for biochemical, cytologic, and tumor marker (eg, carcinoembryonic antigen) analysis. If infection is suspected, a sample should be sent for Gram stain, as well as culture and sensitivity.
4. Contrast filling of the PPC is performed under fluoroscopy to document the size and anatomic boundaries of the cyst. Communication of the cyst with the pancreatic duct may be seen. Filling of the cyst can also be verified by EUS, seen as a visible streamline effect.

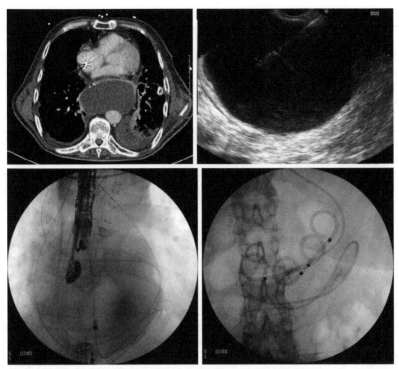

Fig. 1. EUS-guided PPC drainage using a 10F cystostome allowing the insertion of 2 plastic double-pigtail stents of 8.5F and a nasocystic drain.

5. The tract is dilated using an 8-mm balloon over the wire or the 8.5F or 10F cystostome. The main advantage of the cystostome is to create a large cystenterostomy, due to the diffusion of the cautery at the level of the puncturing tract.
6. A chronic cyst with clear liquid contents can be drained with 2 7F or 8.5F double-pigtail stents. An infected cyst mandates irrigation by nasocystic catheter or 2 10F double-pigtail stents, and a nasocystic drain can be placed (see **Fig. 1**). The nasocystic catheter can be removed after 2 or 3 days after a CT examination showing a resolution of the PPC. Pancreatic cysts complicating necrotizing pancreatitis can be managed endoscopically, but require aggressive irrigation and drainage over an extended period of time.

Another technique of EUS-guided PPC drainage has been reported, known as 1-step drainage. For performance of this technique there is a commercially available device for use with large-channel echoendoscopes without the need for any exchanges, using the Needle-Wire Oasis System (NWOA; Cook Medical). This device is an all-in-one stent introduction system, containing a 0.035-in needle-wire suitable for cutting current, a 5.5F guiding catheter, and a pushing catheter with a back-loaded straight stent (8.5F or 10F, 6 cm long). This procedure can be performed with the patient under conscious sedation using standard monitoring in the left lateral position. Intravenous broad-spectrum antibiotics must be used before and after the procedure. The optimal location for performing the procedure is the fluoroscopy suite, because in some cases the radiologic view can be helpful either for insertion of the stent at a better angle or for completing the drainage with cyst irrigation and/or additional stent placement.

First, the cyst is located with the linear array echoendoscope, looking for an optimal contact with the gastric or duodenal wall. Doppler assessment is included to eliminate interposition of large vessels. The needle-wire is then introduced into the intestinal wall, and the cyst wall is penetrated under continuous pressure and cutting current. Once inside the cyst, the internal rigid part of the needle-wire is removed, making it a soft wire that can be easily inserted into the cyst, followed by the dilator catheter and finally the straight plastic endoprosthesis, under endoscopic and ultrasound monitoring.

The single-step technique was first described in 1998 by Vilmann and colleagues[14] and Giovannini and colleagues.[15] In a prospective study, Krüger and colleagues[16] evaluated the 1-step device for drainage of PPCs and abscesses. Endoscopic stent placement was successful in 33 of 35 patients (94%), whereas repeated needle passages were unsuccessful in 2 cases. No procedure-related complications, such as bleeding, perforation, or pneumoperitoneum, were observed. All subsequent complications, such as ineffective drainage (9%), stent occlusion (12%), or cyst infection (12%), were managed endoscopically. The overall resolution rate was 88%, with a recurrence rate of 12%, during a mean follow-up period of 24 months. The investigators concluded that the 1-step EUS-guided technique with a needle-wire device provides safe transmural access and allows effective subsequent endoscopic management of PPCs and abscesses.

Clinical Algorithm

In summary, EUS-guided PPC drainage improves the safety of PPC endoscopic drainage and increases the number of patients suitable for this procedure by avoiding percutaneous and surgical drainage, which are associated with higher morbidity and mortality (**Fig. 2**). Therefore, the EUS-guided procedure seems to be the best and safest technique for transmural endoscopic pseudocyst drainage, and should be considered the first-choice option.

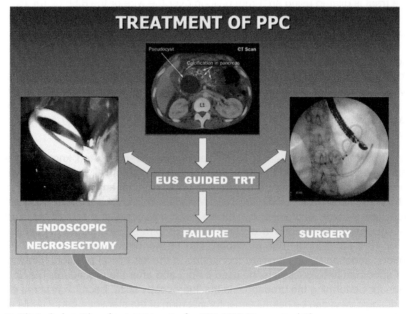

Fig. 2. Clinical algorithm for treatment of a PPC. TRT, Transmural Therapy.

EUS-GUIDED PANCREATICOGASTROSTOMY
Indications

The pain associated with chronic pancreatitis is caused, at least in part, by ductal hypertension. Both surgical and endoscopic treatments can relieve pain by improving ductal drainage. Endoscopic drainage requires transpapillary access to the pancreatic duct during ERCP. The development of interventional EUS has provided better access to the region of the pancreas. Just as pancreatic fluid collections, such as pseudocysts, can be successfully drained from the stomach or duodenum by endoscopic cystenterostomy or cystogastrostomy, the same technique could be used to access a dilated pancreatic duct in cases where the duct cannot be drained by conventional ERCP because of complete obstruction. The main indications are stenosis of pancreaticojejunal or pancreaticogastric anastomosis after Whipple resection that induces recurrent acute pancreatitis, main pancreatic duct stenosis caused by chronic pancreatitis, and post–acute pancreatitis or post–pancreatic trauma after failure of ERCP. EUS-guided pancreaticogastrostomy (EPG) or bulbostomy (EPB) offers an alternative to surgery.

Technical Considerations

By using a linear interventional echoendoscope, the dilated main pancreatic duct (MPD) is well visualized (**Fig. 3**). EPG is then performed under combined fluoroscopic

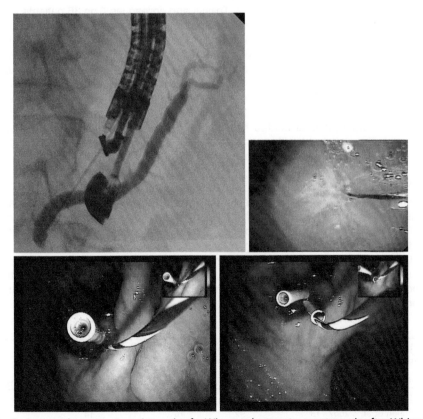

Fig. 3. Pancreaticogastrostomy/stenosis of a Wirsung duct gastroanastomosis after Whipple resection for benign cystic lesion of the head of the pancreas.

and ultrasound guidance, with the tip of the echoendoscope positioned such that the inflated balloon is in the duodenal bulb while the accessory channel remains in the antrum. A needle (19-gauge, EchoTip Ultrasound Needle, EUSN-19-T, or Access needle; Cook Medical) is inserted transgastrically into the proximal pancreatic duct and contrast medium injected. Opacification demonstrates a pancreatogram. The needle is exchanged over a guide wire (0.02-in diameter, Terumo Europe, Leuven, Belgium) for a 6.5F or 8F diathermic sheath (prototype Cysto-Gastro set; EndoFlex, Voerde, Germany), which is then used to enlarge the channel between the stomach and MPD. The sheath is introduced by using a cutting current. After exchange over a guide wire (rigid, 0.035-in diameter), a 7F, 8-cm long pancreaticogastric stent is positioned. This stent will be exchanged for 2 7F stents or 1 8.5F stent 1 month after the first procedure.

The results of the 3 series[17–19] of patients published thus far are much too preliminary in nature to recommend wider use of EPG, which in any case should be restricted to tertiary centers specializing in biliopancreatic therapy. Although pain relief can be accomplished in up to 70% of cases, the complication rate is still high, around 15%, including bleeding, pancreatic collection, and perforation. Nevertheless, the possibility of draining the MPD into the digestive tract through an endoscopically created fistula, with patency maintained by stent placement, might be interesting as an alternative method of drainage without the complication of stent occlusion that is associated with transpapillary drainage.

The largest series was published by Tessier and colleagues[18] on 36 patients. Indications were chronic pancreatitis, with complete obstruction (secondary to a tight stenosis, a stone, or MPD rupture); inaccessible papilla or impossible cannulation (n = 20); anastomotic stenosis after a Whipple procedure (n = 12); complete MPD rupture after acute pancreatitis; or trauma (n = 4). EPG or EPB was unsuccessful in 3 patients; 1 was lost to follow-up. Major complications occurred in 2 patients, and included 1 hematoma and 1 severe acute pancreatitis. The median follow-up was 14.5 months (range 4–55 months). Pain relief was complete or partial in 25 patients (69%, ITT). Eight patients treated had no improvement of their symptoms (4 were subsequently diagnosed with cancer). Stent dysfunction occurred in 20 patients (55%) and required a total of 29 repeat endoscopies.

Clinical Algorithm

It is difficult to determine the place of EUS-guided pancreatic drainage in today's armamentarium. In the author's experience, the best indication is anastomotic stenosis after Whipple procedure for benign pancreatic lesions (cystadenoma, intraductal papillary mucinous neoplasm, neuroendocrine tumor).

EUS-guided pancreatic drainage offers an alternative to surgery, and the best results in the 3 series published (**Table 1**) were shown for this indication. On the other hand, surgery should be considered as the salvage treatment of chronic pancreatitis after failure of the endoscopic route.

Table 1
Studies on EUS-guided pancreaticogastrostomy

References, Year	No. of Patients	Success (%)	Complications (%)	Follow-Up (Months)
Tessier et al,[18] 2007	36	70	11	16.5
Kahaleh et al,[17] 2007	13	92	16	14
Barkay et al,[19] 2010	21	48	2	13

SUMMARY

Curved linear-array echoendoscopes have made transmural pseudocyst puncture under EUS guidance technically possible. With the ability to "see" pseudocysts through the wall of the stomach or duodenum, pseudocysts should be as accessible to the endoscopist as they have been to the radiologist performing percutaneous drainage. Dedicated pseudocyst drainage accessories and large-channel interventional echoendoscopes designed for stent placement will improve the results of EUS-guided pseudocyst drainage. Data in the literature seem to show that the EUS route should be the gold standard for the treatment of pancreatic collection. EUS guidance certainly is mandatory for the nonbulging pseudocyst or in the case of portal hypertension.

Therapeutic EUS with pancreaticogastrostomy and EUS-guided biliary drainage represents today an alternative to surgery or percutaneous biliary drainage when ERCP has failed or is precluded because of previous surgery such as gastrectomy or Whipple resection. These techniques should be performed in a unit experienced in therapeutic endoscopy.

REFERENCES

1. Sahel J, Bastid C, Pellat B, et al. Endoscopic cystoduodenostomy of cysts of chronic calcifying pancreatitis: a report of 20 cases. Pancreas 1987;2:447–53.
2. Cremer M, Deviere J, Engelholm L. Endoscopic management of cysts and pseudocysts in chronic pancreatitis: long-term follow-up after 7 years of experience. Gastrointest Endosc 1989;35:1–9.
3. Binmoeller KF, Seifert H, Sohendra N. Endoscopic pseudo-cyst drainage: a new instrument for simplified cystoenterostomy. Gastrointest Endosc 1994;40:112–3.
4. Binmoeller KF, Sohendra N. Endoscopic ultrasonography in the diagnosis and treatment of pancreatic pseudocysts. Gastrointest Endosc 1995;5(4):805–16.
5. Gerolami R, Giovannini M, Laugier R. Endoscopic drainage of pancreatic pseudocysts guided by endosonography. Endoscopy 1997;29:106–8.
6. Kahaleh M, Shami VM, Conaway MR, et al. Endoscopic ultrasound drainage of pancreatic pseudocyst: a prospective comparison with conventional endoscopic drainage. Endoscopy 2006;38(4):355–9.
7. Yusuf TE, Baron TH. Endoscopic transmural drainage of pancreatic pseudocysts: results of a national and an international survey of ASGE members. Gastrointest Endosc 2006;63(2):223–7.
8. Varadarajulu S, Christein JD, Tamhane A, et al. Prospective randomized trial comparing EUS and EGD for transmural drainage of pancreatic pseudocysts (with videos). Gastrointest Endosc 2008;68(6):1102–11.
9. Park DH, Lee SS, Moon SH, et al. Endoscopic ultrasound-guided versus conventional transmural drainage for pancreatic pseudocysts: a prospective randomized trial. Endoscopy 2009;41(10):842–8.
10. Varadarajulu S, Christein JD, Wilcox CM. Frequency of complications during EUS-guided drainage of pancreatic fluid collections in 148 consecutive patients. J Gastroenterol Hepatol 2011;26(10):1504–8.
11. Varadarajulu S, Wilcox CM, Tamhane A, et al. Role of EUS in drainage of peripancreatic fluid collections not amenable for endoscopic transmural drainage. Gastrointest Endosc 2007;66:1107–19.
12. Vazquez-Sequeiros E. Drainage of peripancreatic-fluid collections: is EUS really necessary? Gastrointest Endosc 2007;66:1120–2.

13. Fockens P, Johnson TG, van Dullemen HM, et al. Endosonographic imaging of pancreatic pseudocysts before endoscopic transmural drainage. Gastrointest Endosc 1997;46:412–6.
14. Vilmann P, Hancke S, Pless T, et al. One-step endosonography-guided drainage of a pancreatic pseudocyst: a new technique of stent delivery through the echo endoscope. Endoscopy 1998;30:730–3.
15. Giovannini M, Bernardini D, Seitz JF. Cystogastrostomy entirely performed under endosonography guidance for pancreatic pseudocyst: results in six patients. Gastrointest Endosc 1998;48:200–3.
16. Krüger M, Schneider AS, Manns MP, et al. Endoscopic management of pancreatic pseudocysts or abscesses after an EUS-guided 1-step procedure for initial access. Gastrointest Endosc 2006;63:409–16.
17. Kahaleh M, Hernandez AJ, Tokar J, et al. EUS-guided pancreaticogastrostomy: analysis of its efficacy to drain inaccessible pancreatic ducts. Gastrointest Endosc 2007;65(2):224–30.
18. Tessier G, Bories E, Arvanitakis M, et al. EUS-guided pancreatogastrostomy and pancreatobulbostomy for the treatment of pain in patients with pancreatic ductal dilatation inaccessible for transpapillary endoscopic therapy. Gastrointest Endosc 2007;65(2):233–41.
19. Barkay O, Sheman S, McHenry L, et al. Therapeutic EUS-assisted endoscopic retrograde pancreatography after failed pancreatic duct cannulation at ERCP. Gastrointest Endosc 2010;7:1166–73.

Endoscopic Ultrasound-Guided Celiac Neurolysis

Michael J. Levy, MD[a],*, Suresh T. Chari, MD[a],
Maurits J. Wiersema, MD[b]

KEYWORDS

• Celiac • Ganglia • Neurolysis • Pancreatic cancer • Pain
• Plexus • Splanchnic

INTRODUCTION

Patients who have pancreatic cancer frequently experience abdominal pain that is often difficult to control. Although initial therapy with nonsteroidal antiinflammatory agents is advocated, the limited efficacy routinely necessitates opioid administration.[1,2] Although opioids may alleviate pain, their use is commonly associated with dry mouth, constipation, nausea, vomiting, drowsiness, delirium, and impaired immune function.[3,4] Celiac neurolysis (CN) may be performed with the goal of improving pain control and quality of life (QOL) and to reduce the risk of drug-induced side effects.

This article reviews the various techniques for performing endoscopic ultrasound (EUS)-guided CN (EUS CN) and considers its role in patients with pancreatic cancer. Given the limited number of EUS CN studies, relevant literature is also discussed pertaining to percutaneous (PQ) and surgical methods for performing CN, which provide some perspective when considering the EUS data.

RELEVANT ANATOMY

A discussion of the relevant anatomy is key to understanding the different approaches to CN. The terms celiac plexus and splanchnic nerves are often used interchangeably. However, they represent anatomically distinct structures.[5–7] The splanchnic nerves are located cephalic to the diaphragm (in a retrocrural position), and anterior to the 12th thoracic vertebra. The celiac plexus is located caudal to the diaphragm (in an antecrural position), surrounds the origin of the celiac trunk, and comprises a dense network of ganglia and interconnecting fibers. Celiac ganglia vary in number (1–5), size (diameter

Financial Relationships: None.
[a] Division of Gastroenterology and Hepatology, Mayo Clinic, 200 First Street SW, Rochester, MN 55905, USA; [b] Private Practice, Lutheran Medical Group, 7900 West Jefferson Boulevard Suite 201, Fort Wayne, IN 46804, USA
* Corresponding author.
E-mail address: levy.michael@mayo.edu

Gastrointest Endoscopy Clin N Am 22 (2012) 231–247
doi:10.1016/j.giec.2012.04.003
1052-5157/12/$ – see front matter © 2012 Elsevier Inc. All rights reserved.

0.5–4.5 cm), and location (T12–L2).[5] The celiac plexus transmits pain sensation for the pancreas and most of the abdominal viscera except the left colon, rectum, and pelvic organs.[8] The neurons that innervate the pancreas[9] can receive nociceptive stimulation and then transmit this pain information to the celiac plexus.[10] Stimuli reach the thalamus and cortex of the brain, inducing the sensation of pain. Descending inhibitory mechanisms may also modulate the ascending pain information.

PQ AND SURGICAL APPROACHES AND OUTCOMES

CN was first performed by Kappis[11] in 1914 via a PQ route. Technical modifications have been introduced, with the goal of improving the precision of needle placement and pain relief and to reduce procedure-related complications. These techniques differ with respect to the route of needle insertion, as well as the use and type of radiologic guidance.

Three meta-analyses have reached conflicting conclusions regarding PQ-guided celiac plexus neurolysis (CPN) (PQ CPN).[12–14] The investigators note the difficulty in analysis given the mostly retrospective and uncontrolled nature of the studies. The evaluation of varied patient populations, including patients with cancer involving the breast, lungs, esophagus, stomach, colon, rectum, liver, gallbladder, bile ducts, adrenal glands, kidneys, and pancreas, also hinders the analysis.[12–14] Lebovits and Lefkowitz[12] concluded that CPN leads to successful relief of pancreatic cancer pain. In contrast, Sharfman and Walsh[13] found the data insufficient to judge the efficacy, long-term morbidity, or cost-effectiveness. Eisenberg and colleagues[14] reviewed 24 studies, of which 2 were randomized controlled trials (RCTs), 1 was prospective, and 21 were retrospective uncontrolled trials. The cancer type was specified in 1117 patients (63% pancreatic, 37% nonpancreatic). Good to excellent pain relief was reported in 89% of patients during the first 2 weeks after CPN. Partial to complete pain relief was reported in about 90% of patients at 3 months and 70% to 90% at the time of death. The investigators concluded that: (1) CPN has long-lasting benefit for 70% to 90% of patients with pancreatic and other intra-abdominal cancers, regardless of the technique used; and (2) adverse effects are common but generally transient and mild.

In a subsequent prospective, randomized, double-blind study of 21 patients with pancreatic cancer the PQ CPN group had a significant reduction in analgesic use and drug-induced side effects compared with patients receiving drug therapy alone.[15] Kawamata and colleagues[16] showed that PQ CPN results in less deterioration in QOL added to morphine therapy versus either morphine or nonsteroidal antiinflammatory drug therapy alone. Improved outcomes were attributed to increased duration of the analgesic effect and reduced opioid side effects.

More recently, Wong and colleagues[17] evaluated 100 patients with unresectable pancreatic cancer to determine the effect of PQ CPN on pain relief, QOL, and survival in a double-blind RCT. Patients underwent either PQ CPN via a posterior approach or received systemic analgesic therapy alone with sham injection. At 1 week after therapy, patients in both groups experienced improved pain control ($P \leq .01$) and QOL ($P < .001$), with an advantage for those randomized to PQ CPN ($P = .005$). The analgesic benefit of PQ CPN over analgesic therapy alone was sustained over the 12-month follow-up or until death. However, opioid consumption, the frequency of opioid-induced adverse effects, QOL, and survival duration were similar between groups.

Yan and Myers[18] subsequently evaluated the non-EUS literature from 1966 to 2005 selecting only RCTs, of which 5 studies were identified. CPN was associated with lower visual analogue scores (VAS) for pain and patient opioid use at 2, 4, and 8 weeks when compared with controls. Although statistically significant, the overall benefit was only a 6% reduction in mean VAS. However, improved pain control resulted in a significant decrease in opioid use (mean reduction 40–80 mg/d) and constipation. Nevertheless, the reduction in opioid use was not associated with a decrease in opioid-associated adverse effects, including nausea, vomiting, and sedation, or an effect on QOL or survival. CPN did not eliminate the requirement for opioids.

CPN may also be performed surgically. Lillemoe and colleagues[19] published a prospective randomized trial in 137 patients with unresectable pancreatic cancer. Neurolysis improved pain control versus placebo at 2, 4, and 6 months' follow-up. When the study stratified treatment groups, patients with preoperative pain had a significant survival advantage after neurolysis versus those patients in the control arm. The reason is unclear, but may relate to reduced opioid-induced side effects, improved nutritional status, and emotional well-being. No study has reproduced these investigators' findings. Potential disadvantages of surgical neurolysis include reduced pain relief reported by some, uncertainty regarding response to therapy because of difficulty differentiating postoperative pain from cancer pain, and limited surgical access that prolongs procedure time.[7,12] In addition, the frequency of surgery for unresectable pancreatic cancer would be expected to decline with more sensitivity of cross-sectional imaging, thereby limiting the population of patients who may benefit from this approach.

EUS TECHNIQUES

EUS CN is usually performed in the outpatient setting, often during the index examination conducted for the purpose of pancreatic cancer diagnosis and staging. The patient is questioned regarding relevant allergies and anticoagulant use. Informed consent is obtained, with a focus on the unique complications associated with neurolysis. In our practice, contraindications to CN include: (1) uncorrectable coagulopathy (international normalized ratio (INR) >1.5), (2) thrombocytopenia (platelets <50,000/L), (3) inadequate sedation, or (4) altered anatomy (eg, gastric bypass or an extensive mass or lymphadenopathy prohibiting visualization or access). Patients are initially hydrated with 500 to 1000 mL normal saline to minimize the risk of hypotension. The procedure is performed with the patent in the left lateral decubitus position under moderate or heavy sedation. Continuous monitoring is necessary during and for 2 hours after the procedure. Before discharge, the blood pressure is rechecked in a supine and erect position to assess for orthostasis.

Described EUS-guided techniques for performing CN include: (1) CPN, (2) celiac ganglia neurolysis (CGN), and (3) broad plexus neurolysis (BPN).

EUS-Guided CPN

The initially described and most widely performed approach to EUS CN involves diffuse injection into the celiac plexus. Linear array imaging from the posterior lesser curve of the gastric fundus allows identification of the aorta, which appears in a longitudinal plane (**Fig. 1**). The aorta is traced distally to the celiac trunk, which is the first major branch below the diaphragm. Targeting is based on the expected location of the celiac plexus relative to the celiac trunk. Doppler may be used to distinguish vascular structures. A 22-gauge needle is primed with the injectate, advanced through the biopsy channel, and affixed to the hub. The needle is inserted under EUS guidance, and the needle tip is placed approximately 5 to 10 mm away from the origin of the celiac trunk (**Fig. 2**). In our practice, we usually inject the entire volume in a single site (unilateral or midline) if possible. Some prefer to inject half the volume on 1 side and the remainder on the opposite side of the aorta (bilateral). Occasionally, altered

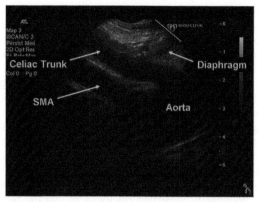

Fig. 1. EUS imaging from the posterior lesser curve of the gastric fundus allows identification of the aorta, which appears in a longitudinal plane.

anatomy resulting from significant lymphadenopathy or bulky tumors may necessitate injection of the entire solution into a single site.

There are limited data regarding the efficacy of single versus bilateral injection. Sahai and colleagues[20] compared unilateral with bilateral injection in a mixed population of patients with pancreatic cancer or chronic pancreatitis. These investigators determined that bilateral CN was significantly more effective than single injection, with a mean pain reduction of 70.4% versus 45.9% ($P = .0016$). Their study offers preliminary data to suggest that bilateral injection may offer enhanced pain relief. These findings were supported by the results of a meta-analysis from Puli and colleagues[21] that revealed that the proportion of patients with pain relief was 84.54% and 45.99% after bilateral versus unilateral EUS-guided CPN (EUS CPN), respectively.

EUS-Guided CGN

Although CPN is considered safe, the degree and duration of pain relief are suboptimal. The limited efficacy may partially be explained by the diffuse injection into the region of the plexus without targeting of the ganglia. Until recently it was believed

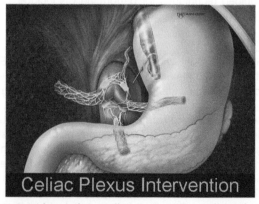

Fig. 2. CPN: under EUS guidance, the needle is inserted immediately adjacent and anterior to the lateral aspect of the aorta at the level of the celiac trunk.

that the celiac ganglia could not be imaged and could be identified only at surgery. The recent recognition that celiac ganglia can be visualized and accessed by EUS allows for direct injection into individual celiac ganglia to perform CGN. This more precise delivery of therapy offers the potential for enhanced efficacy and safety.

A ganglion is defined as a collection of nerve cell bodies and glial cells that are interconnected via a dense network of neural rami and septae of connective tissue. We recently reported the ability to detect the celiac ganglia using EUS.[22,23] Visualized ganglia are typically located adjacent to the celiac artery, anterior to the aorta, and are predominantly oval or almond-shaped, with irregular margins, ranging in size from 2 to 20 mm (**Fig. 3**). Compared with the surrounding retroperitoneal fat, ganglia are echo poor and show similar echogenicity to the adrenal gland. Central echo-rich strands or foci are commonly present with echo-poor threads (presumed neural fibers) extending from ganglia. These threads connect ganglia or course along the anterior surface of the celiac trunk. Color Doppler confirms little or absent flow within these structures.

It was initially unclear how often ganglia could be visualized by EUS. We prospectively evaluated 200 consecutive nonselected patients and documented ganglia detection in 81% of patients. The rate of ganglia detection varied based on the instrument used (radial EUS 79.2% vs linear EUS 85.6%) and among endosonographers (65%–97%).[24] Ganglia detection and appearance did not vary with patient age, alcohol consumption, cigarette use, body mass index (calculated as weight in kilograms divided by the square of height in meters), chronic abdominal pain, or presence of malignancy. The high rate of ganglion visualization and the lack of correlation with other pathologic processes suggested that factors such as edema, fibrosis, inflammation, and malignancy were unnecessary for the visualization of ganglia. Subsequently, a Korean group[25] evaluated 57 consecutive patients using radial EUS, allowing detection in 89% of patients.

The technique for celiac ganglia injection has not been standardized. Our report is the only one thus far to provide any details regarding the specifics of injection.[26] Our general approach for ganglia smaller than 1.0 cm is to position the needle tip within the central point of ganglia and for ganglia 1.0 cm or larger in the needle plane axis, the needle tip is advanced into the deepest point within the ganglia (**Fig. 4**). The injection is then performed as the needle is slowly withdrawn, with care taken to inject the agent evenly throughout each ganglion. As many ganglia as can be identified are injected. Other aspects, such as the total volume injected and volume per ganglion, have not been standardized, as discussed later.

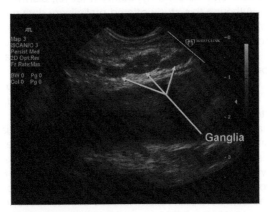

Fig. 3. EUS image of celiac ganglia.

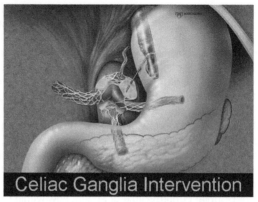

Fig. 4. CGN: under EUS guidance, the needle is inserted directly into a celiac ganglion.

EUS-Guided BPN

Sakamoto and colleagues[27] described the technique of EUS-guided BPN (EUS BPN). The technique involves passing the needle under direct EUS visualization adjacent and anterior to the lateral aspect of the aorta over the level of the superior mesenteric artery (SMA) trunk. There are no other unique aspects to this approach.

EUS Studies

Wiersema and Wiersema[28] published the initial study evaluating EUS CPN and subsequently updated their experience (**Tables 1–4**).[29] The later prospective study, which included the patients from their initial report, involved 58 patients with pain secondary to inoperable pancreatic cancer. Three to 6 mL (0.25%) of bupivacaine and 10 mL (98%) of alcohol were injected into both sides of the celiac trunk. Pain scores were assessed using a standardized 11-point visual analogue scale. Forty-five patients (78%) experienced a decrease ($\geq$1 point) in pain score after EUS CPN. The pain scores were significantly lower ($P<.0001$) 2 weeks after the procedure. On multivariate analysis, sustained pain relief was found for 24 weeks independent of narcotic use or adjuvant therapy. Although opioid use escalated over time, the increase was not statistically significant. There were no major complications. Minor complications were mild and transient and included hypotension (20%), diarrhea (17%), and pain exacerbation (9%). Although this study offered preliminary data suggesting the efficacy and safety of EUS CPN, the small sample size, absence of a placebo control group, and absence of physician or patient blinding limits the strength of the conclusions. In addition, despite 45 patients (78%) experiencing a decrease in pain score, only 31 (54%) experienced a decline of 3 points pr more (or a 50% decrease), which are measures of improvement that some consider necessary to signify efficacy. Furthermore, the efficacy of EUS CPN was relatively short-lived, with escalating pain scores reported at 8 to 12 weeks.

Only 2 studies have been published in nonabstract form that evaluated EUS-guided CGN (EUS CGN) in patients who have pancreatic cancer.[26,30] In the initial study from Levy and colleagues, EUS was used to target as many ganglia as possible, which resulted in therapy for 2.7 ganglia (range 1–6). At 2 to 4 weeks after EUS CGN, partial pain relief was reported in 16 of 17 (94%) patients who have pancreatic cancer; no patient experienced complete pain relief. Narcotic use increased, remained equivalent, and decreased in 2 (12%), 12 (71%), and 3 (18%) patients, respectively. Transient

Table 1 Inclusion and exclusion criteria		
Study	**Inclusion Criteria**	**Exclusion Criteria**

Gunaratnam et al,[29] 2001	Both 1 and 2:
	1. Pancreatic cancer and either
	    a. Unresectable
	    b. Poor operative candidate
	2. Narcotic requiring abdominal pain
		1. PT >18
		2. Platelets <80,000

Levy et al,[26] 2008	Both 1 and 2: 1. Unresectable pancreatic cancer and 2. Moderate/severe narcotic dependent pain	1. INR >1.5 2. Platelets <50,000 3. Inadequate sedation 4. Altered anatomy
Sakamoto et al,[27] 2010	Either 1 or 2: 1. Unresectable pancreatic cancer (n = 60), or 2. Extensive nonpancreatic abdominal cancer (n = 7)	Not stated
Ascunce et al,[30] 2011	Required 1, 2, and 3: 1. Unresectable pancreatic cancer 2. Pain (VAS $\geq$3) 3. >18 years	Not stated
Iwata et al,[31] 2011	1 and either 2 or 3: 1. Pain (VAS $\geq$5), with or without narcotic use 2. Unresectable pancreatic cancer (n = 40) or 3. Nonpancreatic abdominal cancer (n = 7)	1. INR >1.5 2. Platelets <50,000 3. Esophageal or gastric cardia varices

postural hypotension was experienced by 6 of 17 patients (35%). Patients noted marked (n = 2) and mild (n = 2) improvement in their underlying constipation, and diarrhea did not develop in any patient. When immediate intraprocedural discomfort or pain was excluded, subsequent initial pain exacerbation in the recovery room or soon thereafter was experienced by 36%, of either 2.2 or 1.1 days' duration for neurolysis or blockade, respectively. Patients who developed an initial pain exacerbation tended to subsequently experience greater pain relief at follow-up, with 7 of 7 (100%) patients who had an initial pain exacerbation reporting eventual efficacy of CGN versus 9 of 11 (81%, P = .23). There was no evidence of other complications, and specifically no patient described any neurologic deficits. The retrospective, noncontrolled nature of this study, which includes a limited enrollment and inadequate measure of pain monitoring, provides inadequate power to permit firm conclusions and raises as many questions as it answers. Recognizing these limitations, the data suggest the safety and short-term efficacy of direct EUS CGN in patients with moderate to severe pain resulting from unresectable pancreatic carcinoma.

A subsequent study from Ascunce and colleagues[30] retrospectively evaluated the efficacy of EUS CN in 64 patients with pancreatic cancer. EUS CGN (n = 40) was performed whenever ganglia could be identified, with a median of 2.0 ganglia (range 1–4)

Table 2
Study design, enrollment, and injection data

Study	Design	No. of Patients	Site of Injection	Injectate (Total Volumes)
Gunaratnam et al,[29] 2001	Prospective	58	Celiac plexus-bilateral around celiac artery (n = 58)	Bupivacaine (0.25%, 6–12 mL) Alcohol (98%, 20 mL)
Levy et al,[26] 2008	Retrospective	17[a]	Celiac ganglia (n = 17)	Bupivacaine (0.25%, 8.3 mL) Alcohol (99%, 12.7 mL)
Sakamoto et al,[27] 2010	Retrospective	67	Celiac plexus-bilateral around celiac artery (n = 34) Broad plexus-bilateral around superior mesenteric artery (n = 33)	Lidocaine (1%, 3 mL) Alcohol (9 mL) Contrast (1 mL)
Ascunce et al,[30] 2011	Retrospective	64	Celiac plexus-bilateral around celiac artery (n = 24) Celiac ganglia (n = 40)	Lidocaine (1%, 10 mL) Alcohol (98%, 20 mL)
Iwata et al,[31] 2011	Retrospective	47	Celiac plexus-multiple injections	Bupivacaine (2–3 mL) Alcohol (≤20 mL)

[a] Excluded 1 patient with pancreatic cancer who underwent celiac block with steroids rather than CN with alcohol.

injected. Standard bilateral EUS CPN (n = 24) was performed when ganglia could not be visualized. One week after CN, 32 patients (50%) had a symptomatic response. Pain relief was reported in 26 of 40 (65%) and 6 of 24 (25%) patients undergoing CGN and CPN, respectively (P<.002). For the group as a whole, there was a significant (P<.0001) reduction of 2.1 points in pain score from a mean of 6.7 at baseline to 4.5 at 1 week. When excluding 2 patients lost to follow-up, persistent pain relief (measured at 4 weeks) was reported in 23 of 30 (77%) initial responders, but only 23 of 62 patients (37%) overall.

These results are further disappointing when considering that the threshold for pain response (decreased VAS of 2 or more) is less than most consider necessary to define pain relief. In addition, although the study enrolled patients with initial pain of 3 or greater on the VAS, 21 patients (33%) had not yet taken any narcotic analgesics at the time of EUS. Transient diarrhea developed in 15 (23%) patients. One patient experienced a transient pain exacerbation within a few hours of therapy, which returned to baseline at 24 hours. This patient ultimately experienced a pain response. One (2%) patient developed transient hypotension, which responded to intravenous fluids. The investigators concluded that EUS CN was modestly effective for palliation of pain in pancreatic cancer. The 50% and 37% response rates at 1 and 4 weeks, respectively, and the soft threshold for pain response raise concern regarding the usefulness of EUS CN.

Sakamoto and colleagues[27] compared EUS BPN (n = 33) with EUS CPN (n = 34) in patients with unresectable pancreatic cancer (n = 60) or extensive nonpancreatic abdominal cancers (n = 7). Analgesic use and pain scores were recorded 7 and 30 days after therapy. For both procedures, 3 mL of 1% lidocaine was injected followed

Table 3
Measures of pain response and pain relief

Study	Measures of Pain Response	Pain Relief

Gunaratnam et al,[29] 2001	Measured in 2 ways:
	1. VAS and calculate either:
	  a. VAS (decrease by ≥1 point) or
	  b. VAS (decrease by ≥3 points)
		2 wk:
		45/58 (78%); VAS decrease any degree (≥1 point)
		31/58 (54%); VAS decrease ≥3 points

Levy et al,[26] 2008	One of the following: 1. Complete response 2. Partial response 3. No response	2–4 wk: 00/17 (00%); complete pain relief 16/17 (94%); partial pain relief
Sakamoto et al,[27] 2010	One criterion: 1. VAS (decrease by ≥3 points)	30 d: 43/67 (64%); entire group 17/34 (50%); CGN 25/33 (76%); BPN
Ascunce et al,[30] 2011	Required all 3 of the following: 1. Feeling better 2. VAS (decrease ≥2 points) 3. Narcotics dose not increased	1 wk: 32/64 (50%); entire group 26/40 (65%); CGN 06/24 (25%); CPN 4 wk: 23/62 (37%)[a]; entire group
Iwata et al,[31] 2011	Successful pain relief defined by: 1. VAS ≤3 2. Narcotic dose not increased Complete pain relief defined by: 1. VAS 0 or 1 2. Narcotic dose not increased	1 wk: 14/47 (36%); complete pain relief 32/47 (68%); successful pain relief

[a] 2 patients lost to follow-up.

by bilateral injection of a mixture of 9 mL of alcohol and 1 mL of contrast. A decrease by 3 points or more on the VAS was considered good pain relief. For the EUS CPN group, the mean VAS initially and 7 and 30 days after the procedure were 7.8, 3.9, and 4.8, respectively. The equivalent scores for the EUS BPN group were 7.8, 2.5, and 3.4, respectively, with EUS BPN providing significantly greater pain relief on days 7 and 30 ($P<.05$). At 30 days, pain relief was reported in 25 of 33 (76%) patients undergoing BPN versus 17 of 34 (50%) after CPN. Because of technical limitations or patient-related factors, 3 of 37 (8%) patients undergoing CPN and 6 of 39 (15%) patients undergoing BPN were excluded from analysis. The exclusion of these patients affects the data and an intention-to-treat approach would have been favored.

Patients underwent immediate computed tomography to correlate pain relief with the pattern and extent of alcohol infiltration. The assessment was made in the frontal plane of the celiac, superior, and inferior mesenteric arteries, and the anatomy was divided into 6 regions, namely left and right (upper, middle, and lower regions). A higher proportion of patients in the BPN group had contrast spread to all 6 (42%) or 5 (28%) areas compared with CPN, which had no patients with contrast spread to all 6 areas and only 9% with spread to 5 areas. On day 30, patients with contrast in 4 or 5 areas had a significantly greater reduction in VAS versus those with contrast

Table 4 Complications	
Study	**Complications**
Gunaratnam et al,[29] 2001	Hypotension, n = 12 (20%); transient Diarrhea, n = 10 (17%); transient (<48 h; n = 9); one patient had diarrhea for 7 d Pain exacerbation, n = 5 (09%); transient (<48 h)
Levy et al,[26] 2008	Pain exacerbation, n = 7 (41%); mean 2.2 d, correlated with improved pain relief Hypotension, n = 6 (35%); transient
Sakamoto et al,[27] 2010	No major complications Minor complications were not addressed
Ascunce et al,[30] 2011	Diarrhea, n = 15 (23%); transient Pain exacerbation, n = 1 (02%); transient, subsequently responded to therapy Hypotension, n = 1 (02%); transient and responded to intravenous fluids
Iwata et al,[31] 2011	Diarrhea, n = 11 (23%); transient, controlled with medication, resolve in 4 d (range 1–7 d) Hypotension, n = 8 (17%); transient Inebriation, n = 4 (09%)

in 3 areas or fewer. Of the 14 patients with contrast spread to all 6 areas, 13 (93%) showed good long-term pain relief. Patients with contrast in only 1 or 2 areas did not have significant reductions in VAS at 7 or 30 days. Overall, patients in the BPN group had a greater decrease in narcotic use compared with the CPN group.

Most recently, Iwata and colleagues[31] published their retrospective experience after EUS CPN among 47 patients with unresectable pancreatic cancer (n = 4) or non-pancreatic abdominal cancer (n = 7). These investigators performed CPN with a median of 2 (range 2–4) needle insertions and injections, and therefore the technique is most analogous to the bilateral versus unilateral approach. A total of 2 to 3 mL of bupivacaine was injected followed by a median of 20 mL (range 15–20 mL) of alcohol. Successful or complete pain relief required a stable dose of narcotics and a VAS of 3 or less versus a score of 1 or less, respectively. At 1 week, 14 of 47 patients (36%) had complete pain relief versus 32 of 47 (68%) patients with successful pain relief.

OTHER TECHNICAL CONSIDERATIONS

Regardless of the technique used, other aspects of EUS CN must be considered, including the volume and concentration of the drugs injected, whether to administer them separately or as a combined compound, ideal needle caliber, and whether to use a standard end-hole or multisidehole injection needle. At this point, these decisions are not data driven, but rather are based on personal experience or historical norms. Most studies of CPN in patients who have pancreatic cancer have administered a local anesthetic (bupivacaine or lidocaine) and neurolytic agent (phenol or alcohol). The local anesthetic reduces the discomfort caused by the neurolytic agent. Phenol produces minimal pain because of its local anesthetic effect. Although direct comparisons between alcohol and phenol have not been performed, alcohol is favored because it induces greater neurolysis and presumably greater pain relief.[32] In our practice, we typically inject a premixed solution containing 10 mL of bupivacaine (0.25%) and 10 mL of alcohol (98%). We use standard end-hole 22-gauge needles and have not found larger or smaller caliber or multisidehole needles to be of any greater usefulness.

COMPLICATIONS OF CN

In a review of the pooled data from 5 RCTs of the PQ CPN literature, Yan and Myers[18] reported a low rate of adverse events: diarrhea (9%), transient hypotension (8%), constipation (40%), nausea and vomiting (41%), and lethargy (49%). No serious adverse events were reported. Severe complications were reported in 13 of 628 patients (2%) in the meta-analysis from Eisenberg and colleagues,[14] including neurologic (lower extremity weakness or paresthesia, epidural anesthesia, and lumbar puncture) as well as pain (chest, pleuritic, shoulder), pneumothorax, hiccupping, and hematuria. In the same meta-analysis, the most common side effects of PQ CPN included local pain (96%), diarrhea (44%), and hypotension (38%) and were generally mild and transient.[14]

Neurologic complications are believed to develop secondary to ischemia or direct injury to the spinal cord or somatic nerves. Spinal cord ischemia may result from thrombosis or spasm of the artery of Adamkiewicz, which is located to the left of the spine between T8 and L4 and perfuses the lower two-thirds of the spinal cord.[33,34] Despite theoretic advantages of certain methods (eg, anterior approaches), it is thought that the risk of neural dysfunction is not influenced by the route of therapy. Paraplegia has been reported with each PQ method regardless of the use of radiologic guidance. There are even reports of paraplegia associated with the most direct approach (surgical neurolysis).[35]

Although the reported complication and efficacy rates of EUS CPN have been similar to PQ methods, the lack of comparative studies does not allow the assumed equivalence to be verified.[36] Serious complications (such as paraplegia) have never been reported with EUS. This situation is likely because PQ methods are used more often than EUS, as much as because of any difference in the inherent risk for a particular procedure. However, EUS is an anterior approach and thereby avoids the retro-crural space and may reduce the risk of neurologic dysfunction and pulmonary complications. Furthermore, as opposed to the PQ anterior approach, with EUS the needle traverses only the gastric wall, presumably eliminating complications resulting from inadvertent penetration of surrounding organs. Although it is impossible to substantiate, we assume that the complication risk would be similar for EUS and PQ approaches.

EVALUATION OF EUS DATA

Despite the presence of only 5 full-length published studies, 2 meta-analyses have been conducted evaluating the usefulness of EUS CN in patients with pancreatic cancer pain. At the time of the meta-analysis from Kaufman and colleagues,[37] only 2 full articles[26,29] and 1 abstract[38] had been published. Based on these 3 reports, these investigators found EUS CN to be 72% effective in managing pancreatic cancer pain, without distinction of the role of CPN versus CGN. They concluded that EUS CN is a reasonable option for patients developing tolerance to narcotic analgesics. Puli and colleagues[21] conducted a meta-analysis in which they considered the findings of 8 studies. However, most reports were published in abstract form and the investigators also included trials that provided updated data from initial pilot studies, thereby including duplicate data. The investigators found that 80% of the pooled proportion of patients with pancreatic cancer showed pain relief. Based on their review, they concluded that EUS CN offers a safe and important alternative for pain relief in patients who have pancreatic cancer.

With respect to the investigators of the meta-analyses, the statistics tell only 1 side of the story. As stated by Henry Clay, "Statistics are no substitute for judgment." A superficial look at the data and study conclusions suggests that EUS CN is a reasonable option and safe and important alternative for pain relief in patients who have pancreatic cancer. However, a closer review of the published literature (see **Tables 1–4**), excluding abstracts, may lead some to view the role of EUS CN alternatively to that expressed in the meta-analyses. The body of literature includes only 253 patients who have cancer (239 with pancreatic cancer). The studies are too varied to allow careful examination and determination of the usefulness of any one approach. However, a pain response was reported in only 145 of 251 (58%) patients. Documentation of a complete pain response occurred in only 14 of 64 (22%) patients. The findings are further disappointing because efficacy was determined only 1 to 4 weeks after therapy and some investigators used less stringent criteria to define a pain response. Furthermore, virtually all patients continued to require the same or greater narcotic dose. In addition, the beneficial effect of chemoradiation that many patients likely received would have accounted for some of the perceived pain relief. These studies, including the ones from our center, also share another important feature, namely insufficient methodology to permit accurate determination of the usefulness of EUS CN. Concerns regarding EUS CN are supported by the results of a recent prospective double-blind, randomized trial published in abstract form reporting a similar pain response for EUS CPN and a sham procedure.[39] Although short-term, modest pain relief is of value to patients suffering from often-debilitating pancreatic cancer pain, existing data are discouraging. Although EUS CN provides a statistical benefit in terms of pain relief, we only cautiously accept its role as an adjunct approach to standard pain management and do not consider it effective as a single method to control pain in patients with unresectable pancreatic cancer. The lack of comparative trials prohibits accurate comparison of EUS with non-EUS methods of CN, but it is likely that the limitations of CN are not restricted to EUS.

CLINICAL ALGORITHM

Given the marginal benefit of CN, it is reasonable to wonder if this technique should even be included in the algorithm of pancreatic cancer pain management, and if so, at what point in the disease process. We consider CN in patients who have pancreatic cancer only after failure of initial opioid administration or patients with intolerable opioid-induced side effects. This approach is in keeping with that advocated by the World Health Organization.[40] There are several potential advantages of EUS versus PQ techniques for performing CN. The proximity of the posterior lesser curve of the stomach to the region, ability to detect the ganglia, use of continuous real-time visualization of the target area, and availability of Doppler to assess the vasculature all facilitate accurate needle placement. By doing so, EUS may theoretically improve pain relief and reduce complications. The lack of well-designed comparative trials prohibits verification of these assumptions. However, review of available data suggests that EUS and PQ CN offer similar efficacy and side effect profile. Furthermore, there are no compelling data to suggest that any of the EUS and PQ technical modifications enhance pain relief or safety. This view is supported by the results of a meta-analysis, which found that the efficacy of PQ CPN was independent of the use or means of radiologic guidance.[14] One might assume that enhanced methods for radiologic guidance would improve the outcomes. Instead, patients who underwent blind PQ injection (without imaging guidance) were more likely to achieve pain relief (95%) compared with the use of various imaging modalities (86%–91%, $P > .05$). Theoretic advantages of direct ganglia injection have yet to be substantiated in well-designed studies. Prospective, controlled, and comparative trials are needed to confirm the findings of initial retrospective studies favoring EUS CGN over EUS CPN. Until then, we do not advocate this approach within routine clinical practice.

If EUS guidance offers no advantage in terms of pain relief or safety, then one may question its role in performing CN. The major disadvantage of EUS CPN is the inherent cost associated with the endoscopy that is further heightened in patients requiring anesthesia-assisted sedation. The ability to perform EUS CN at the time of tumor biopsy and staging combines diagnostic and therapeutic modalities, thereby simplifying patient care and reducing cost. We perform CN under EUS guidance in patients undergoing EUS for another reason, including the need for diagnosis or staging and when disease spread precludes a satisfactory PQ approach.

Pancreatic cancer pain is a multifactorial process. This factor likely explains that although CN offers some degree of pain relief, it rarely eliminates pain and nearly all patients continue to require opioid use. When counseling patients, it is important to provide a realistic goal, which is not to eliminate pain, but rather to optimize oral pharmacologic therapy and minimize narcotic-induced side effects. The timing of the neurolysis relative to the onset of pain may predict response. In 1 study, CPN was more effective when performed early after pain onset rather than late in its course.[6] This finding may be explained by the fact that early pancreatic cancer pain seems to derive mainly from the celiac plexus. However, we consider these data insufficient to justify CN for patients with mild or absent pain. The short duration of pain relief may also suggest a need to delay CN until it is more clearly clinically indicated. Furthermore, this approach may also be supported by the study from Ascunce and colleagues,[30] who found that higher baseline pain levels were weakly associated with an improved pain response. Likewise, the number of times that CN should be performed and stopping rules have not been established. In our practice, we may repeat CN in patients who have an adequate response based on the intensity of pain relief ($\geq$3-point or $\geq$50% decrease in VAS) and for sufficient duration ($\geq$1 month).

Despite the theoretic advantages of EUS CPN, the absence of comparative data prohibits any assessment of the relative safety and efficacy. An even great experience has been developed with modifying PQ approaches since first reported by Kappis and colleagues in 1914.[11] Since then investigators have used innumerable technical variations in terms of access sites, routes of delivery, method of guidance, in addition to altering the composition, volume, and concentrate of the injectate. In parallel, some have sought to identify the procedural and patient-specific factors that predict treatment success. As usual, the presence of many options indicates some controversy and a lack of any meaningful progress. If 1 particular method were clearly superior, the other techniques would have become obsolete.

Predictors of Response

The tumor location may predict a therapeutic response. Studies by both Catalano and colleagues[38] and Ascunce and colleagues[30] reported that CPN was more effective in patients with pancreatic cancer located in the pancreatic body or tail versus those within the pancreatic head. Rykowski and Hilgier[41] evaluated the effectiveness of PQ CPN based on the pancreatic cancer location and reached an opposing view. After PQ CPN, 37 of 50 patients (74%) had effective pain relief during the first 3 months or until death. Effective pain relief was seen in 33 of 36 (92%) versus 4 of 14 (29%) patients with a cancer located in the pancreatic head versus body/tail, respectively.

In a study by Sakamoto and colleagues,[27] a subgroup analysis was performed in which the cancers were categorized as upper cancers (those not spread beyond the SMA) and lower cancers (tumors that expanded beyond the SMA). For patients with upper cancers, CPN and BPN provided similar rates of long-term pain relief (78% [14/18] and 72% [10/14], respectively). However, for patients with lower cancer, BPN was more effective, because 79% (15/19) achieved good long-term pain control compared with only 19% (3/16) for CPN. A similar study by De Ciccio and colleagues[42] evaluated the pattern of spread and corresponding efficacy of pain relief in 53 patients who had undergone PQ CPN. The patients were divided into 2 groups (caudal or cephalad to the celiac artery) based on needle tip position. The injection pattern was evaluated by dividing the frontal plane of the celiac region into 4 quadrants. Three or 4 quadrants contained contrast in 79% when the needle tip was placed cephalad to the celiac trunk compared with only 38% when the needle tip was placed in a caudal position ($P<.01$). Patients in the group with the cephalad needle position had superior short-term and long-term pain relief. Although the findings of the 2 studies are in direct contrast to one another, methodologic variation prohibits accurate comparison between studies.

In the study by Ascunce and colleagues,[30] a multivariate analysis was performed, revealing that ganglia visualization best predicted a pain response. A baseline pain score of greater than 7 also correlated with therapeutic benefit. Patient age, gender, tumor size and location, baseline narcotic use, existing versus pending tissue diagnosis, and number of ganglia visualized did not correlate with outcomes. Iwata and colleagues[31] evaluated various clinical and radiographic features to determine their potential impact on pain response, including gender, age, initial VAS, initial narcotic use, tumor location, tumor type, presence of ascites, distant metastasis, direct invasion of the celiac plexus, and distribution of alcohol (on both sides of the celiac artery vs the left side only). On multivariate analysis, the only features that significantly correlated with lesser pain response included direct tumor invasion of the celiac plexus (present in 20 of 47 patients) ($P = .005$) and distribution of alcohol limited to the left side of the aorta (occurring in 9 of 47 patients) ($P = .0025$). These investigators also compared patients who had previously taken narcotics (n = 18) versus those who had never taken narcotics (n = 29) and there was no significant difference among groups. The findings may suggest that initial pain severity poorly predicts treatment response.

SUMMARY

Patients with pancreatic cancer commonly develop pain that is poorly managed with oral analgesic therapy. Current use of CN exceeds our understanding of the efficacy, and the ideal role has not been established. The literature pertaining to PQ approaches to CN is fraught with small, poorly designed trials that typically yield data of unclear clinical relevance. The same limitations exist within the EUS literature, with even fewer quality studies. The varied study limitations prohibit one from making firm conclusions regarding the safety or efficacy. Although some have reported statistical benefit of CN, a careful review of the literature raises concern whether the statistically significant benefit equates to a clinically significant benefit. Despite the noted concerns, EUS CN maintains a role in our practice as an adjunct to pain management because of the limited options in patients suffering from often-debilitating pain and because of the safety and nominal cost when performed during the initial diagnostic and staging EUS examination. Clear and rationale patient counseling is key in moderating expectations.

Although the lack of comparative trials prohibits accurate comparison of EUS with non-EUS methods of CN, it is likely that the limitations of CN are not restricted to EUS approaches. Well-designed trials are needed to determine: (1) optimal method and timing of CN, (2) composition of the injectate, (3) cost, (4) patient preference, (5) influence on QOL, and (6) impact on survival. Only then can we establish the efficacy and safety of CN and identify the optimal means of delivery to clarify the role of CN and offer therapy in a more scientific manner.

IMPORTANT POINTS

- Patients who have pancreatic cancer frequently experience abdominal pain that is often difficult to control.
- Oral pharmacologic therapies often insufficiently manage pancreatic cancer pain and side effects commonly develop.
- EUS CN diminishes pain associated with pancreatic cancer in approximately 60% of patients over the first 1 to 4 weeks after therapy.
- Although direct comparative trials are lacking, there are no convincing data that any 1 method, or technical variations of a given method, provides superior pain relief.
- When performed, consider EUS-guided approaches to CN during the initial diagnostic and staging EUS examination. When EUS is not otherwise indicated, PQ approaches are likely favored.
- Well-designed trials are needed to verify the efficacy and safety of CN and to select the optimal approach for treating pancreatic cancer pain.

REFERENCES

1. Ventafridda GV, Caraceni AT, Sbanotto AM, et al. Pain treatment in cancer of the pancreas. Eur J Surg Oncol 1990;16:1–6.
2. Lankisch PG. Natural course of chronic pancreatitis. Pancreatology 2001;1:3–14.
3. Ventafridda V, Tamburini M, Caraceni A, et al. A validation study of the WHO method for cancer pain relief. Cancer 1987;59:850–6.
4. Yeager MP, Colacchio TA, Yu CT, et al. Morphine inhibits spontaneous and cytokine-enhanced natural killer cell cytotoxicity in volunteers. Anesthesiology 1995;83:500–8.
5. Ward EM, Rorie DK, Nauss LA, et al. The celiac ganglia in man: normal anatomic variations. Anesth Analg 1979;58:461–5.
6. Ischia S, Ischia A, Polati E, et al. Three posterior percutaneous celiac plexus block techniques. A prospective, randomized study in 61 patients with pancreatic cancer pain. Anesthesiology 1992;76:534–40.
7. Brown DL, Moore DC. The use of neurolytic celiac plexus block for pancreatic cancer: anatomy and technique. J Pain Symptom Manage 1988;3:206–9.
8. Plancarte R, Velasquez R, Patt R. Neurolytic blocks of the sympathetic axis. In: Patt R, editor. Cancer Pain. Philadelphia: Lippincott; 1993. p. 377.
9. Nagakawa T, Mori K, Nakano T, et al. Perineural invasion of carcinoma of the pancreas and biliary tract. Br J Surg 1993;80:619–21.
10. Gebhardt GF. Visceral pain mechanisms. In: Chapman CR, Foley KM, editors. Current and emerging issues in cancer pain. New York: Raven Press; 1993. p. 99–111.
11. Kappis M. Erfahrungen mit local Anasthesie bie Bauchoperationen. Vehr Dtsch Gesellsch Chir 1914;43:87–9 [in German].

12. Lebovits AH, Lefkowitz M. Pain management of pancreatic carcinoma: a review. Pain 1989;36:1–11.
13. Sharfman WH, Walsh TD. Has the analgesic efficacy of neurolytic celiac plexus block been demonstrated in pancreatic cancer pain? Pain 1990;41:267–71.
14. Eisenberg E, Carr DB, Chalmers TC. Neurolytic celiac plexus block for treatment of cancer pain: a meta-analysis [Erratum appears in Anesth Analg 1995;1(81):213]. Anesth Analg 1995;80:290–5.
15. Polati E, Finco G, Gottin L, et al. Prospective randomized double-blind trial of neurolytic coeliac plexus block in patients with pancreatic cancer. Br J Surg 1998;85:199–201.
16. Kawamata M, Ishitani K, Ishikawa K, et al. Comparison between celiac plexus block and morphine treatment on quality of life in patients with pancreatic cancer pain. Pain 1996;64:597–602.
17. Wong GY, Schroeder DR, Carns PE, et al. Effect of neurolytic celiac plexus block on pain relief, quality of life, and survival in patients with unresectable pancreatic cancer: a randomized controlled trial. JAMA 2004;291:1092–9.
18. Yan BM, Myers RP. Neurolytic celiac plexus block for pain control in unresectable pancreatic cancer. Am J Gastroenterol 2007;102:430–8.
19. Lillemoe KD, Cameron JL, Kaufman HS, et al. Chemical splanchnicectomy in patients with unresectable pancreatic cancer. A prospective randomized trial. Ann Surg 1993;217:447–55 [discussion: 456–7].
20. Sahai AV, Lemelin V, Lam E, et al. Central vs. bilateral endoscopic ultrasound-guided celiac plexus block or neurolysis: a comparative study of short-term effectiveness. Am J Gastroenterol 2009;104:326–9.
21. Puli SR, Reddy JBK, Bechtold ML, et al. EUS-guided celiac plexus neurolysis for pain due to chronic pancreatitis or pancreatic cancer pain: a meta-analysis and systematic review. Dig Dis Sci 2009;54:2330–7.
22. Levy MJ, Topazian M, Keeney G, et al. Preoperative diagnosis of extrapancreatic neural invasion in pancreatic cancer. Clin Gastroenterol Hepatol 2006;4:1479–82.
23. Levy MJ, Rajan E, Keeney G, et al. Neural ganglia visualized by endoscopic ultrasound. Am J Gastroenterol 2006;101:1787–91.
24. Gleeson FC, Levy MJ, Papachristou GI, et al. Frequency of visualization of presumed celiac ganglia by endoscopic ultrasound. Endoscopy 2007;39:620–4.
25. Ha TI, Kim GH, Kang DH, et al. Detection of celiac ganglia with radial scanning endoscopic ultrasonography. Korean J Intern Med 2008;23:5–8.
26. Levy MJ, Topazian MD, Wiersema MJ, et al. Initial evaluation of the efficacy and safety of endoscopic ultrasound-guided direct Ganglia neurolysis and block. Am J Gastroenterol 2008;103:98–103.
27. Sakamoto H, Kitano M, Kamata K, et al. EUS-guided broad plexus neurolysis over the superior mesenteric artery using a 25-gauge needle. Am J Gastroenterol 2010;105:2599–606.
28. Wiersema MJ, Wiersema LM. Endosonography-guided celiac plexus neurolysis. Gastrointest Endosc 1996;44:656–62.
29. Gunaratnam NT, Sarma AV, Norton ID, et al. A prospective study of EUS-guided celiac plexus neurolysis for pancreatic cancer pain. Gastrointest Endosc 2001;54:316–24.
30. Ascunce G, Ribeiro A, Reis I, et al. EUS visualization and direct celiac ganglia neurolysis predicts better pain relief in patients with pancreatic malignancy (with video). Gastrointest Endosc 2011;73:267–74.
31. Iwata K, Yasuda I, Enya M, et al. Predictive factors for pain relief after endoscopic ultrasound-guided celiac plexus neurolysis. Dig Endosc 2011;23:140–5.

32. Mercadante S, Nicosia F. Celiac plexus block: a reappraisal [comment]. Reg Anesth Pain Med 1998;23:37–48.
33. De Conno F, Caraceni A, Aldrighetti L, et al. Paraplegia following coeliac plexus block [comment]. Pain 1993;55:383–5.
34. van Dongen RT, Crul BJ. Paraplegia following coeliac plexus block. Anaesthesia 1991;46:862–3.
35. Hayakawa J, Kobayashi O, Murayama H. Paraplegia after intraoperative celiac plexus block. Anesth Analg 1997;84:447–8.
36. Levy MJ, Wiersema MJ. EUS-guided celiac plexus neurolysis and celiac plexus block. Gastrointest Endosc 2003;57:923–30.
37. Kaufman M, Singh G, Das S, et al. Efficacy of endoscopic ultrasound-guided celiac plexus block and celiac plexus neurolysis for managing abdominal pain associated with chronic pancreatitis and pancreatic cancer. J Clin Gastroenterol 2010;44:127–34.
38. Catalano M, Ahmed U, Chauhan S. Celiac plexus neurolysis (CPN) in the treatment of refractory pain of pancreatic cancer (PCA): site specific response to therapy. Gastrointest Endosc 2005;1:A273.
39. Wallace MB, Woodward TA, Hoffman BJ, et al. A prospective double blind randomized controlled trial of EUS guided celiac neurolysis vs sham for pancreatic cancer pain. Gastrointest Endosc 2010;71:A224.
40. World Health Organization. Cancer pain relief. Geneva: WHO; 2006.
41. Rykowski JJ, Hilgier M. Efficacy of neurolytic celiac plexus block in varying locations of pancreatic cancer: influence on pain relief. Anesthesiology 2000;92:347–54.
42. De Cicco M, Matovic M, Balestreri L, et al. Single-needle celiac plexus block: is needle tip position critical in patients with no regional anatomic distortions? Anesthesiology 1997;87:1301–8.

Endoscopic Ultrasonography-Guided Biliary Drainage: Rendezvous Technique

Takuji Iwashita, MD, PhD[a,b], John G. Lee, MD[a,*]

KEYWORDS

- Endoscopic ultrasonography
- Endoscopic retrograde cholangiopancreatography
- Biliary access • Biliary drainage • Rendezvous
- Failed cannulation

INTRODUCTION

Endoscopic retrograde cholangiopancreatography (ERCP) has been widely used as the main therapeutic technique for biliary diseases. Therapeutic ERCP requires deep cannulation into the common bile duct (CBD). The success rate of deep cannulation is high but still not perfect, even with the use of advanced cannulation techniques such as precut sphincterotomy.[1–3] In particular, periampullary diverticula,[4–7] tumor infiltration,[8,9] or altered surgical anatomy[10,11] occasionally complicates biliary cannulation. Alternatives if deep biliary cannulation fails include repeat ERCP on a different day by the same or a more experienced endoscopist,[12–15] or other alternatives such as percutaneous transhepatic biliary drainage (PTBD)[16,17] or surgical intervention.[18] However, a patient's condition often may not allow waiting for another ERCP session on a different day, and both PTBD and surgical intervention are associated with considerable morbidity and occasional mortality.[16–18]

Over the past decade, the development of the linear-array echoendoscope has enabled various endoscopic ultrasonography (EUS)-related diagnostic and therapeutic techniques such as fine-needle aspiration (FNA),[19,20] pancreatic pseudocyst drainage,[21–23] and celiac plexus neurolysis.[24–26] The use of EUS-guided cholangiography was first reported in 1996.[27] Following this report, an initial case report of EUS-guided

a Division of Gastroenterology and Hepatology, H.H. Chao Comprehensive Digestive Disease Center, University of California, Irvine Medical Center, 101 The City Drive, Building 22C, First Floor, Orange, CA 92868, USA; b First Department of Internal Medicine, Gifu University Hospital, Gifu, Japan
* Corresponding author.
E-mail address: jglee@uci.edu

Gastrointest Endoscopy Clin N Am 22 (2012) 249–258
doi:10.1016/j.giec.2012.04.018
1052-5157/12/$ – see front matter © 2012 Elsevier Inc. All rights reserved.

giendo.theclinics.com

biliary duct puncture followed by transduodenal stent placement after failed ERCP was published in 2001[28] and, more recently, the EUS-guided rendezvous (EUS-RV) technique has emerged as a salvage technique for failed cannulation in ERC.

EUS-RV
Indications for EUS-RV

After failed deep biliary cannulation using conventional techniques, the choice to perform EUS-RV should be cautiously made, based on comprehensive consideration for the reason behind biliary cannulation failure, the patient's condition, and the available alternatives. EUS-RV should be performed by endoscopists who are experienced with both ERCP and EUS in an endoscopic facility featuring both fluoroscopy and EUS capabilities. If EUS-RV fails, immediate availability of the percutaneous approach is important in minimizing the risk of bile leakage from the punctured biliary duct. The authors recommend administration of broad-spectrum antibiotics before EUS-RV as prophylaxis against potential spillage of infected bile.

EUS-RV Technique

After failed biliary cannulation in ERC, EUS is performed using a linear scanning video echoendoscope and processor with color Doppler function. Following EUS examination of the biliary system including evaluation of the regional vasculature using color Doppler, the bile duct is punctured from the gut under EUS guidance using a 19-gauge or 22-gauge FNA needle that has been primed with contrast agent (**Fig. 1**A). Aspiration

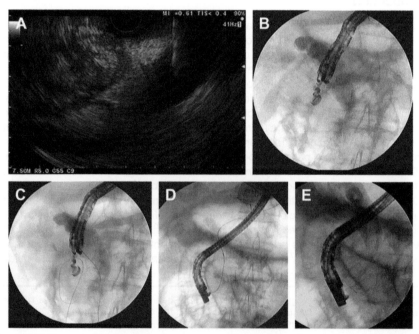

Fig. 1. (A) The extrahepatic bile duct was punctured from the second portion of the duodenum under EUS guidance. (B) A cholangiogram was taken through the needle to determine the configuration of the biliary ducts. (C) A guide wire was placed though the needle, biliary duct, obstruction, and ampulla, deeply into the duodenum. (D) Deep biliary cannulation was achieved over the guide wire. (E) A metallic stent was deployed at the stricture.

of bile confirms proper puncture of the biliary duct; next, limited cholangiography is performed to delineate the biliary obstruction (see **Fig. 1**B).

Once the bile duct configuration and the level of the obstruction are identified, a 0.018- to 0.035-in guide wire is advanced through the needle and manipulated antegradely into the small bowel via the native ampulla or surgical anastomosis (see **Fig. 1**C). A 22-gauge FNA needle accommodates a 0.018-in guide wire, and a 19-gauge FNA needle can accommodate a guide wire diameter of up to 0.035 in. The needle and the echoendoscope are withdrawn while keeping the guide wire in place. An appropriate endoscope dependent on the anatomy is then reinserted along-side the guide wire. Biliary cannulation is again attempted beside the antegradely placed guide wire (see **Fig. 1**D). If this attempt fails, the distal end of the EUS-placed guide wire is grasped with forceps or a snare. The guide wire is pulled out through the mouth with the endoscope or through the accessory channel of the endoscope. A duodenoscope is then back-loaded over the guide wire and advanced again to the ampulla or anastomosis, if the guide wire is pulled through the mouth. Deep biliary cannulation is then performed over the EUS-placed guide wire (see **Fig. 1**E). Following deep biliary cannulation, appropriate treatment is provided (see **Fig. 1**F).

In Cases with Failed EUS-RV

The authors recommend an immediate repeat attempt at conventional ERCP if EUS-RV fails, especially in case the ampulla or orifice cannot be detected for some reason. EUS cholangiography can help to identify the biliary orifice and the configuration of the distal bile duct, which can facilitate repeat ERCP and increase the chance of its success. If this also fails, alternative biliary decompression, such as PTBD, should be considered to minimize the risk of bile leak.

LITERATURE REVIEW

Mallery and colleagues[29] first reported the use of EUS-guided biliary puncture with subsequent RV technique for 2 cases of malignant distal biliary obstruction after failed ERCP in 2004. Since then, several groups[8,9,30–34] have reported that EUS-RV is an effective salvage technique to obtain deep biliary cannulation after failed ERCP (**Table 1**).

Table 1
Success rates of the EUS-guided rendezvous technique

	Authors	Year	Ref.	Overlapping Articles	No. of Patients	No. of Accessed Biliary Ducts		Overall Success Rate
						EHBD	IHBD	
1	Tarantino et al	2008	33	—	8	4/8 (50%)	—	50% (4/8)
2	Maranki et al	2009	34	31,32	49	8/14[a] (57%)	26/40 (65%)	63% (34/54)
3	Kim et al	2010	8	29,30	15	12/15 (80%)	—	80% (12/15)
4	Iwashita et al	2012	9	—	40	25/31 (81%)	4/9 (44%)	73% (29/40)

Abbreviations: EHBD, extrahepatic bile duct; IHBD, intrahepatic bile duct.
[a] Including 5 patients converted from IHBD.

Selection of Device

Either 19-gauge or 22-gauge FNA needles can be used for this technique. Although only a 0.018-in guide wire is applicable for a 22-gauge needle, a 19-gauge needle allows larger guide wires (0.018–0.035 in) to pass through the needle. Theoretically, the usage of a 22-gauge needle can make needle puncture easier, especially in the transduodenal approach, and reduce the risk of bile leakage or bleeding because of the smaller caliber and more flexible needle of the needle itself. However, Maranki and colleagues[34] reported that a 19-gauge needle was better despite being less maneuverable, because a 0.035-in guide wire provided better control than a 0.018-in guide wire. Kim and colleagues[8] noted that the larger needle caliber permitted freer passage of different guide wires and decreased the risk of shredding the guide wire coating by the sharp needle edge. Kim and colleagues[8] prefer using a combination of the 19-gauge needle with a 0.020-in or 0.021-in guide wire as the initial devices, with change to a 22-gauge needle with a 0.018-in guide wire if they have technical difficulty in using a 19-gauge needle. The authors prefer using a 19-gauge needle and a 0.035-in guide wire because of the improved maneuverability, visibility, stiffness, and ease of handling of the larger guide wire. In addition, using a larger needle allows the use of a smaller-caliber guide wire, whereas using a 22-gauge FNA needle limits one to using a 0.018-in guide wire.

Selection of Biliary Ducts for Puncture

EUS-RV can be divided into intrahepatic bile duct (IHBD) and extrahepatic bile duct (EHBD) approaches in terms of access to the biliary tree. Maranki and colleagues[34] reported their experience with a predominantly IHBD approach for interventional EUS cholangiography. Their series included EUS-RV cases as well as patients who underwent hepaticogastrostomy, choledochoduodenostomy, and antegrade treatment via choledochoenteral fistula as salvage for failed EUS-RV. In this study, EUS-RV was defined as successful on the basis of manipulating the guide wire across the obstruction. IHBD was chosen as the access route in 40 of 49 patients because the investigators believed IHBD to have less risk of bile leak.[32] This approach failed in 5 patients, because of the inability to advance the guide wire into the IHBD in 4 patients and inability to puncture the IHBD in 1 patient; these 5 patients underwent repeat attempts using the EHBD approach. The investigators successfully passed the guide wire into the small intestine in 26 of 40 patients with the IHBD approach, followed by stent placement in 25 of these 26 patients and balloon dilation of an anastomotic stricture in the remaining patient. A gastrohepatic stent was placed in 3 of the remaining 9 patients because of the inability to advance the guide wire across the obstruction, and the final 6 patients experienced failure resulting from inability to advance the guide wire. Therefore, the EUS-RV success rate with the IHBD approach was 65% (26/40).

In the authors' recent series, the EHBD approach was used in the majority of patients with failed biliary cannulation.[9] The EHBD approach (antegrade) was chosen for patients with distal obstruction to maximize the maneuverability of the guide wire and minimize the length of manipulation needed. The authors used the IHBD approach typically in patients with hilar strictures or surgically altered anatomy. EUS-RV with the IHBD approach was performed in 9 patients with successful EUS cholangiography obtained in all patients, but with failure to pass the guide wire through the stricture in 5 patients, for a success rate of 44% (4/9).

Kim and colleagues[8] reported their retrospective experience with EUS-RV with only the EHBD approach in 15 patients after failed ERCP. Successful bile duct puncture followed by guide-wire placement into the biliary duct was obtained in all patients. However, the guide wire could not pass into the duodenum because of its inability to traverse a stricture in 2 patients and the dissection of a choledochocele in 1 patient. Thus, the overall success rate of EUS-RV was 80% (12/15). The authors have reported a success rate of 81% (25/31), with failures resulting from inability to pass the guide wire into the intestine. Maranki and colleagues[34] reported the success rate of the EHBD approach to be 57% (8/14; 5 of whom converted from the IHBD approach), but did not report the reasons for the failures except in 4 patients who underwent transenteric biliary stent placement after failed advancement of the guide wire across the stricture.

These studies highlight that guide-wire manipulation is one of the most challenging aspects of EUS-RV. In this technique the guide wire has to pass through a long rigid needle, biliary ducts, obstruction, and ampulla or anastomosis into the small intestine. For this reason, the authors maintain that the EHBD approach is preferred over the IHBD approach because the shorter wire length maximizes the maneuverability and propulsive force of the wire at the tip. Although the authors were able to access the biliary system using the IHBD approach in all cases, it was more difficult to puncture smaller-caliber bile ducts. Perhaps for this reason, Maranki and colleagues[34] failed to achieve IHBD access in 5 of 40 patients (13%). These observations suggest that the EHBD approach is preferable for EUS-RV whenever anatomically and technically possible. Although some theorize that the EHBD approach itself may increase the risk of bile leak, the authors believe that adequacy of the drainage is the most important risk factor to prevent bile leaks. In addition, there are no actual data to show that the EHBD approach is associated with a greater risk of bile leak.

Selection of Intestinal Locations for Biliary Duct Puncture

In EUS-RV with the IHBD approach, the biliary ducts in the left lobe are only approached from the stomach in patients with normal anatomy or the small intestine in cases with surgically altered anatomy. In the EHBD approach, the biliary duct is normally punctured from the bulb or the second portion of the duodenum. Kim and colleagues[8,29,30] stated that the goal of biliary access is to puncture the biliary ducts with the long axis of the needle directed as close as possible, and in a parallel plane to the long axis of the duct with the needle tip directed toward the point of obstruction, because such an approach limits buckling of the guide wire and allows greater force to be exerted against the obstruction. This procedure is only possible from the second portion of the duodenum in most patients with normal anatomy, because the needle usually points to the liver hilum when passed from the duodenal bulb. Unfortunately, it may not be possible to perform the needle puncture from the second portion because of obstruction, tumor, or inability to visualize the needle and the bile duct in one plane, especially if the bile duct is not dilated near the ampulla. The authors recommend first trying to access the bile duct from the second portion of the duodenum using a 19-gauge FNA needle, with the approach from the bulb reserved for patients with failed access.

Complications

EUS-RV includes both ERCP and EUS-guided biliary access, and can cause complications resulting from both aspects. Reported complications associated with EUS-guided biliary access include abdominal pain, cholangitis, biloma, sepsis, bleeding, pneumoperitoneum, and bile peritonitis.[8,9,28,32–54] EUS-RV requires only needle puncture and temporary guide-wire placement in contrast to EUS-guided enterobiliary

Table 2
Complication rates of the EUS-guided rendezvous technique

Authors	Year	Ref.	Overlapping Articles	No. of Accessed Biliary Ducts, Details		Overall Complication Rate
				EHBD	IHBD	
1 Tarantino et al	2008	33	—	1/8 (13%) Death due to LC 1[a]	—	13% (1/8)
2 Maranki et al	2009	34	31,32	3/14[b] (21%) Abdominal pain 1 Pneumoperitoneum 1 Biliary peritonitis 1	5/35 (14%) Bleeding 1 Pneumoperitoneum 3 Aspiration pneumonia 1	16% (8/49)
3 Kim et al	2010	8	29,30	2/15 (13%) Pancreatitis 1 Sepsis 1	—	13% (2/15)
4 Iwashita et al	2012	9	—	4/31 (13%) Pancreatitis 2 Abdominal pain 1 Sepsis/death 1[a]	1/9 (11%) Pneumoperitoneum 1	13% (5/40)

Abbreviations: EHBD, extrahepatic bile duct; IHBD, intrahepatic bile duct; LC, laparoscopic cholecystectomy.
[a] Assessed unrelated to the procedure.
[b] Including 5 patients converted from IHBD approach.

fistulotomy or antegrade treatment, both of which require creation and dilation of a biliary enteric fistula. Although theoretically the risks of EUS-RV causing complications associated with biliary access should be lower than those of other EUS-guided biliary access techniques, bile peritonitis and pneumoperitoneum have been reported (**Table 2**).[8,9,33,34] Therefore, the prompt availability of alternative biliary drainage is very important in minimizing the potential risks of complications, especially in cases with unrelieved biliary obstruction.[9,34] Another major factor in minimizing procedure-associated risk is to ensure adequate expertise of the endoscopist in the EUS and ERCP procedures.[29]

SUMMARY

EUS-RV is a feasible and safe salvage technique with which to achieve deep biliary cannulation after failed ERCP, although further studies are needed to compare it with alternative techniques. Prompt PTBD should be available to minimize potential complications for patients with unrelieved biliary obstruction.

REFERENCES

1. Artifon EL, Sakai P, Cunha JE, et al. Guide wire cannulation reduces risk of post-ERCP pancreatitis and facilitates bile duct cannulation. Am J Gastroenterol 2007; 102:2147–53.
2. Bailey AA, Bourke MJ, Williams SJ, et al. A prospective randomized trial of cannulation technique in ERCP: effects on technical success and post-ERCP pancreatitis. Endoscopy 2008;40:296–301.
3. Lee TH, Park do H, Park JY, et al. Can wire-guided cannulation prevent post-ERCP pancreatitis? a prospective randomized trial. Gastrointest Endosc 2009; 69:444–9.
4. Lobo DN, Balfour TW, Iftikhar SY. Periampullary diverticula: consequences of failed ERCP. Ann R Coll Surg Engl 1998;80:326–31.
5. Fogel EL, Sherman S, Lehman GA. Increased selective biliary cannulation rates in the setting of periampullary diverticula: main pancreatic duct stent placement followed by pre-cut biliary sphincterotomy. Gastrointest Endosc 1998;47:396–400.
6. Huang CH, Tsou YK, Lin CH, et al. Endoscopic retrograde cholangiopancreatography (ERCP) for intradiverticular papilla: endoclip-assisted biliary cannulation. Endoscopy 2010;42(Suppl 2):E223–4.
7. Garcia-Cano J. ERCP cannulation of a hidden papilla within a duodenal diverticulum. Endoscopy 2008;40(Suppl 2):E53.
8. Kim YS, Gupta K, Mallery S, et al. Endoscopic ultrasound rendezvous for bile duct access using a transduodenal approach: cumulative experience at a single center. A case series. Endoscopy 2010;42:496–502.
9. Iwashita T, Lee JG, Shinoura S, et al. Endoscopic ultrasound guided rendezvous technique for biliary access after failed cannulation. Endoscopy 2012;44(1):60–5.
10. Wright BE, Cass OW, Freeman ML. ERCP in patients with long-limb Roux-en-Y gastrojejunostomy and intact papilla. Gastrointest Endosc 2002;56:225–32.
11. Koornstra JJ, Fry L, Monkemuller K. ERCP with the balloon-assisted enteroscopy technique: a systematic review. Dig Dis 2008;26:324–9.
12. Ramirez FC, Dennert B, Sanowski RA. Success of repeat ERCP by the same endoscopist. Gastrointest Endosc 1999;49:58–61.
13. Kevans D, Zeb F, Donnellan F, et al. Failed biliary access following needle knife fistulotomy: is repeat interval ERCP worthwhile? Scand J Gastroenterol 2010; 45:1238–41.

14. Kumar S, Sherman S, Hawes RH, et al. Success and yield of second attempt ERCP. Gastrointest Endosc 1995;41:445–7.
15. Choudari CP, Sherman S, Fogel EL, et al. Success of ERCP at a referral center after a previously unsuccessful attempt. Gastrointest Endosc 2000;52:478–83.
16. Doctor N, Dick R, Rai R, et al. Results of percutaneous plastic stents for malignant distal biliary obstruction following failed endoscopic stent insertion and comparison with current literature on expandable metallic stents. Eur J Gastroenterol Hepatol 1999;11:775–80.
17. Beissert M, Wittenberg G, Sandstede J, et al. Metallic stents and plastic endoprostheses in percutaneous treatment of biliary obstruction. Z Gastroenterol 2002;40:503–10.
18. Smith AC, Dowsett JF, Russell RC, et al. Randomised trial of endoscopic stenting versus surgical bypass in malignant low bile duct obstruction. Lancet 1994;344:1655–60.
19. Chang KJ, Albers CG, Erickson RA, et al. Endoscopic ultrasound-guided fine needle aspiration of pancreatic carcinoma. Am J Gastroenterol 1994;89:263–6.
20. Wiersema MJ, Vilmann P, Giovannini M, et al. Endosonography-guided fine-needle aspiration biopsy: diagnostic accuracy and complication assessment. Gastroenterology 1997;112:1087–95.
21. Grimm H, Binmoeller KF, Soehendra N. Endosonography-guided drainage of a pancreatic pseudocyst. Gastrointest Endosc 1992;38:170–1.
22. Yasuda I, Iwata K, Mukai T, et al. EUS-guided pancreatic pseudocyst drainage. Dig Endosc 2009;21(Suppl 1):S82–6.
23. Wiersema MJ. Endosonography-guided cystoduodenostomy with a therapeutic ultrasound endoscope. Gastrointest Endosc 1996;44:614–7.
24. Wiersema MJ, Wiersema LM. Endosonography-guided celiac plexus neurolysis. Gastrointest Endosc 1996;44:656–62.
25. Levy MJ, Topazian MD, Wiersema MJ, et al. Initial evaluation of the efficacy and safety of endoscopic ultrasound-guided direct ganglia neurolysis and block. Am J Gastroenterol 2007;103:98–103.
26. Sahai AV, Lemelin V, Lam E, et al. Central vs. bilateral endoscopic ultrasound-guided celiac plexus block or neurolysis: a comparative study of short-term effectiveness. Am J Gastroenterol 2009;104:326–9.
27. Wiersema MJ, Sandusky D, Carr R, et al. Endosonography-guided cholangiopancreatography. Gastrointest Endosc 1996;43:102–6.
28. Giovannini M, Moutardier V, Pesenti C, et al. Endoscopic ultrasound-guided bilioduodenal anastomosis: a new technique for biliary drainage. Endoscopy 2001;33:898–900.
29. Mallery S, Matlock J, Freeman ML. EUS-guided rendezvous drainage of obstructed biliary and pancreatic ducts: report of 6 cases. Gastrointest Endosc 2004;59:100–7.
30. Lai R, Freeman ML. Endoscopic ultrasound-guided bile duct access for rendezvous ERCP drainage in the setting of intradiverticular papilla. Endoscopy 2005;37:487–9.
31. Kahaleh M, Wang P, Shami VM, et al. EUS-guided transhepatic cholangiography: report of 6 cases. Gastrointest Endosc 2005;61:307–13.
32. Kahaleh M, Hernandez AJ, Tokar J, et al. Interventional EUS-guided cholangiography: evaluation of a technique in evolution. Gastrointest Endosc 2006;64:52–9.
33. Tarantino I, Barresi L, Repici A, et al. EUS-guided biliary drainage: a case series. Endoscopy 2008;40:336–9.

34. Maranki J, Hernandez AJ, Arslan B, et al. Interventional endoscopic ultrasound-guided cholangiography: long-term experience of an emerging alternative to percutaneous transhepatic cholangiography. Endoscopy 2009;41:532–8.
35. Burmester E, Niehaus J, Leineweber T, et al. EUS-cholangio-drainage of the bile duct: report of 4 cases. Gastrointest Endosc 2003;57:246–51.
36. Puspok A, Lomoschitz F, Dejaco C, et al. Endoscopic ultrasound guided therapy of benign and malignant biliary obstruction: a case series. Am J Gastroenterol 2005;100:1743–7.
37. Yamao K, Sawaki A, Takahashi K, et al. EUS-guided choledochoduodenostomy for palliative biliary drainage in case of papillary obstruction: report of 2 cases. Gastrointest Endosc 2006;64:663–7.
38. Bories E, Pesenti C, Caillol F, et al. Transgastric endoscopic ultrasonography-guided biliary drainage: results of a pilot study. Endoscopy 2007;39:287–91.
39. Will U, Thieme A, Fueldner F, et al. Treatment of biliary obstruction in selected patients by endoscopic ultrasonography (EUS)-guided transluminal biliary drainage. Endoscopy 2007;39:292–5.
40. Artifon EL, Chaves DM, Ishioka S, et al. Echoguided hepatico-gastrostomy: a case report. Clinics (Sao Paulo) 2007;62:799–802.
41. Fujita N, Noda Y, Kobayashi G, et al. Histological changes at an endosonography-guided biliary drainage site: a case report. World J Gastroenterol 2007;13:5512–5.
42. Itoi T, Itokawa F, Sofuni A, et al. Endoscopic ultrasound-guided choledochoduodenostomy in patients with failed endoscopic retrograde cholangiopancreatography. World J Gastroenterol 2008;14:6078–82.
43. Hanada K, Iiboshi T, Ishii Y. Endoscopic ultrasound-guided choledochoduodenostomy for palliative biliary drainage in cases with inoperable pancreas head carcinoma. Dig Endosc 2009;21(Suppl 1):S75–8.
44. Park H, Koo JE, Oh J, et al. EUS-guided biliary drainage with one-step placement of a fully covered metal stent for malignant biliary obstruction: a prospective feasibility study. Am J Gastroenterol 2009;104:2168–74.
45. Brauer BC, Chen YK, Fukami N, et al. Single-operator EUS-guided cholangiopancreatography for difficult pancreaticobiliary access (with video). Gastrointest Endosc 2009;70:471–9.
46. Iwamuro M, Kawamoto H, Harada R, et al. Combined duodenal stent placement and endoscopic ultrasonography-guided biliary drainage for malignant duodenal obstruction with biliary stricture. Dig Endosc 2010;22:236–40.
47. Nguyen-Tang T, Binmoeller KF, Sanchez-Yague A, et al. Endoscopic ultrasound (EUS)-guided transhepatic anterograde self-expandable metal stent (SEMS) placement across malignant biliary obstruction. Endoscopy 2010;42:232–6.
48. Park H, Song TJ, Eum J, et al. EUS-guided hepaticogastrostomy with a fully covered metal stent as the biliary diversion technique for an occluded biliary metal stent after a failed ERCP (with videos). Gastrointest Endosc 2010;71:413–9.
49. Hara K, Yamao K, Niwa Y, et al. Prospective clinical study of EUS-guided choledochoduodenostomy for malignant lower biliary tract obstruction. Am J Gastroenterol 2011;106:1239–45.
50. Artifon EL, Okawa L, Takada J, et al. EUS-guided choledochoantrostomy: an alternative for biliary drainage in unresectable pancreatic cancer with duodenal invasion. Gastrointest Endosc 2011;73:1317–20.
51. Komaki T, Kitano M, Sakamoto H, et al. Endoscopic ultrasonography-guided biliary drainage: evaluation of a choledochoduodenostomy technique. Pancreatology 2011;11(Suppl 2):47–51.

52. Prachayakul V, Aswakul P, Kachintorn U. EUS-guided choledochoduodenostomy for biliary drainage using tapered-tip plastic stent with multiple fangs. Endoscopy 2011;43(Suppl 2):E109–10.

53. Horaguchi J, Fujita N, Noda Y, et al. Endosonography-guided biliary drainage with one-step placement of a newly designed fully covered metal stent for malignant biliary obstruction. Dig Endosc 2011;23:207.

54. Belletrutti PJ, Dimaio CJ, Gerdes H, et al. Endoscopic ultrasound guided biliary drainage in patients with unapproachable ampullae due to malignant duodenal obstruction. J Gastrointest Cancer 2011;42:137–42.

Endoscopic Ultrasound-Guided Choledochoduodenostomy for Malignant Lower Biliary Tract Obstruction

Kenji Yamao, PhD, MD[a],*, Kazuo Hara, PhD, MD[a],
Nobumasa Mizuno, PhD, MD[a], Susumu Hijioka, MD[a],
Hiroshi Imaoka, PhD, MD[a], Vikram Bhatia, MD[b],
Yasuhiro Shimizu, PhD, MD[c]

KEYWORDS

- Interventional EUS • EUS biliary drainage • EUS-BD
- EUS-guided choledochoduodenostomy • EUS-CDS

Endoscopic biliary drainage (EBD) may be unsuccessful in some patients because of failed biliary cannulation or tumor infiltration limiting endoscopic access to the major papilla.[1,2] The salvage technique of percutaneous transhepatic biliary drainage has a risk of complications such as bleeding and intra-abdominal or extra-abdominal bile leakage.[3]

Recently, endoscopic ultrasound (EUS)-guided biliary stent placement has been described in patients with malignant biliary obstruction in many review articles.[4–18] Technically, EUS-guided biliary drainage (EUS-BD) is possible via a transgastric or transduodenal route or through the small intestine with direct access or rendezvous technique. The following section evaluates the current evidence and potential role of EUS-guided choledochoduodenostomy (EUS-CDS), that is, direct stent insertion from duodenum, to relieve jaundice caused by lower end obstruction of the extrahepatic bile duct.

Financial support: None.
Potential competing interests: None.
[a] Department of Gastroenterology, Aichi Cancer Center Hospital, 1-1 Kanokoden, Chikusa-Ku, Nagoya 464-8681, Japan; [b] Department of Medical Hepatology, Institute of Liver and Biliary Sciences, D-1, Vasant Kunj, Delhi 110070, India; [c] Department of Gastrointestinal Surgery, Aichi Cancer Center Hospital, 1-1, Kanokoden, Nagoya 464-8681, Japan
* Corresponding author.
E-mail address: kyamao@aichi-cc.jp

TECHNIQUE OF EUS-CDS
Technique of EUS-CDS for Initial Stent Insertion

The method of EUS-CDS with electrocautery is described in a later section.[16,17] A convex linear array echoendoscope positioned in the duodenal bulb usually displays a markedly dilated extrahepatic bile duct in the setting of a lower bile duct obstruction. For optimal visualization, the echoendoscope should be in a long (looped) position, with the tip of the echoendoscope directed toward the hepatic hilum (**Figs. 1** and **2**). Under real-time EUS guidance, a 22-gauge needle is inserted transduodenally into the extra-hepatic bile duct. A cholangiogram is obtained to display the dilated intrahepatic and extrahepatic biliary ducts proximal to the obstruction, under fluoroscopy. Although it is possible to proceed without fluoroscopic guidance, cholangiography and fluoro-scopic guidance are useful to choose the most appropriate puncture site for EUS-CDS and to direct the guidewire deep into the intrahepatic ducts. After the removal of the needle for cholangiogram EUS-guided puncture of the dilated extrahepatic bile duct is performed with a needle knife (Zimmon papillotomy knife; Cook Endoscopy, Winston-Salem, NC, USA), followed by a 0.035-in guidewire placement (Jag wire, 450 cm length; Microvasive, Boston Scientific Corp, Natick, MA, USA) through the outer sheath of the needle knife. Tapered biliary dilation catheters of sizes 6F, 7F, and 9F (Soe-hendra biliary dilation catheters [SBDC-6, SBDC-7, and SBDC-9], Wilson-Cook, NC, USA) are used to sequentially dilate the punctured tract, over the intrabiliary guidewire. Finally, an 8.5F straight biliary stent (Tannenbaum, Wilson-Cook, NC, USA, or Flexma, Microvasive, Boston Scientific Corp, Natick, MA, USA) is inserted through the choledo-choduodenostomy opening into the extrahepatic bile duct over the guidewire (**Figs. 3** and **4**). When a 9F biliary dilator cannot be passed, a 7F straight biliary stent (Tannen-baum, Wilson-Cook, NC, USA) is inserted. The authors have also used a partially covered metal stent (WallFlex Biliary RX Stent, 10-mm diameter, 4 cm or 6 cm long, Boston Scientific Corp, Natick, MA, USA) instead of a plastic stent for EUS-CDS (**Fig. 5**).

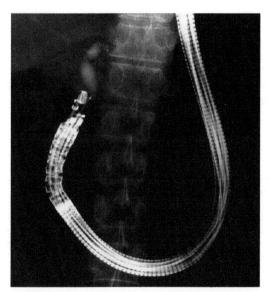

Fig. 1. Cholangiogram obtained by EUS-guided puncture with the tip of the convex trans-ducer directed to the hepatic hilum. The echoendoscope was observed in the long/pushing scope position.

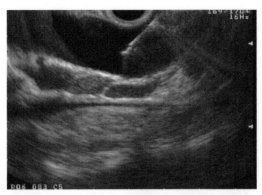

Fig. 2. Convex echoendoscope, located in the apex of the duodenal bulb, clearly displayed the extrahepatic bile duct, cystic duct, and puncture needle.

The technique of EUS-CDS without using the electrocautery is as follows. EUS-guided puncture of the dilated extrahepatic bile duct from the duodenal bulb is performed with a 19-gauge puncture needle (Echo Tip19; Cook Endoscopy, Winston-Salem, NC, USA). A 0.025- or 0.035-in guidewire (Jag wire, 450 cm long; Microvasive, Boston Scientific Corp, Natick, MA, USA) is placed through the fine-needle aspiration (FNA) needle deeply into the bile duct. A biliary balloon dilator catheter of 5F diameter (Max Force; Microvasive, Boston Scientific Corp, Natick, MA, USA) and/or a tapered biliary dilation catheter is used to dilate the tract over the guidewire. When it is difficult to dilate the fistula using these devices, a fistulotome over the guidewire may be useful. Finally, a 7F straight biliary stent (Flexma, Microvasive, Boston

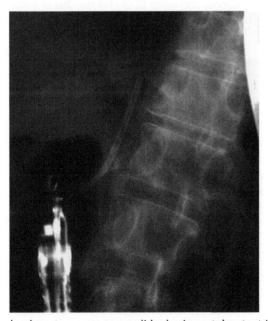

Fig. 3. Choledochoduodenostomy was accomplished using a tube stent in the apex of the duodenal bulb.

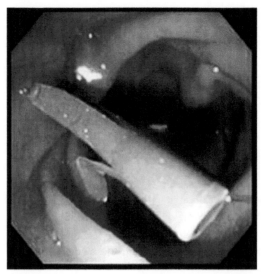

Fig. 4. Duodenoscope showed an 8.5F biliary stent in the first portion of the duodenum.

Scientific Corp, Natick, MA, USA) is inserted through choledochoduodenostomy into the extrahepatic duct over the guidewire.

No standardized method for EUS-CDS has yet been established, and researchers have performed the procedures in their own individual ways (**Table 1**).[18–40] For the extrahepatic bile duct puncture, a needle knife or fistulotome was used in 7 institutions, 19- and 22-gauge EUS-FNA needles in 5 institutions, EUS-FNA needles followed by a needle knife in 4 institutions, and either EUS-FNA needles or a needle knife in 2 institutions. Using an EUS-FNA needle to access the bile duct seems safer, although it is

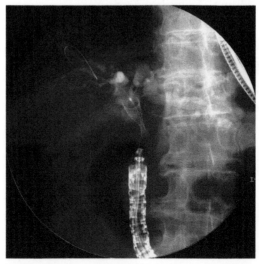

Fig. 5. Choledochoduodenostomy was accomplished using a metal stent in the apex of the duodenal bulb, using a forward-viewing echoendoscope.

Table 1
Overview of the reported cases on EUS-CDS

Authors	Year	Number of Cases	Device for Puncture	Technical Success (%)	Treatment Success (%)	Initial Stent (Number of Cases)	Early Complication (Number of Cases)
Giovanini et al[20]	2001	1	NK (1)	1/1 (100)	1/1 (100)	10F PS	None
Brumester et al[21]	2003	2	19G FT (2)	1/2 (50)	1/1 (100)	8.5F PS	Bile peritonitis (1)
Puspok et al[24]	2005	5	NK (5)	4/5 (80)	4/4 (100)	7F–10F PS	None
Kahaleh et al[23]	2006	1	19G FN (1)	1/1 (100)	1/1 (100)	10-mm MS	Pneumoperitoneum (1)
Yamao et al[16,25,26]	2006, 2006, and 2008[a]	5	NK (5)	5/5 (100)	5/5 (100)	7F–8.5F PS	Pneumoperitoneum (1)
Ang et al[27]	2007	2	NK (2)	2/2 (100)	2/2 (100)	7F PS	Pneumoperitoneum (1)
Fujita et al[28]	2007[a]	1	19G FN (1)	1/1 (100)	1/1 (100)	7F PS	None
Tarantino et al[29]	2008	4	19G, 22G FN/NK (4)	4/4 (100)	4/4 (100)	PS[b]	None
Itoi et al[30]	2008	4	NK (2), 19G FN (2)	4/4 (100)	4/4 (100)	7F PS (3), NBD (1)	Bile peritonitis (1)
Brauer et al[31]	2009	3	19G, 22G FN (3)	3/3 (100)	3/3 (100)	7F PS	Pneumoperitoneum (1)
Nguyen-Tang et al[32]	2009	2	NK (2)	1/2 (50)	1/1 (100)	10-mm MS	Pneumoperitoneum (1)
Horaguchi et al[33]	2009[a]	7	19G FN (7)	7/7 (100)	7/7 (100)	7F PS (6), 6F NBD (1)	Peritonitis (1)
Hanada et al[34]	2009	4	19G FN (4)	4/4 (100)	4/4 (100)	6F–7F PS	None
Park et al[35]	2009	4	19G FN/NK (4)	4/4 (100)	4/4 (100)	10-mm FCMS	None
Iwamuro et al[36]	2010	5	NK (5)	5/5 (100)	5/5 (100)	7F PS	Severe abdominal pain (1)
Hara et al[37]	2011	18	NK (18)	17/18 (94)	17/17 (100)	7F PS (2), 8.5F PS (15)	Bile peritonitis (2), hemobilia (1)
Siddiqui et al[38]	2011	8	19G FN/NK (8)	8/8 (100)	8/8 (100)	10-mm FCMS	Stent migration/duodenal perforation (1)
Fabbri et al[39]	2011	13	19G FN/NK (13)	9/13 (69)	9/9 (100)	PCMS[b]	Pneumoperitoneum (1)
Komaki et al[40]	2011	15	NK (9), 19G FN (6)	14/15 (93)	14/14 (100)	7F PS	None
Total	—	104	—	96/104 (92)	96/96 (100)	—	14/104 (13)

Abbreviations: FCMS, fully covered metal stent; FN, fine needle; FT, fistolotome; G, gauge; MS, metal stent; NBD, nasobiliary drainage; NK, needle knife; PCMS, partially covered metal stent; PS, plastic stent.
a Excluding the overlapping cases.
b Stent diameter is not described.

more difficult to sufficiently dilate the fistula for insertion of a biliary stent. Using a needle with electrocautery seems more risky, but it is easier and quicker to dilate the fistula large enough to insert a bigger stent. The site of needle equipped with the present over-the-guide wire needle knife is different from the site of the guide wire channel, so the needle knife seems to have a risk not to make the appropriate fistula for stenting.

Method for Exchanging an Occluded Stent Placed at EUS-CDS

In cases where the EUS-CDS stent has been in situ for a long time, the occluded stent is simply removed by using a Dormia basket through a duodenoscope. The choledo-choduodenal fistula is usually mature by 2 or 3 weeks after the stent insertion. After stent removal, the choledochoduodenal fistula is cannulated using an endoscopic retrograde cholangiopancreatography (ERCP) catheter (Tandem 3-lumen ERCP catheter; Microvasive Endoscopy, Boston Scientific Corp, Natick, MA, USA) followed by placement of a 0.035-in guidewire (Jag wire, 450 cm, Microvasive Endoscopy, Boston Scientific Corp, Natick, MA, USA) deeply into the intrahepatic biliary ducts. A new 8.5F straight biliary stent (Tannenbaum stent, Wilson-Cook, NC, USA) is then inserted over the guidewire.

In cases where the EUS-CDS stent has been inserted for only a short time, a mature choledochoduodenal fistula tract would not have formed. Hence, alternate techniques of exchanging the occluded stent of EUS-CDS should be adapted.[19] A 0.035-in guidewire is carefully inserted into the bile duct through the occluded stent using an ERCP catheter (**Fig. 6**). The occluded stent is then removed by using a snare keeping the guidewire in place, through the biopsy channel of the duodenoscope (**Fig. 7**). A new 8.5F straight biliary stent is then inserted over the guidewire.

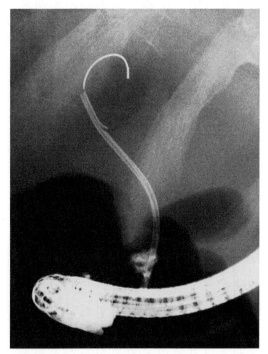

Fig. 6. A 0.035-in guidewire was inserted into the bile duct through an occluded stent using an ERCP catheter.

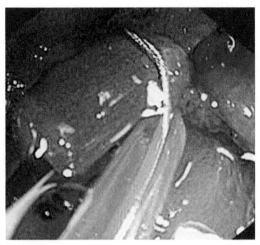

Fig. 7. The occluded stent is then removed by using a snare with the guidewire in place, through the biopsy channel of the duodenoscope.

SUCCESS RATE AND LIMITATIONS

Nineteen retrospective studies and 2 prospective studies describing 104 cases of EUS-CDS have been reported to date.[16,20–40] An overview of 104 cases of EUS-CDS, including the 81 cases in published articles along with the authors' published 23 cases, is shown in **Table 1**.

Technical and Functional Success Rate

Although the procedure was unsuccessful in 8 patients, transduodenal stents were successfully inserted in the remaining 96 patients (96/104, 92%). Among the 8 failed cases, Fabbri and colleagues[39] reported technical failure due to instability of the scope in the duodenal bulb in 1 case, stent impaction at the site of the choledocho-duodenostomy puncture in 1 case, and failure to create a fistula with the needle knife in 2 cases. In the remaining 4 cases, the causes of technical failure included hemobilia at the time of initial puncture with a 22-gauge needle for obtaining a cholangiogram[37] and failure to create a fistula because of sclerosing cholangitis[40] in one case each. The cause for the procedural failure has not been described in detail in the remaining 2 cases. Among the 96 cases with technical success, functional success was achieved in all the 96 cases (96/96, 100%).

The advantage of the EUS-CDS technique is that the puncture site is very close to the extrahepatic bile duct and away from the obstructing tumor.[16] No large intervening blood vessels lie between the duodenal wall and extrahepatic bile duct. The echoendoscope is stable in this position, and the direction of puncture is upward toward the hepatic hilum. To prevent dislocation of the guidewire and dilator, an appropriate puncture site should be selected aiming at the extrahepatic bile duct between the upper margin of the pancreas and hepatic hilum.

Complications

Early complications of this technique include pneumoperitoneum in 6 patients,[23,26,27,31,32,39] (bile) peritonitis in 5 cases,[21,30,33,37] stent migration followed by duodenal perforation in 1 case,[38] hemobilia in 1 case,[37] and severe abdominal pain in 1 case.[36] Bile peritonitis may not occur if a stent is promptly placed after the dilation of the fistula between the duodenum and bile duct. To prevent the dislocation of the guidewire and the dilator, an appropriate puncture site should be selected aiming at the extrahepatic bile duct between the upper margin of the pancreas and hepatic hilum. A one-step method with direct puncture of the bile duct, as is reported for EUS-guided pseudocyst drainage,[41] may reduce the risk of guidewire dislocation while the instruments are exchanged.

Although comparatively high rates of complications (13%) have been reported, complications in all patients except in one with stent migration[38] improved with conservative treatment. EUS-guided rendezvous technique is probably safe, but the success rate of drainage is comparatively low.[14] The usefulness and indications of the direct choledochoduodenostomy versus rendezvous technique need to be clarified in future studies.

FOLLOW-UP RESULTS

Stent patency rates in patients who underwent EUS-CDS have been reported in some articles. The authors have previously reported long-term follow-up data on stent patency in patients who underwent EUS-CDS.[26] The mean duration of stent patency was 211.8 days using Kaplan-Meier method. In a prospective study by the authors, duration of stent patency was 272 days and longer than previously reported.[37] Tarantino and colleagues[29] described that biliary stents were exchanged at day 180 in 3 patients with EUS-CDS. In another case of EUS-CDS, the plastic stent was exchanged for a metal stent after 1 month, with total stent patency duration of 240 days after the initial stent insertion. Horaguchi and colleagues[33] reported that initial plastic stent insertion followed by metal stent exchange provided stent patency durations of 27 days, 151 days, and 165 days among 3 cases of malignant lower biliary obstruction. Hanada and colleagues[34] reported that the stent patency duration ranged from 65 to 120 days in 4 cases of EUS-CDS with plastic stent insertion. Iwamuro and colleagues[36] also reported that stent patency ranged from 4.9 to 46.4 weeks in 5 cases of EUS-CDS combined with duodenal stents. The comparatively long patency of EUS-CDS achieved in the authors' patients was superior to that in those with transpapillary plastic stents and uncovered metallic stent and inferior to that in those with covered metallic stent in patients with lower biliary obstruction. In addition, the stent used for EUS-CDS is significantly cheaper and can be exchanged unlike a covered metallic stent. The authors speculate that EUS-CDS can prevent stent clogging and tumor ingrowth and/or overgrowth by creating a fistula away from the obstructing tumor.

Park and colleagues[35] recently reported 4 cases of EUS-BD with 1-step placement of a fully covered self-expandable metal stent. Although the follow-up periods were short (range, 2–7 months), only 1 reintervention was required because of stent migration. Fabbri and colleagues[39] reported that 6 patients died during follow-up (range, 140–189 days) with a partially covered metal stent still functioning. They also reported that the stent patency was 195, 205, and 230 days in 3 survivors with EUS-CDS. Longer stent patency using a fully or partially covered metal stent can thus be expected.

SUMMARY

EUS-CDS performed from the first portion of the duodenum is technically feasible without any serious complications, offering clinically effective drainage in almost all patients with a comparatively long patency period. As more experience is gained, investigators have to decide which of the following are more effective than their alternatives: (1) transduodenal approach versus transgastric approach, (2) direct access versus rendezvous technique, (3) fistulotome versus fine needle for duct puncture, (4) tapered biliary dilators versus balloon dilation, (5) plastic stent versus (covered) metal stent, (6) straight stent versus pigtail stent, (7) 8.5 French stent versus larger or smaller size stent, and on other issues related to trouble shooting early and late complications. Prospective randomized studies are needed in the near future to compare the efficacy and safety of EUS-CDS with EBD and EUS-rendezvous and EUS-HGS. As the earlier-mentioned issues are resolved, we envision that the technique of EUS-CDS will be gradually standardized and new dedicated endoscopic devices will be developed.

REFERENCES

1. Ponchon T. Diagnostic endoscopic retrograde cholangiopancreatography. Endoscopy 2000;32:200–8.
2. Schofl R. Diagnostic endoscopic retrograde cholangiopancreatography. Endoscopy 2001;33:147–57.
3. Winick AB, Waybill PN, Venbrux AC. Complications of percutaneous transhepatic biliary interventions. Tech Vasc Interv Radiol 2001;4:200–6.
4. Itoi T, Yamao K, EUS 2008 Working Group. EUS 2008 Working Group document: evaluation of EUS-guided choledochoduodenostomy (with video). Gastrointest Endosc 2009;69:S8–12.
5. Püspök A. Biliary therapy: are we ready for EUS-guidance? Minerva Med 2007; 98:379–84.
6. Buchner AM, Wallace MB. New frontiers in therapeutic EUS: dreams, style exercises or actual possibilities. Minerva Med 2007;98:287–98.
7. Shami VM, Kahaleh M. Endoscopic ultrasonography (EUS)-guided access and therapy of pancreatico-biliary disorders: EUS-guided cholangio and pancreatic drainage. Gastrointest Endosc Clin N Am 2007;17:581–93, vii-viii.
8. Ramesh J, Varadarajulu S. Interventional endoscopic ultrasound. Dig Dis 2008; 26:347–55.
9. Gleeson FC, Levy MJ. Endoscopic ultrasound (EUS) guided access and therapy of pancreatico-biliary disorders. Minerva Gastroenterol Dietol 2008;54: 151–60.
10. Ashida R, Chang KJ. Interventional EUS for the treatment of pancreatic cancer. J Hepatobiliary Pancreat Surg 2009;16:592–7.
11. Kitano M, Sakamoto H, Komaki T, et al. Present status and future perspective of EUS-guided drainage. Dig Endosc 2009;21:S66–70.
12. Irisawa A, Hikichi T, Shibukawa G, et al. Pancreatobiliary drainage using the EUS-FNA technique: EUS-BD and EUS-PD. J Hepatobiliary Pancreat Surg 2009;16: 598–604.
13. Kida M, Itoi T. Current status and future perspective of interventional endoscopic ultrasound in Japan. Dig Endosc 2009;21:S50–2.
14. Yamao K, Hara K, Mizuno N, et al. EUS-guided biliary drainage. Gut Liver 2010;4: S67–75.
15. Itoi T, Sofuni A, Itokawa F, et al. Endoscopic ultrasonography-guided biliary drainage. J Hepatobiliary Pancreat Sci 2010;17:611–6.
16. Yamao K, Sawaki A, Takahashi K, et al. EUS-guided choledochoduodenostomy for palliative biliary drainage in case of papillary obstruction: report of 2 cases. Gastrointest Endosc 2006;64:663–7.

17. Hara K, Yamao K, Mizuno N, et al. Endoscopic ultrasound-guided choledocho-duodenostomy. Dig Endosc 2010;22:147–50.
18. Itoi T, Isayama H, Sofuni A, et al. Stent selection and tips on placement technique of EUS-guided biliary drainage: transduodenal and transgastric stenting. J Hepatobiliary Pancreat Sci 2011;18:664–72.
19. Hara K, Yamao K, Mizuno N, et al. Interventional endoscopic ultrasonography for pancreatic cancer. World J Clin Oncol 2011;2:108–14.
20. Giovannini M, Moutardier V, Pesenti C, et al. Endoscopic ultrasound-guided bilio-duodenal anastomosis: a new technique for biliary drainage. Endoscopy 2001; 33:898–900.
21. Burmester E, Niehaus J, Leineweber T, et al. EUS-cholangio-drainage of the bile duct: report of 4 cases. Gastrointest Endosc 2003;57:246–51.
22. Kahaleh M, Yoshida C, Kane L, et al. Interventional EUS cholangiography: a report of five cases. Gastrointest Endosc 2004;60:138–42.
23. Kahaleh M, Hernandez AJ, Tokar J, et al. Interventional EUS-guided cholan-giography: evaluation of a technique in evolution. Gastrointest Endosc 2006;64: 52–9.
24. Puspok A, Lomoschitz F, Dejaco C, et al. Endoscopic ultrasound guided therapy of benign and malignant biliary obstruction: a case series. Am J Gastroenterol 2005;100:1743–7.
25. Yamao K, Mizxuno N, Takahashi K, et al. A case of duodenoscopic ultrasound guided transduodenal biliary drainage in a case of carcinoma of papilla of Vater. Suizo 2006;21:353–7.
26. Yamao K, Bhatia V, Mizuno N, et al. EUS-guided choledochoduodenostomy for palliative biliary drainage in patients with malignant biliary obstruction: results of long-term follow-up. Endoscopy 2008;40:340–2.
27. Ang TL, Teo EK, Fock KM. EUS-guided transduodenal biliary drainage in unre-sectable pancreatic cancer with obstructive jaundice. JOP 2007;9:438–43.
28. Fujita N, Noda Y, Kobayashi G, et al. Histological changes at an endosonography-guided biliary drainage site: a case report. World J Gastroenterol 2007;13:5512–5.
29. Tarantino I, Barresi L, Repici A, et al. EUS-guided biliary drainage: a case series. Endoscopy 2008;40:336–9.
30. Itoi T, Itokawa F, Sofuni A, et al. Endoscopic ultrasound-guided choledochoduo-denostomy in patients with failed endoscopic retrograde cholangiopancreatogra-phy. World J Gastroenterol 2008;14:6078–82.
31. Brauer BC, Chen YK, Fukami N, et al. Single-operator EUS-guided cholangiopan-creatography for difficult pancreaticobiliary access (with video). Gastrointest Endosc 2011;73:251–6.
32. Nguyen-Tang T, Binmoeller KF, Sanchez-Yague A, et al. Endoscopic ultrasound (EUS)-guided transhepatic anterograde self-expandable metal stent (SEMS) placement across malignant biliary obstruction. Endoscopy 2010;42:232–6.
33. Horaguchi J, Fujita N, Noda Y, et al. Endosonography-guided biliary drainage in cases with difficult transpapillary endoscopic biliary drainage. Dig Endosc 2009; 21(4):239–44.
34. Hanada K, Iiboshi T, Ishii Y. Endoscopic ultrasound-guided choledochoduode-nostomy for palliative biliary drainage in cases with inoperable pancreas head carcinoma. Dig Endosc 2009;21:S75–8.
35. Park HE, Koo JE, Oh J, et al. EUS-guided biliary drainage with one-step place-ment of a fully covered metal stent for malignant biliary obstruction: a prospective feasibility study. Am J Gastroenterol 2009;104:2168–74.

36. Iwamuro M, Kawamoto H, Harada R, et al. Combined duodenal stent placement and endoscopic ultrasonography-guided biliary drainage for malignant duodenal obstruction with biliary stricture. Dig Endosc 2010;22(3):236–40.

37. Hara K, Yamao K, Niwa Y, et al. Prospective clinical study of EUS-guided chole-dochoduodenostomy for malignant lower biliary tract obstruction. Am J Gastroen-terol 2011;106:1239–45.

38. Siddiqui AA, Sreenarasimhaiah J, Lara LF, et al. Endoscopic ultrasound-guided transduodenal placement of a fully covered metal stent for palliative biliary drainage in patients with malignant biliary obstruction. Surg Endosc 2011;25: 549–55.

39. Fabbri C, Luigiano C, Fuccio L, et al. EUS-guided biliary drainage with placement of a new partially covered biliary stent for palliation of malignant biliary obstruc-tion: a case series. Endoscopy 2011;43:438–41.

40. Komaki T, Kitano M, Sakamoto H, et al. Endoscopic ultrasonography-guided biliary drainage: evaluation of a choledochoduodenostomy technique. Pancrea-tology 2011;11(Suppl 2):47–51.

41. Krüger M, Schneider AS, Manns MP, et al. Endoscopic management of pancre-atic pseudocysts or abscesses after an EUS-guided 1-step procedure for initial access. Gastrointest Endosc 2006;63(3):409–16.

Endoscopic Ultrasonography-Guided Hepaticogastrostomy

Do Hyun Park, MD, PhD

KEYWORDS

- EUS-guided biliary drainage
- EUS-guided hepaticogastrostomy • Biliary obstruction
- Percutaneous transhepatic biliary drainage
- Endoscopic retrograde cholangiopancreatography

INTRODUCTION

Endoscopic retrograde cholangiopancreatography (ERCP) is the standard procedure for biliary drainage in patients with benign or malignant biliary obstruction, with a success rate of approximately 90% to 97% and a risk of complications less than 10%.[1–3] Alternative biliary accesses are percutaneous transhepatic biliary drainage (PTBD) or surgical bypass. PTBD is successful in 87% to 100% of cases, with a post-procedure adverse event rate of 9% to 33% and a mortality rate of 2% to 15%.[4–6] Surgical bypass may also be considered an alternative, but this procedure can have relatively high postprocedure adverse event and mortality rates.[7] To date, PTBD has been considered the most appropriate salvage of biliary access after failed ERCP.[6] Since endoscopic ultrasonography (EUS)-guided bile duct puncture was first described in 1996,[8] sporadic case reports of EUS-guided biliary drainage (EUS-BD) have suggested it as an alternative to PTBD after failed ERCP.[1,8–23] The potential benefits of EUS-BD include that it is a 1-stage procedure, as with ERCP, and internal drainage, avoiding long-term external drainage in cases where external PTBD drainage catheters cannot be internalized; this can significantly improve the quality of life of terminally ill patients and possibly result in lower morbidity than PTBD or surgery.[2,23–25]

EUS-guided hepaticogastrostomy (EUS-HG) is one form of EUS-BD. This method of access allows biliary drainage from the intrahepatic bile duct to the stomach. Previously, percutaneous hepaticogastrostomy was attempted, and achieved a high technical

The author has no financial relationship relevant to this publication.

Division of Gastroenterology, Department of Internal Medicine, University of Ulsan College of Medicine, Asan Medical Center, 88, Olympic-Ro 43 Gil, Songpa-gu, Seoul 138-736, Korea

E-mail address: dhpark@amc.seoul.kr

Gastrointest Endoscopy Clin N Am 22 (2012) 271–280
doi:10.1016/j.giec.2012.04.009

success rate but with 2 mortalities. This 2-stage approach, using fluoroscopic, laparoscopic, and endoscopic assistance, places a temporary fenestrated gastrostomy tube through the liver with the bumper in the stomach for 2 weeks, followed by a replacement metal biliary stent between the left biliary system and the stomach.[25–27] Because of the complexity of the procedure and mortalities, this approach has not been widely used. Since EUS-HG with transluminal stenting was first reported by Burmester and colleagues[12] in 2003, a few case series regarding this technique have been reported. Compared with percutaneous hepaticogastrostomy, EUS-HG can be performed as a 1-stage procedure in the same endoscopic session after failed ERCP.[2]

This article describes the indications, techniques, and outcomes of published data on EUS-HG.

INDICATIONS FOR EUS-HG

Indications for EUS-HG include patients with proximal bile duct obstruction, surgically altered anatomy such as Roux-en-Y anastomosis, and duodenal bulb invasion after failed ERCP.[2] In patients with an occluded biliary metal stent inserted after a hilar bilateral metal stent or a combined duodenal and biliary insertion of a metal stent, EUS-HG may be also considered as an alternative to PTBD after failed ERCP.[22]

Compared with other EUS-BD techniques such as EUS-choledochoduodenostomy or rendezvous, EUS-HG with transluminal stenting (EUS-HGS) may be most appropriate in patients with surgically altered anatomy after failed ERCP, because of the difficult and often prolonged effort in passing the guide wire into the duodenum or small bowel with the EUS-guided rendezvous technique. Furthermore, EUS-HGS can eliminate the need for deep enteroscopy (in patients with surgically altered anatomy) to grasp the antegrade-placed guide wire placed via the EUS-HG rendezvous technique.[2] The intent of EUS-HGS is to provide a permanent biliary diversion, whereas EUS-HG with the rendezvous technique is intended to facilitate access to the bile duct. Thus, EUS-HGS is most appropriate for palliative biliary drainage. In right-sided intrahepatic biliary obstruction or complex hilar biliary strictures such as Klatskin tumor Bismuth type III or IV, EUS-HGS may not be effective for such circumstances because EUS-HGS offers only left-sided biliary decompression (**Box 1**).[25]

Box 1
Indications for EUS-HG

1. Proximal bile duct obstruction[a] after failed ERCP

2. Surgically altered anatomy such as Roux-en-Y anastomosis after failed ERCP

3. Duodenal bulb invasion after failed ERCP

4. In patients with occluded biliary metal stent after a hilar bilateral metal stent[b] placement or after a combined duodenal and biliary metal stent placement, as an alternative to PTBD after failed ERCP

Notes:
1, 3, and 4: palliative biliary drainage for malignant biliary obstruction.

2: Benign or malignant biliary obstruction. Consider EUS-HGS or EUS-HG with rendezvous technique.

[a] Common hepatic duct or mid–common bile duct obstruction. Klatskin tumor Bismuth type ≥III may not be feasible.
[b] Left-sided hilar stricture (especially dilated bile duct segment 3 due to segmental tumor progression).

TECHNIQUE OF EUS-HG

After administration of prophylactic antibiotics, EUS-HG is performed using a linear-array echoendoscope, and the tip of the echoendoscope is placed at the cardia or lesser curvature of the stomach. EUS-HG is formed by puncturing dilated left intrahepatic biliary system with a 19-gauge needle. After removal of the stylet, bile is aspirated, and radiopaque contrast is injected to visualize the biliary system under fluoroscopy. A 0.035-in or 0.021-in guide wire is then passed via the needle into the left intrahepatic system. Every attempt should be made to pass the wire into the duodenum across the biliary stricture so that rendezvous ERCP drainage can be undertaken with transpapillary biliary stent placement. If this is not possible, the wire can be coiled in the liver hilum for transluminal stent placement. Transluminal stenting is performed in most cases because the passage of a transhepatically placed guide wire into the duodenum across the biliary stricture is technically challenging. For dilation of the transmural tract, a graded dilation can be used as in EUS-guided pseudocyst drainage (**Fig. 1**). In brief, an ERCP cannula ultra-tapered to 4F is inserted over the guide wire. Then 6F and 7F biliary dilator catheters are inserted over the guide wire and removed, in that order, to dilate the tract. If there is resistance to the advancement of the 6F dilator catheter, a triple-lumen needle-knife with a 7F shaft diameter or a cystotome is gently inserted over the guide wire to dilate the tract using a brief burst of pure cutting current. A plastic stent or an expandable metal stent is then transgastrically deployed into the left intrahepatic system (**Figs. 2 and 3**).[2,25]

TECHNICAL TROUBLESHOOTING OF EUS-HG

When selecting the intrahepatic bile duct to puncture, dilated bile duct segment 3 (B3) is the preferred puncture site over B2 for transgastric stenting. The B3 puncture is usually made in the lesser curve of the stomach body, and when deploying the stent, the stent tip in the stomach can be checked, and complications such as stent migration prevented.[22,28]

By contrast, B2 puncture is made in the cardia or the esophageal gastric junction, whereby it is difficult to visualize stent deployment under direct endoscopic imaging. In addition, the puncture is often made via the transesophageal route rather than the transgastric route. However, puncture to B2 is more feasible than B3 puncture for the

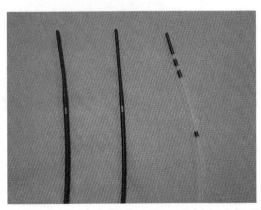

Fig. 1. Endoscopic devices for graded dilation. From right to left: 4F ERCP cannula, 6F bougie dilator, 7F bougie dilator.

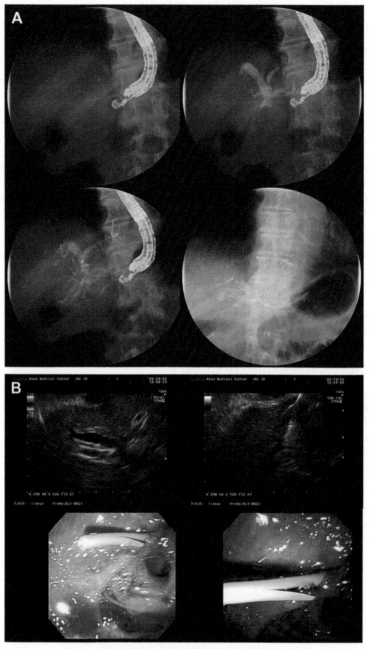

Fig. 2. (*A*) EUS-guided hepaticogastrostomy was performed in this 69-year-old male patient with distal gastrectomy and Roux-en-Y anastomosis after failed ERCP. The bile duct (segment 3) puncture was performed with a 19-gauge needle. To confirm successful biliary access, contrast medium was injected under fluoroscopy to demonstrate biliary opacification. A 0.035-in guide wire was introduced through the EUS needle and advanced in an antegrade fashion. After graded dilation, a plastic stent was placed. (*B*) In the intrahepatic approach, the linear-array echoendoscope was placed in the lesser curvature of the stomach and was oriented to view the left intrahepatic system. Bile duct puncture was performed with a 19-gauge needle. Because intrahepatic bile duct was not significantly dilated, a plastic stent was placed under echoendoscopic and fluoroscopic view.

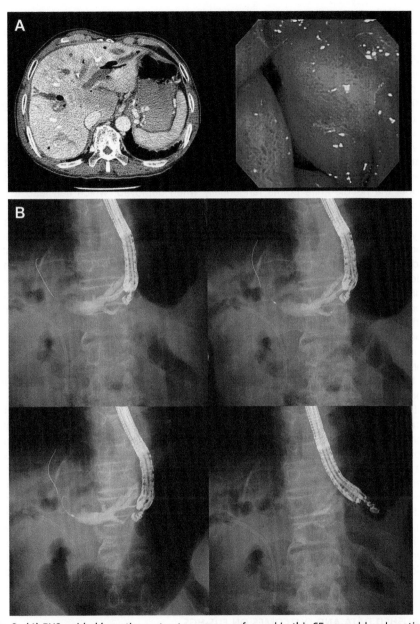

Fig. 3. (A) EUS-guided hepaticogastrostomy was performed in this 65-year-old male patient with a hilar cholangiocarcinoma and occluded biliary plastic stent. Because of accompanying duodenal invasion, ERCP was unsuccessful. A computed tomography scan showed marked left intrahepatic ductal dilatation. (B) The bile duct (segment 3) puncture was performed with a 19-gauge needle. To confirm successful biliary access, contrast medium was injected under fluoroscopy to demonstrate biliary opacification. A 0.035-in guide wire was introduced through the EUS needle and advanced in an antegrade fashion. After graded dilation with a 4F ERCP catheter and 6F and 7F bougie dilators, a fully covered self-expandable metal stent was placed.

rendezvous technique because the direction of the guide wire in B2 is relatively straight and acutely angled compared with B3, resulting in easy passage of the guide wire into the duodenum or small bowel.[22,28,29]

For graded dilation, an appropriate plane for passing the dilator catheter should be identified (in-line guide wire) and maintained as in EUS-guided pseudocyst drainage with noncautery entry.[30] If graded dilation with ERCP catheter and bougie dilator is difficult, repeated graded dilation in the sequence 4F ERCP catheter, 6F bougie dilator, 7F bougie dilator, needle-knife or cystotome may be helpful. The drawback of using a needle-knife or cystotome for fistula dilation is the higher probability of adverse events compared with graded dilation. The location of the EUS-HG is such that it is accessed from the gastric cardia or the fundus of the stomach. When a catheter is deployed at these locations, because of the acute angulation of the echoendoscope, the needle-knife points tangentially when deployed, which can lead to an undesirable incision with a chance of pneumoperitoneum or bleeding.[2,31]

The deployment of a stent under fluoroscopic and endoscopic guidance is mandatory, as in stent placement in EUS-guided drainage of pseudocysts. In transgastric stenting through B3, scope position will be backward for identification of the distal end of the deploying stent, and a stent will eventually be placed in a more inner side of the intrahepatic duct during stent deployment (especially in a J-shaped stomach).[28] This placement may result in proximal stent migration after stent deployment. Therefore, a longer stent, 8 or 10 cm in length, is best used to prevent this complication. With respect to choosing a metal stent, a covered Wallstent (Boston Scientific, Natick, MA) may shorten after stent deployment compared with a covered nitinol metal stent.[32] Thus, a fully covered self-expandable metal stent (FCSEMS) with nitinol wire may be better for EUS-HGS.[1,2,13,18,22] If the placed metal stent appears to be too short for the transmural tract, another metal stent can be placed in a stent-in-stent manner.

If the intrahepatic duct is not significantly dilated, placement of a plastic stent can be considered.[2] For stent revision with over-the-guide-wire technique, a straight plastic stent may be preferable to a single pigtail stent. Most plastic stents (except Flexima [Boston Scientific]) have push-type stent deployment. It is important to anticipate the length of stent before deployment, as changing the plastic stent during deployment is impossible. With respect to choosing the length of the stent, therefore, choose the longest stent possible (at least 6 cm). Otherwise, fully covered or partially covered self-expandable metal stents may be considered for EUS-HG with transgastric stenting. During the follow-up period following EUS-HGS, some patients may need a stent revision for various reasons, such as stent clogging. In a previous study,[2] a 7F plastic stent revision with over-the-guide-wire technique proved difficult compared with EUS-guided choledochoduodenostomy with plastic stenting. Contrary to plastic stents, the revision of EUS-HG with metal stents seems to be more technically feasible.

PUBLISHED DATA AND OUTCOMES ON EUS-HGS

Compared with EUS-HG with rendezvous techniques, EUS-HGS may involve a higher chance of adverse events because of its procedural complexity.[2] In EUS-HGS, the technical success rate is 91% to 100% and the clinical success rate is 75% to 100% (**Table 1**). The overall rate of postprocedure adverse events is 25%.[1,2,11,12,16,19,20,33,34] Postprocedure adverse events include stent migration, bile leaks, pneumoperitoneum, and cholangitis.[2] Even though complications such as bile peritonitis or pneumoperitoneum occur during or after placement of an FCSEMS, EUS-BDS with an FCSEMS may prevent the degree of these complications, because

Table 1
Technical and clinical success rates and adverse event rates in published cases using EUS-HGS

References, Year	No. of Patients	Technical Success (%)	Clinical Success (%)	Postprocedure Adverse Events (%)	Profiles of Postprocedure Adverse Events
Burmester et al,[12] 2003	1	1/1 (100)	1/1 (100)	0	—
Kahaleh et al,[16] 2006	2	2/2 (100)	2/2 (100)	0	—
Will et al,[20] 2007	4	4/4 (100)	3/4 (75)	1/4 (25)	Cholangitis
Bories et al,[11] 2007	11	10/11 (91)	10/10 (100)	4/11 (36.4)	Ileus, biloma, stent migration, and cholangitis in each case
Artifon et al,[34] 2007	1	1/1 (100)	1/1 (100)	0	—
Ramirez-Luna et al,[36] 2011	2	2/2 (100)	2/2 (100)	1/2 (50)	Distal stent migration
Park et al,[2] 2011	31	31/31 (100)	27/31 (87)	6/31 (19)	Self-limited pneumoperitoneum (4), mild bleeding (2)
Total	52	51/52 (98)	46/52 (88)	13/52 (25)	—

Abbreviation: EUS-HGS, EUS-guided hepaticogastrostomy with transluminal stenting.

the dilated fistulous tract can be immediately sealed using an FCSEMS.[1,2] However, proximal stent migration to the liver is possible if the distal end of the stent in the stomach is not adequate. In this complication, delayed bile peritonitis may develop.[32] Therefore, an adequate length of the distal stent in the stomach (at least 1.5 cm) should be secured. EUS-HGS may have a minimal rate of distal stent migration compared with EUS-CD.[1,2] In recent a prospective follow-up study,[2] EUS-HGS had similar technical and functional success to EUS-CDS. Both techniques offer durable and comparable stent patency.

FUTURE PROSPECTS FOR EUS-HG

The traverse of an antegrade-inserted guide wire to the duodenum or small bowel in EUS-HG with rendezvous technique is challenging, because it tends to pass into the right intrahepatic system during guide-wire manipulation.[25] In EUS-HGS, there remains a risk of losing access, because only a short length of the guide wire remains coiled within the intrahepatic system during exchange of accessories.[25] Furthermore, the use of a needle-knife for fistula dilation was a risk factor for postprocedure adverse events after EUS-BD in a recent prospective study.[2] Therefore, development of dedicated endoscopic devices for fistula dilation and guide-wire manipulation in EUS-HG may be warranted. Following this development, the standardized technique of EUS-HG will then become an available and popular interventional EUS procedure.

In various benign and malignant conditions, such as intrahepatic ductal stones, anastomotic biliary strictures, or hilar biliary strictures, previous case series suggest the route of EUS-HGS may serve as a conduit for various interventional endoscopic procedures.[29,35] Therefore, indications for EUS-HG may be extended after dedicated endoscopic devices for EUS-HG are launched and the safety and efficacy of this technique validated.

Prospective randomized trials on EUS-HG and PTBD are also needed to confirm that this approach can serve as a valid alternative to PTBD after failed ERCP.

REFERENCES

1. Park DH, Koo JE, Oh J, et al. EUS-guided biliary drainage with one-step placement of a fully covered metal stent for malignant biliary obstruction: a prospective feasibility study. Am J Gastroenterol 2009;104:2168–74.
2. Park DH, Jang JW, Lee SS, et al. EUS-guided biliary drainage with transluminal stenting after failed ERCP: predictors of adverse events and long-term results. Gastrointest Endosc 2011;74(6):1276–84.
3. Schofl R. Diagnostic endoscopic retrograde cholangiopancreatography. Endoscopy 2001;33:147–57.
4. Beissert M, Wittenberg G, Sandstede J, et al. Metallic stents and plastic endoprostheses in percutaneous treatment of biliary obstruction. Z Gastroenterol 2002;40:503–10.
5. Doctor N, Dick R, Rai R, et al. Results of percutaneous plastic stents for malignant distal biliary obstruction following failed endoscopic stent insertion and comparison with current literature on expandable metallic stents. Eur J Gastroenterol Hepatol 1999;11:775–80.
6. Kuhn JP, Busemann A, Lerch MM, et al. Percutaneous biliary drainage in patients with nondilated intrahepatic bile ducts compared with patients with dilated intrahepatic bile ducts. AJR Am J Roentgenol 2010;195:851–7.
7. Bornman PC, Harries-Jones EP, Tobias R, et al. Prospective controlled trial of transhepatic biliary endoprosthesis versus bypass surgery for incurable carcinoma of head of pancreas. Lancet 1986;1:69–71.
8. Wiersema MJ, Sandusky D, Carr R, et al. Endosonography-guided cholangiopancreatography. Gastrointest Endosc 1996;43:102–6.
9. Ang TL, Teo EK, Fock KM. EUS-guided transduodenal biliary drainage in unresectable pancreatic cancer with obstructive jaundice. JOP 2007;8:438–43.
10. Artifon EL, Okawa L, Takada J, et al. EUS-guided choledochoantrostomy: an alternative for biliary drainage in unresectable pancreatic cancer with duodenal invasion. Gastrointest Endosc 2011;73(6):1317–20.
11. Bories E, Pesenti C, Caillol F, et al. Transgastric endoscopic ultrasonography-guided biliary drainage: results of a pilot study. Endoscopy 2007;39:287–91.
12. Burmester E, Niehaus J, Leineweber T, et al. EUS-cholangio-drainage of the bile duct: report of 4 cases. Gastrointest Endosc 2003;57:246–51.
13. Fabbri C, Luigiano C, Fuccio L, et al. EUS-guided biliary drainage with placement of a new partially covered biliary stent for palliation of malignant biliary obstruction: a case series. Endoscopy 2011;43(5):438–41.
14. Giovannini M, Moutardier V, Pesenti C, et al. Endoscopic ultrasound-guided bilioduodenal anastomosis: a new technique for biliary drainage. Endoscopy 2001;33:898–900.
15. Itoi T, Itokawa F, Sofuni A, et al. Endoscopic ultrasound-guided choledochoduodenostomy in patients with failed endoscopic retrograde cholangiopancreatography. World J Gastroenterol 2008;14:6078–82.
16. Kahaleh M, Hernandez AJ, Tokar J, et al. Interventional EUS-guided cholangiography: evaluation of a technique in evolution. Gastrointest Endosc 2006;64:52–9.

17. Kim YS, Gupta K, Mallery S, et al. Endoscopic ultrasound rendezvous for bile duct access using a transduodenal approach: cumulative experience at a single center. A case series. Endoscopy 2010;42:496–502.

18. Siddiqui AA, Sreenarasimhaiah J, Lara LF, et al. Endoscopic ultrasound-guided transduodenal placement of a fully covered metal stent for palliative biliary drainage in patients with malignant biliary obstruction. Surg Endosc 2011;25:549–55.

19. Will U, Meyer F, Schmitt W, et al. Endoscopic ultrasound-guided transesophageal cholangiodrainage and consecutive endoscopic transhepatic Wallstent insertion into a jejunal stenosis. Scand J Gastroenterol 2007;42:412–5.

20. Will U, Thieme A, Fueldner F, et al. Treatment of biliary obstruction in selected patients by endoscopic ultrasonography (EUS)-guided transluminal biliary drainage. Endoscopy 2007;39:292–5.

21. Yamao K, Sawaki A, Takahashi K, et al. EUS-guided choledochoduodenostomy for palliative biliary drainage in case of papillary obstruction: report of 2 cases. Gastrointest Endosc 2006;64:663–7.

22. Park DH, Song TJ, Eum J, et al. EUS-guided hepaticogastrostomy with a fully covered metal stent as the biliary diversion technique for an occluded biliary metal stent after a failed ERCP (with videos). Gastrointest Endosc 2010;71:413–9.

23. Brauer BC, Chen YK, Fukami N, et al. Single-operator EUS-guided cholangiopancreatography for difficult pancreaticobiliary access (with video). Gastrointest Endosc 2009;70:471–9.

24. Ang TL. Current status of endosonography-guided biliary drainage. Singapore Med J 2010;51:762–6.

25. Savides TJ, Varadarajulu S, Palazzo L. EUS 2008 Working Group document: evaluation of EUS-guided hepaticogastrostomy. Gastrointest Endosc 2009;69:S3–7.

26. Soulez G, Gagner M, Therasse E, et al. Malignant biliary obstruction: preliminary results of palliative treatment with hepaticogastrostomy under fluoroscopic, endoscopic, and laparoscopic guidance. Radiology 1994;192:241–6.

27. Soulez G, Therasse E, Oliva VL, et al. Left hepaticogastrostomy for biliary obstruction: long-term results. Radiology 1997;204:780–6.

28. Itoi T, Isayama H, Sofuni A, et al. Stent selection and tips on placement technique of EUS-guided biliary drainage: transduodenal and transgastric stenting. J Hepatobiliary Pancreat Sci 2011;18:664–72.

29. Park DH, Jang JW, Lee SS, et al. EUS-guided transhepatic antegrade balloon dilation for benign bilioenteric anastomotic strictures in a patient with hepaticojejunostomy. Gastrointest Endosc 2012;75(3):692–3.

30. Park DH, Lee SS, Moon SH, et al. Endoscopic ultrasound-guided versus conventional transmural drainage for pancreatic pseudocysts: a prospective randomized trial. Endoscopy 2009;41:842–8.

31. Varadarajulu S. EUS followed by endoscopic pancreatic pseudocyst drainage or all-in-one procedure: a review of basic techniques (with video). Gastrointest Endosc 2009;69:S176–81.

32. Martins FP, Rossini LG, Ferrari AP. Migration of a covered metallic stent following endoscopic ultrasound-guided hepaticogastrostomy: fatal complication. Endoscopy 2010;42(Suppl 2):E126–7.

33. Yamao K, Hara K, Mizuno N, et al. EUS-guided biliary drainage. Gut Liver 2010;4(Suppl 1):S67–75.

34. Artifon EL, Chaves DM, Ishioka S, et al. Echoguided hepatico-gastrostomy: a case report. Clinics (Sao Paulo) 2007;62:799–802.

35. Eum J, Park DH, Ryu CH, et al. EUS-guided biliary drainage with a fully covered metal stent as a novel route for natural orifice transluminal endoscopic biliary interventions: a pilot study (with videos). Gastrointest Endosc 2010;72:1279–84.
36. Ramirez-Luna MA, Tellez-Avila FI, Giovannini M, et al. Endoscopic ultrasound-guided biliodigestive drainage is a good alternative in patients with unresectable cancer. Endoscopy 2011;43:826–30.

Endoscopic Ultrasound-Guided Abscess Drainage

Ganapathy A. Prasad, MD[a], Shyam Varadarajulu, MD[b],*

KEYWORDS

- Endoscopic ultrasound • Drainage • Pelvic abscess
- Abdominal abscess • Therapeutic EUS

Areas adjacent to the gastrointestinal (GI) tract that can be easily accessed for drainage by endoscopic ultrasound (EUS) include the subphrenic space, perihepatic regions (left lobe of the liver), lesser sac, areas adjacent to the esophagus (posterior mediastinum), proximal small bowel, left colon, and the perirectal space. Most of the literature and well-designed trials involve drainage of pancreatic fluid collections (PFCs) in the lesser sac,[1–3] which is discussed elsewhere in this supplement. This article discusses the existing data, techniques, limitations, and safety profile of the EUS-based approach for drainage of other abdominal and pelvic abscesses.

Most abdominal abscesses are post-surgical in nature or secondary to organ perforation and hence benign in etiology. Patients typically present with fever and abdominal pain. The objective of treatment is to evacuate the abscess and enable irrigation of the cavity to facilitate resolution of infection. EUS has the following advantages over conventional endoscopy: (1) it enables access to abscess cavities that do not cause a luminal compression, (2) drainage can be performed real time under sonographic guidance, (3) intervening vasculature can be avoided, and (4) an alternative diagnosis can be established in a small subset of patients.

INSTRUMENTS AND MATERIALS

A clear understanding of the anatomy of the abdomen or pelvis and its relationship to the abscess is important before embarking on drainage. In all patients, a dedicated magnetic resonance imaging or computed tomographic (CT) imaging should initially

Disclosures: Ganapathy Prasad: None. Shyam Varadarajulu: Consultant, Boston Scientific Corporation and Olympus Medical Systems Corporation.
[a] Division of Gastroenterology-Hepatology, Mayo Clinic, 200 1st Street SW, Rochester, MN 55905-0002, USA; [b] Division of Gastroenterology, Department of Medicine, Basil I. Hirschowitz Endoscopic Center of Excellence, University of Alabama at Birmingham School of Medicine, 1530-3rd Avenue South, Birmingham, AL 35294, USA
* Corresponding author.
E-mail address: svaradarajulu@yahoo.com

Gastrointest Endoscopy Clin N Am 22 (2012) 281–290
doi:10.1016/j.giec.2012.04.002
1052-5157/12/$ – see front matter
giendo.theclinics.com

be performed to ascertain their underlying nature and confirm that these abscesses are in close proximity to the GI lumen. Abscesses that are multiloculated measure less than 4 cm in size, have immature walls (without a definitive rim), are located at the level of the dentate line (pelvic abscess) or greater than 2 cm from the EUS transducer, should be managed by alternative techniques. Laboratory parameters must be checked to ensure that patients are not coagulopathic or thrombocytopenic. Patients should be administered prophylactic antibiotics before the intervention and continued on oral antibiotics for 3 to 5 days. Drainage procedures are best performed in a unit with fluoroscopy set up to enable visualization of wire exchanges and stent or drain placement within the abscess. In patients with pelvic abscess, a preparation in the form of an enema and/or polyethylene glycol is mandatory to minimize the chances of contamination and for adequate visualization. Also, patients should be instructed to void urine before the procedure because a distended bladder may impair visualization of a small pelvic abscess during EUS. A sample of the abscess contents should routinely be sent for gram stain and culture in all patients.

Echoendoscopes

Linear array echoendoscopes offering a working channel of at least 3 mm should be used; this includes the FG 38UX (Pentax Precision Instruments Corp., Orangeburg, NY, USA), the EG 38UT (Pentax Precision Instruments Corp., Orangeburg, NY, USA), and the GF-UCT140/180 (Olympus Medical System Corporation, Center Valley, PA, USA). The EG 38UT and the GF-UCT 140, which are used with working channels of 3.8 and 3.7 mm, respectively, both allow placement of a 10F stent. On the other hand, the FG 38X has a working channel of 3.2 mm, which only permits placement of an 8.5F stent. If only echoendoscopes with smaller working channels are available, then after EUS-guided passage of a guidewire, the echoendoscope must be exchanged for a therapeutic gastroscope or duodenoscope, over the previously placed guidewire, to perform abscess drainage.[4]

Accessories

A 19-gauge EUS–fine-needle aspiration (FNA) needle is required to pass a stiff 0.035-in guidewire into the abscess cavity (**Box 1**). An over-the-wire needle knife catheter is required to puncture the wall of the abscess to facilitate stent or drain placement. Alternatively, in patients who are at high risk for bleeding, a standard 4.5F endoscopic retrograde cholangiopancreatography (ERCP) cannula can be passed over the guidewire to gradually 'burrow' the wall of the abscess cavity to achieve the same effect. A through-the-scope balloon (6–15 mm) is needed to further dilate the tract between the abscess cavity and GI lumen. Double pigtail plastic stents (7/8.5F or 10F) and/or catheter are required to facilitate drainage of the abscess cavity.

Box 1
Requisite materials for EUS-guided abscess drainage

- Echoendoscope with a biopsy channel greater than 3.7 mm
- 19-gauge FNA needle
- 0.035 in guidewire
- 4.5F ERCP cannula or an over-the-wire needle-knife catheter
- Over-the-wire balloon dilators
- 7F or 10F double-pigtail plastic stents and/or drainage catheter

---

Procedural Technique

Graded dilation technique for drainage of abdominal abscess

Once the echoendoscope is advanced to the duodenum, a gradual withdrawal is performed with back and forth torque to identify the abscess cavity. Caution must be exercised to differentiate a gallbladder from the abscess. Inadvertent puncture of the gallbladder with a 19-gauge needle can lead to biliary peritonitis. Once the abscess is identified, after excluding the presence of vasculature in the path of the needle using color Doppler ultrasound, a 19-gauge FNA needle is used to puncture the cavity under EUS guidance (**Fig. 1**A). A 0.035-in guidewire is then introduced through the needle and coiled within the abscess cavity (see **Fig. 1**B) under fluoroscopic guidance. The tract is then sequentially dilated by first passing a 4.5F ERCP cannula over the guidewire. Further dilation is then undertaken using a 6- to 15-mm over-the-wire biliary balloon dilator (see **Fig. 1**C). After dilation, two 7 or 10F double-pigtail stents are deployed within the abscess under fluoroscopic guidance (see **Fig. 1**D). Multiple stents and a 7 or 10F nasocystic drainage catheter has to be deployed in some patients for periodic flushing and evacuation of the abscess contents.

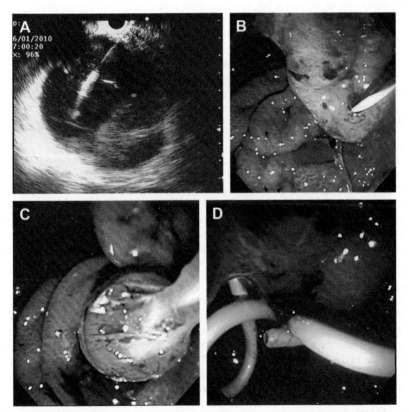

Fig. 1. (*A*) The intra-abdominal abscess is accessed under EUS guidance using a 19-gauge FNA needle. (*B*) A 0.035-in guidewire is then coiled within the abscess cavity. (*C*) The transmural tract is sequentially dilated to 15 mm with drainage of abscess contents. (*D*) Two 7F 4-cm double-pigtail stents are deployed for decompression of abscess contents.

Technical tips

A major advantage of the graded dilation technique is that electrocautery is not used during any step of the procedure. Although there are no data on abdominal abscess drainage, in the largest series reported to date on EUS-guided drainage of PFCs using the graded dilation technique, bleeding or perforation was encountered in only about 1% of patients.[5] In patients with a thick abscess wall, the ERCP cannula may "bounce off" if not aligned properly. It is important that the cannula be in line with the guidewire when it exits the echoendoscope so as to penetrate the abscess perpendicularly. Once within the cavity, the cannula should be withdrawn into the echoendoscope, and repeated penetration of the abscess should be attempted so as to dilate the transmural tract further.

Needle-Knife Technique for Abdominal Abscess Drainage

After coiling a guidewire within the abscess cavity using a 19-gauge FNA needle, the transmural tract can be dilated using electrocautery administered via an over-the-wire needle-knife catheter (rather than dilating the tract with an ERCP cannula). Another alternative includes the use of a dedicated commercially available cystotome. The cystotome is a modified needle-knife papillotome that consists of an inner wire with a needle-knife tip, a 5F inner catheter, and a 10F outer catheter equipped with a diathermy ring at its distal tip. The proximal end of this device includes a handle with connectors for administration of electrocautery. The abscess is punctured with the cystotome using the knife tip of the inner catheter, by administration of electrocautery, and then entered with the inner catheter. The metal part of the inner catheter is then withdrawn, and a 0.035-in guidewire is passed through the inner catheter into the cavity. The outer 10F sheath of the cystotome that is equipped with a diathermy ring is advanced through the puncture site using electrocautery. The cystotome is then removed leaving the guidewire in the cyst cavity. The trasmural tract is then dilated followed by stent deployment.

Technical tips

An advantage of the needle-knife technique is that it penetrates the abscess wall with relative ease. The main disadvantage of the technique is that perforation has been reported as a complication in several series evaluating drainage of PFCs.[6–10] When an abscess is approached via the gastric cardia or the fundus of the stomach, because of acute angulation of the echoendoscope, the deployed needle knife may point tangentially leading to an undesirable incision. Maintaining a degree of tension on the guidewire keeps the needle-knife catheter in plane with the guidewire as it exits the echoendoscope and can possibly minimize the risk of perforation.

Post-procedure follow-up

Although there are no formal recommendations, a follow-up CT is performed within 2 to 3 days. If the abscess has decreased in size by more than 50% and the patient is afebrile with improved symptoms, the drainage catheter is discontinued before patient discharge from the hospital. Another CT is then obtained within 6 to 8 weeks to ascertain resolution of the abscess. If the abscess has resolved, the transmural stent is removed by endoscopy. If the abscess is persistent, additional stents are deployed or the patient is referred for surgery.

Pelvic abscess drainage

First, the abscess must be located using a curved linear array echoendoscope. It can sometimes be challenging to differentiate a urinary bladder from pelvic abscess. Unlike an abscess, the urinary bladder generally does not have sediment at its base. Also, as most patients with pelvic abscess are bed bound with a foley catheter in place, the presence of a catheter in the bladder can help make this distinction. If the urinary bladder is accidentally punctured, it generally does not lead to a complication (provided one has not attempted dilation). Once located, intervening vasculature must be excluded using color Doppler. Under EUS guidance, a 19-gauge FNA needle is used to puncture the abscess cavity (**Fig. 2**A). The stylet is removed, and the needle is flushed with saline and aspirated to evacuate as much pus as possible. If there is no return of abscess contents on applying suction, one must irrigate 20 mL normal saline via the FNA needle and then apply suction again. It is likely that the abscess content is thick or the lumen of the needle is clogged with mucosa or debris. A 0.035-in guidewire is then passed through the needle and coiled within the abscess cavity

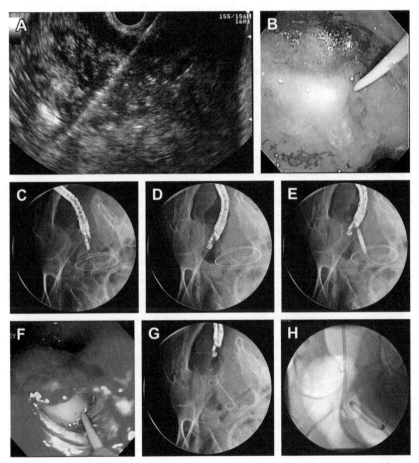

Fig. 2. (*A*) Passage of a 19-gauge FNA needle into the pelvic abscess under EUS guidance. (*B, C*) A 0.035-in guidewire is then coiled within the abscess cavity (*B*, endoscopy view), and this can be confirmed by fluoroscopy (*C*). (*D–F*) Fluoroscopy view revealing dilation of the tract by using an ERCP cannula (*D*) and an over-the-wire balloon dilator (*E*). Pus is seen to extrude following dilation of the transmural tract (*F*). (*G*) Fluoroscopic view revealing the presence of a stent within the pelvic abscess cavity. (*H*) In patients with large pelvic abscess (>8 cm), an additional transrectal drainage catheter is deployed to facilitate short-term drainage of the abscess contents as seen on fluoroscopic image.

(see **Fig. 2**B, C). The needle is then exchanged over the guidewire for a 4.5F ERCP cannula or a needle-knife catheter to dilate the tract between the rectum and the abscess cavity (see **Fig. 2**D). The tract is then further dilated using an 8-mm over-the-wire balloon dilator (see **Fig. 2**E, F). Once the tract is dilated, one or two 7F/10F double-pigtail transmural stents are deployed (see **Fig. 2**G). The decision to place one or more stents is based on the viscosity of the abscess contents: one if the fluid flowed smoothly and more if the contents were thicker. In patients with abscesses that measure 8 cm or more in size and in those abscesses that do not drain well despite placement of transmural stents, an additional translumenal drainage catheter is deployed (see **Fig. 2**H). The abscess cavity is accessed again with a 5F ERCP cannula to pass another 0.035-in guidewire. A 10F, 80-cm single-pigtail drain is then deployed over the guidewire. This drain will exit the anus and remain secured to the patient's gluteal region using tape. This drain is then flushed with 30 to 50 mL of normal saline every 4 hours until the aspirate is clear.

Post-procedure follow-up

Follow-up CT should be obtained at 36 to 48 hours to ensure the fluid collection has decreased in size. If there is greater than 50% reduction in size of the abscess cavity, the drainage catheter can be removed and the patient discharged home. The remaining stents can continue to assist with drainage and be removed in 2 weeks with sigmoidoscopy as long as a repeat CT of the pelvis shows complete abscess resolution.

Technical Considerations

Which is the best technique to dilate the wall of the abscess cavity: needle-knife versus "burrowing" with catheters?

In the absence of comparative data, this question is difficult to answer. Perforation has been reported as a complication during EUS-guided drainage of PFCs using the needle-knife technique. It can sometimes be challenging to control the direction of the cut when using needle-knife catheters. Although this could be minimized by using an over-the-wire needle-knife, the needle when deployed often points in a tangential angle because of its thin caliber, leading to an undesirable incision. The authors sequentially dilate the wall of the abscess cavity using a 4.5F ERCP cannula and then a balloon dilator. Our technical outcomes and safety profile using this technique has been excellent.[5] The decision to undertake either technique should be based on expertise of the endoscopist and availability of resources.

Is there a limit to the degree of transmural dilation that can be performed?

Currently, there is no evidence to provide definitive recommendations (**Table 1**). In general, large transmural dilation leads to better drainage of abscess contents. Large

Table 1
Recommended dilation for transmural drainage procedures

Route	Diameter (mm)
Esophagus	6
Stomach	
Large abscess (>6 cm)	12–15
Small abscess (<6 cm)	8–10
Duodenum	8–10
Jejunum	6–8
Rectum	6–8

abscesses abut a larger surface area of the gastric wall and therefore can be safely dilated to 12 to 15 mm. If the size of the abscess is small, then the area of abutment to the gastric wall will be minimal as well. In these patients, performing a large dilation has the potential to cause perforation or leak. Under such circumstances, an 8 to 10 mm dilation is suffice. Likewise, when performing transduodenal drainage, the dilation is maintained to between 8 and 10 mm. Transesophageal drainage has the potential to cause pneumomediastinum.[11] Most of these patients remain asymptomatic despite the presence of mediastinal air. In the experience of these authors, 6-mm dilation is safe in the esophagus with less chance for pneumomediastinum.[12] Also, 6- to 8-mm dilation has been shown to be sufficient for performing transjejunal drainage procedures.[13] For transrectal drainages, a dilation of 6 to 8 mm has been shown to be effective in most patients.[14–16]

Which is the best technique to drain abscesses: stent versus drainage catheter placement?

There are no studies comparing outcomes between both techniques. However, because of its small caliber, when draining pelvic abscesses, transrectal stents can potentially get clogged easily by fecal matter and when left long term can cause perirectal pain or migrate spontaneously. Placing a drainage catheter enables continued access to the abscess cavity for flushing and draining of the infected fluid collection. Also, the chance of infecting a sterile abscess is remote with transrectal drain placement than with stenting. Moreover, the drain can be removed in a shorter period of time as continued irrigation will potentially resolve the abscess faster.

Limitations

Drainage of GI abscess cannot be undertaken when the wall of the abscess cavity is greater than 20 mm from the EUS transducer. Also, the presence of multiple cavities in an abscess precludes successful drainage. It is important to perform a helical CT scan before embarking on this procedure because poorly defined or multilocular fluid collections are not suitable for this nonsurgical method of drainage. The best outcomes are usually in patients with a unilocular cavity. Currently, EUS-guided drainage procedures require the use of multiple accessories, and one must be familiar with therapeutic ERCP to perform EUS-guided abscess drainage. Dedicated one-step devices are needed to further advance the role of EUS for performing therapeutic interventions.

Outcomes

Most clinical outcomes on EUS-guided abscess drainage pertain to the management of PFCs. **Table 2** provides a summary of published literature on EUS-guided abscess drainage that does not encompass PFCs. It is readily apparent that a bulk of the literature is on drainage of pelvic abscesses and postoperative fluid collections. Pelvic abscess occurs as a complication of surgery or medical conditions like inflammatory bowel disease, diverticulitis, and ischemic colitis.[16] In a study of 12 patients with deep pelvic abscesses in whom EUS-guided transrectal stent (8.5/10F) placement was attempted, Giovannini and colleagues[17] reported a technical success rate of 75% with resolution of abscess in 8 of 12 patients. In 3 patients, stenting was not possible because of the distance between the abscess and the rectal wall (>20 mm). The mean duration of stenting was 4.3 months. With the exception of 2 patients (largest abscess measured 85 × 83 mm), others had a pelvic abscess that was smaller than 60 mm. The outcome was unsuccessful in the patient with largest abscess, and he eventually required surgical drainage. No complications were encountered in this study. In a prospective study, the authors performed EUS-guided drainage of pelvic abscesses

Table 2
Published data on EUS-guided drainage of abscesses other than pancreatic fluid collections

Author (References)	Abscess Location	Number of Cases	Clinical Outcomes
Baron & Wiersema,[11] 2000	Mediastinum	1	Success
Varadarajulu & Drelichman,[14] 2007	Pelvic	4	75% success
Trevino & Drelichman,[15] 2008	Pelvic	4	100% success
Varadarajulu & Drelichman,[16] 2009	Pelvic	25	96% success
Giovannini et al,[17] 2003	Pelvic	12	75% success
Varadarajulu,[18] in press	J-pouch	1	Success
Shami et al,[19] 2008	Biloma	5	100% success
Piraka et al,[20] 2009	Pelvic (n = 3) Biloma (n = 2) Peri-gastric (n = 2)	7	100% success
Itoi T et al,[21] 2011	Liver	1	Success
Ang et al,[22] 2009	Liver	1	Success
Seewald et al,[23] 2004	Subphrenic	1	Success
Lee et al,[24] 2006	Spleen	1	Success
Varadarajulu & Decker,[26] 2011	Intra-abdominal	1	Success

Abbreviation: n, number.

in 4 patients who were not amenable for drainage by the percutaneous route.[14] The mean size of the abscess in these 4 patients was 68 × 72 mm. All patients had successful placement of a 10F drainage catheter into the abscess cavity under EUS guidance. The abscesses resolved spontaneously within a mean duration of 6 days, and there was no recurrence at 3-month follow-up. Although 1 patient died of worsening heart failure, no procedure-related complications were encountered. However, drainage catheters are prone to accidental dislodgement, and their management mandates a prolonged inpatient hospital stay. A combined technique was then developed by using both EUS-guided transrectal drainage catheter and stent placement for management of patients with pelvic abscesses.[15] Although the drainage catheter provided access for short-term (36 hours) management of the abscess, the stents were left in place for medium-term (2 weeks) drainage. In a pilot trial, treatment was successful both in the short- and medium-term in all 4 patients, and the mean duration of the post-procedure hospital stay was only 2 days.[15] At a mean follow-up of 221 days, all 4 patients were doing well, without any symptoms of pelvic-abscess recurrence. This strategy was then subsequently validated in 25 patients with successful clinical outcomes in 24 (96%) patients.[16] Management of pelvic abscess in patients with a J-pouch construction for Crohn disease can be technically challenging given the altered surgical anatomy.[17] In a recent technical note, the authors reported the successful outcomes with EUS-guided approach in one such patient with a J-pouch and pelvic abscess.[18] Management of pelvic abscess using EUS guidance in the setting of inflammatory bowel disease remains a prime area for clinical research.

The management of abdominal abscesses under EUS-guidance is an area of interest that continues to evolve. Most of these abscesses are postsurgical in nature and hence best treated noninvasively. In 2 reports, bilomas were treated successfully in 7 patients with good clinical outcomes.[19,20] Other drainage procedures undertaken include abscesses involving the liver, spleen, subphrenic area, and mediastinum.[11,21–24] The procedure is particularly effective in critically ill patients, such as, in the post-transplant setting, where drainage can be accomplished at patient bedside using a mobile EUS cart.[25] In one patient who developed abdominal abscess following a liver transplantation, EUS was effective in draining the abscess with excellent clinical outcomes.[26]

SUMMARY

EUS-guided drainage is an effective treatment modality for the management of abdominal or pelvic abscesses that are not amenable to conventional therapy and in critically ill patients. The preliminary data are promising, and the safety profile of the technique appears excellent. Dedicated one-step devices are needed to make EUS the mainstream treatment modality for management of these complex patients.

REFERENCES

1. Varadarajulu S, Tamhane A, Blakely J. Graded dilation technique for EUS-guided drainage of peripancreatic fluid collections: an assessment of outcomes and complications and technical proficiency (with video). Gastrointest Endosc 2008;68:656–66.
2. Varadarajulu S, Christein JD, Tamhane A, et al. Prospective randomized trial comparing EUS and EGD for transmural drainage of pancreatic pseudocysts (with videos). Gastrointest Endosc 2008;68:1102–11.
3. Varadarajulu S, Wilcox CM, Tamhane A, et al. Role of EUS in drainage of peripancreatic fluid collections not amenable for endoscopic transmural drainage. Gastrointest Endosc 2007;66:1107–19.
4. Varadarajulu S. EUS followed by endoscopic pancreatic pseudocyst drainage or all-in-one procedure: a review of basic techniques (with video). Gastrointest Endosc 2009;69:S176–81.
5. Varadarajulu S, Christein JD, Wilcox CM. Frequency of complications during EUS-guided drainage of pancreatic fluid collections in 148 consecutive patients. J Gastroenterol Hepatol 2011;10:1504–8.
6. Kahaleh M, Shami VM, Conaway MR, et al. Endoscopic ultrasound drainage of pancreatic pseudocyst: a prospective comparison with conventional endoscopic drainage. Endoscopy 2006;38:355–9.
7. Antillon MR, Shah RJ, Stiegmann G, et al. Single-step EUS-guided transmural drainage of simple and complicated pancreatic pseudocysts. Gastrointest Endosc 2006;63(6):797–803.
8. Azar RR, Oh YS, Janec EM, et al. Wire-guided pancreatic pseudocyst drainage by using a modified needle knife and therapeutic echoendoscope. Gastrointest Endosc 2006;63:688–92.
9. Giovannini M, Pesenti CH, Rolland AL, et al. Endoscopic ultrasound guided drainage of pancreatic pseudo-cyst and pancreatic abscess using a therapeutic echoendoscope. Endoscopy 2001;33:473–7.
10. Will U, Wegener C, Graf KI, et al. Differential treatment and early outcome in the interventional endoscopic management of pancreatic pseudocysts in 27 patients. World J Gastroenterol 2006;12:4175–8.
11. Baron TH, Wiersema MJ. EUS-guided transesophageal pancreatic pseudocyst drainage. Gastrointest Endosc 2000;52:545–9.
12. Trevino JM, Christein JD, Varadarajulu S. EUS-guided transesophageal drainage of peripancreatic fluid collections. Gastrointest Endosc 2009;70:793–7.
13. Trevino JM, Varadarajulu S. Endoscopic Ultrasound-guided transjejunal drainage of a pancreatic pseudocyst. Pancreas 2010;39:419–20.

14. Varadarajulu S, Drelichman ER. EUS-guided drainage of pelvic abscess. Gastrointest Endosc 2007;66:372–6.
15. Trevino JM, Drelichman ER, Varadarajulu S. Modified technique for EUS-guided drainage of pelvic abscess (with video). Gastrointest Endosc 2008;68:1215–9.
16. Varadarajulu S, Drelichman ER. Effectiveness of EUS in drainage of pelvic abscesses in 25 consecutive patients (with video). Gastrointest Endosc 2009; 70:1121–7.
17. Giovannini M, Bories E, Moutardier V, et al. Drainage of deep pelvic abscesses using therapeutic echo endoscopy. Endoscopy 2003;35:511–4.
18. Varadarajulu S. Endoscopic ultrasound-guided drainage of a pelvic abscess via a J-pouch. Endoscopy 2012;(44 Suppl 2 UCTN):E92–3.
19. Shami VM, Talreja JP, Mahajan A, et al. EUS-guided drainage of bilomas: a new alternative? Gastrointest Endosc 2008;67:136–40.
20. Piraka C, Shah RJ, Fukami N, et al. EUS-guided transesophageal, transgastric, and transcolonic drainage of intra-abdominal fluid collections and abscesses. Gastrointest Endosc 2009;70:786–92.
21. Itoi T, Ang TL, Seewald S, et al. Endoscopic ultrasonography-guided drainage for tuberculous liver abscess drainage. Dig Endosc 2011;23(Suppl 1):158–61.
22. Ang TL, Seewald S, Teo EK, et al. EUS-guided drainage of ruptured liver abscess. Endoscopy 2009;41(Suppl 2):E21–2.
23. Seewald S, Brand B, Omar S, et al. EUS-guided drainage of subphrenic abscess. Gastrointest Endosc 2004;59:578–80.
24. Lee DH, Cash BD, Womeldorph CM, et al. Endoscopic therapy of a splenic abscess: definitive treatment via EUS-guided transgastric drainage. Gastrointest Endosc 2006;64:631–4.
25. Varadarajulu S, Eloubeidi MA, Wilcox CM. The concept of bedside EUS. Gastrointest Endosc 2008;67:1180–4.
26. Decker C, Varadarajulu S. EUS-guided drainage of an intra-abdominal abscess after liver transplantation. Gastrointest Endosc 2011;73:1056–8.

Endoscopic Ultrasound-Guided Pancreatic Cyst Ablation

John DeWitt, MD

KEYWORDS

- Endoscopic ultrasonography • Cyst • Pancreas • Ablation
- Ethanol • Paclitaxel • Mucinous cystic neoplasm
- Intraductal papillary mucinous neoplasm

PANCREATIC CYSTIC NEOPLASMS
Classification

Cysts within the pancreas may be broadly classified as (1) those complicating acute or chronic pancreatitis (acute fluid collections and pseudocysts) and (2) neoplasms lined by epithelium. Because acute fluid collections and pseudocysts are not lined by epithelium, they are uniformly benign with no malignant potential. The epithelium that outlines pancreatic cystic neoplasms (PCNs) may have negligible malignant potential (serous cystadenomas) or represent either premalignant (ie, intraductal papillary mucinous neoplasms [IPMNs] or mucinous cystadenomas [MCNs]) or malignant (ie, invasive IPMNs or mucinous cystadenocarcinomas) tumors.[1]

MCNs are usually associated with the production of extracellular mucin and variable degrees of cyst wall epithelial atypia. These cysts are characterized by the presence of ovarian stroma underlying the mucinous columnar cyst epithelium, which differentiates MCNs from IPMNs.[2] IPMNs are mucinous cystic lesions that arise from the main pancreatic duct (MD-IPMN), one of its side branches (SB-IPMN), or both sites (mixed IPMN). Unlike MCN, these cysts are distinctively associated with ductal ectasia and intraductal papillary growth.[3]

Pancreatic Cysts: Asymptomatic and Symptomatic

Pancreatic cysts are encountered in clinical practice either as asymptomatic lesions found incidentally on imaging studies or as lesions initially noted during evaluation

---

Consultant: Cook Medical, Inc.; Boston-Scientific Inc.
Research Support: Red Path Integrated Technologies, Inc.
Division of Gastroenterology and Hepatology, Indiana University Medical Center, 550 North University Boulevard, UH 4100, Indianapolis, IN 46202, USA
E-mail address: jodewitt@iupui.edu

Gastrointest Endoscopy Clin N Am 22 (2012) 291–302
doi:10.1016/j.giec.2012.04.001
1052-5157/12/$ – see front matter © 2012 Elsevier Inc. All rights reserved.

of symptoms such as abdominal pain, weight loss, and jaundice. The routine use of abdominal imaging studies for symptoms such as nonspecific abdominal pain has led to increased recognition of pancreatic cysts; however, the exact prevalence of pancreatic cysts is unknown. Recent magnetic resonance imaging (MRI)[4,5] and computerized tomography (CT) studies[6] indicate a prevalence of pancreatic cysts ranging between 2.4% and 14%.

Surgery or Surveillance?

Consensus guidelines and expert opinion recommend surgical resection of mucinous pancreatic cysts (ie, MCNs and IPMNs) that are symptomatic, larger than 3 cm in diameter, possess mural nodules, or involve the main pancreatic duct (ie, MD-IPMN).[7–10] However, even at experienced centers, reported surgical morbidity and mortality rates for PCNs are 20% to 40% and up to 2%, respectively.[11–15] Because of operative risk, there has been increasing interest within the last decade to evaluate the feasibility of nonoperative surveillance of low-risk PCNs (particularly SB-IPMNs[16–22]), which do not meet definite criteria for surgical resection. These studies evaluating the surveillance of low-risk PCNs have demonstrated that patients with asymptomatic SB-IPMNs measuring less than 3 cm in diameter and without mural nodules can be safely followed by using a combination of close follow-up of patient symptoms and imaging studies (ie, MRI or endoscopic ultrasonography) performed at least annually. This practice has been adopted by most physicians who treat these patients.

Are There Alternatives?

Although surgery or surveillance alone may be optimal management for most patients with PCNs, there has been increased interest in a minimally invasive technique to treat these lesions. Pancreatic cyst ablation, a minimally invasive technique, may be an attractive option to some patients, particularly for patients with multiple preoperative comorbidities deemed high-risk for surgical intervention. The purpose of this review is to summarize the rationale, technique, and available data for pancreatic cyst ablation.

POTENTIAL BENEFITS AND RISKS FOR PANCREATIC CYST ABLATION
Benefits

Decreased malignant potential
Endoscopists routinely perform polypectomy on colon adenomas to arrest their potential neoplastic transformation, and studies have documented that this technique decreases subsequent risk of development and death from colon cancer. A similar but largely unproven rationale underlies the endoscopic therapy for Barrett neoplasia to prevent esophageal cancer. The malignant potential of PCNs, such as MCNs and IPMNs, arise from the cyst epithelial lining. Hence, the destruction of the epithelial lining of PCNs may abate or completely remove the neoplastic potential. However, this hypothesis of the potential benefit of nonoperative therapy for PCNs remains only theoretical.

Decreased costs over time
Surveillance of pancreatic cysts is most commonly performed every 1 to 2 years with imaging studies, such as CT or MRI. However, this surveillance is expensive. If ablation could be documented to be effective and durable, surveillance intervals could theoretically be lengthened or completely stopped. However, the technique of pancreatic cyst ablation is still in its infancy and whether the other still evolving nonoperative surveillance patterns of PCNs can be changed following ablation is still unknown.

Psychological benefit to the patient

In some patients, knowledge that they possess a premalignant cyst can provoke significant anxiety. This anxiety can be augmented if the cyst does not meet the criteria for surgical resection or the patient is not a candidate for surgery because of comorbidities. In these patients, cyst ablation may allay some fears and provide some hope that an attempted intervention is performed for the lesion.

Risks

Complications

Adverse events associated with endoscopic pancreatic cyst ablation may include outcomes from either endoscopy or injection of ablative agents. The incidence and management of these outcomes are discussed subsequently.

Incomplete ablation

During colonoscopy, endoscopic polypectomy may be incomplete and leave residual adenoma. Similarly, ablation of Barrett esophagus may not completely destroy the metaplastic intestinal epithelium. After pancreatic cyst ablation, some epithelium may remain untreated and therefore continue to harbor malignant potential.

High initial treatment costs

If a decision is made to ablate a pancreatic cyst, then there will be increased upfront costs associated with 1 or more endoscopies in the first year during attempted cyst eradication. If surveillance is chosen, then it is possible that no further expenses will be incurred until a follow-up imaging study is performed 1 year later.

CHOICE OF ABLATIVE AGENT
Ethanol

The ideal choice for pancreatic cyst ablation should be cheap, widely available, locally destructive, and easy to use. Many ablative agents, such as acetic acid or tetracycline, have been applied percutaneously or intraoperatively to various anatomic sites, but ethanol is most commonly used. Ethanol is hypothesized to induce cell death by membrane lysis, protein denaturation, and vascular occlusion[23] and has been used for the destruction of solid liver or adrenal tumors[24,25] as well as cystic lesions of the liver,[26,27] kidney,[28,29] thyroid gland,[30] and various other sites.[31–33] It is therefore not surprising that ethanol was the initial agent used for endoscopic ablation of PCNs. In addition to fulfilling all of the criteria for an ideal choice listed above, ethanol also possesses thin viscosity, which permits easy injection through a 22-gauge needle used in endoscopic ultrasound-guided fine-needle aspiration (EUS-FNA).

Paclitaxel

The only other agent used to date for endoscopic pancreatic cyst ablation is paclitaxel. Paclitaxel is a hydrophobic, viscous chemotherapeutic agent that inhibits cell processes that are dependent on microtubule turnover.[34]

HOW TO PERFORM PANCREATIC CYST ABLATION
Linear Endosonography

The advent of linear endoscopic ultrasound (EUS) transformed EUS from a purely diagnostic to also a therapeutic technique. Linear EUS permits EUS-FNA by placement of a needle into various anatomic sites to sample tumors or lymph nodes. EUS-FNA may also aspirate and drain pancreatic cysts and other fluid collections. Because of the close apposition between the endoscope and the pancreas, EUS is an ideal minimally invasive technique for guiding therapeutic interventions, such as pseudocyst drainage, tissue ablation, and cyst ablation in the pancreas. Endosonographers desiring to perform pancreatic tumor ablation should be competent in all aspects of EUS-FNA.

Technique

All studies to date describing EUS-guided pancreatic cyst ablation have used a 22-gauge needle.[35–41] The safety of any 19-gauge needle or 20-gauge celiac neurolysis needle (Cook Medical, Inc., Winston-Salem, NC, USA) for this technique has not been evaluated. Therefore these 2 needles are not recommended for use at present. Use of a stylet before cyst ablation is not essential. After transgastric or transduodenal passage of a 22-gauge FNA needle into a cyst, a syringe is attached to the proximal end of the needle and near-complete evacuation of the cyst should be attempted. If fluid is present within the syringe, it may be used for cyst analysis if required. The amount of aspirated fluid, the viscosity, and the color should be noted. To ensure that the cyst is not completely collapsed, the needle remains within the cyst before injection of the ablative agent. If the cyst fluid is viscous, it may not be possible to evacuate the cyst contents as much as desired. Hence, 0.5 to 1.0 mL of saline is injected into the cyst to decrease the viscosity of cyst fluid or expand the small cyst cavity to confirm proper needle placement. With the needle in the nearly collapsed cyst, ethanol is injected in the cyst using a volume equal to that initially aspirated from the cyst. If the cyst fluid is not viscous and 3 to 4 mL is aspirated, then an equal volume of alcohol (3–4 mL) of ethanol is used in the initial injection. Studies to date have performed cyst lavage for 5 minutes, alternately filling and emptying the cavity. For cysts with viscous fluid, this is performed as 3 to 4 lavages over the 5-minute period. When cyst fluid is thin then 7 to 8 lavages are done over the same period. At the conclusion of the lavage, the ethanol-cyst fluid mixture should be completely drained of fluid as much as possible. When used, paclitaxel is injected into the cyst after alcohol lavage and left in place.[37,40]

CYSTS CONSIDERED ELIGIBLE FOR ABLATION
Size

In published studies, the treated cysts are usually suspected clinically as mucinous cysts (ie, MCNs and IPMNs) that measure between 1 and 6 cm in maximal diameter **(Table 1)**. Macrocystic (diameter >2 cm) serous cysts have also been ablated; however, these should generally be avoided because of their very low malignant potential. Intentional treatment of other pancreatic cysts such as neuroendocrine tumors or lymphoepithelial cysts has not been reported.

Baseline cyst size may be predictive of treatment success. Oh and colleagues[40] found that an initial cyst size of less than 35 mm was predictive of complete radiologic resolution after ablation with ethanol and paclitaxel. However, in a smaller study, DeWitt and colleagues[38] found that a size of less than 25 mm did not predict resolution after ethanol injection, but these results may only reflect an inadequate sample size to detect a difference. Nevertheless, it seems intuitive that a nonviscous injectate will have less contact with a cyst wall during ablation as baseline cyst size increases.

Morphology

The ideal cyst for treatment is unilocular and most MCNs maintain this morphology. Branched duct IPMNs (BD-IPMNs) may be unilocular yet they often have a tortuous septated configuration or have a narrow 1- to 2-mm duct that forms the side branch

Table 1
Trial design and cyst characteristics in studies on EUS-guided pancreatic cyst ablation

References	Design	N	Lavage Used	Median size, mm (range)	Septations	Cyst Location Head	Cyst Location Body/Tail	Clinical Diagnosis
Gan et al,[35] 2005	Prospective, Cohort	25	Increasing concentrations of ethanol	19.4 (6–30)	Second half of study	32%	68%	MCN 52% IPMN 16% Indeterminate 32%
Oh et al,[36] 2008	Prospective, Cohort	14	Ethanol and Paclitaxel	25.5 (17–52)	Not stated	7.1%	92.9%	MCN 52% IPMN 16% Indeterminate 32%
Oh et al,[37] 2009[a]	Prospective, Cohort	10	Ethanol and Paclitaxel	29.5 (20–68)	All patients	40%	60%	MCN 30% IPMN 0% Indeterminate 70%
DeWitt et al,[38] 2009	Prospective, DBRCT	42	Saline vs Ethanol	22.4 (10–58)	≤5	81%	19%	MCN 41% IPMN 41% Indeterminate 18%
Oh et al,[40] 2011[b]	Prospective, Cohort	52	Ethanol and Paclitaxel	31.8 (17–68)	1–5	31%	69%	MCN 17% SCA 19% PC 4% Indeterminate 50%

Abbreviations: PC, pseudocyst; SCA, serous cystadenoma.
[a] Includes patients from reference.[36]
[b] Includes patients from reference.[36,37]

throughout the cyst. These changes make treatment of some BD-IPMNs difficult if not impossible because the injected ablative agent may not safely come in contact with the entire cyst. Ablation should only be considered in cysts in which the endosonographer thinks that morphology favors safe ablation of the entire cyst epithelium.

Septations

The presence of septations within the cyst is not considered an absolute contraindication to therapy. Studies to date[37,38,40] have reported treatment of cysts with up to 5 to 6 septations internally. In these septated cysts, ablation may be performed initially in 1 locule of the cyst. The needle then pierces each septation sequentially and ablation continues until the cyst is completely treated. Microcystic serous cysts are not considered treatable because of the presence of up to hundreds of small cysts, which do not permit uniform application or retention of a liquid ablative agent.

Clinical Diagnoses

Given the limitations of nonoperative diagnosis of pancreatic cysts, endosonographers must combine results from available clinical, radiologic, morphologic, and cyst fluid analysis data to arrive at a suspected diagnosis. However, even after EUS, between 18% and 70% of cysts ablated in published series are classified as indeterminate cystic lesions (see **Table 1**). Clinically suspected mucinous cysts (ie, cyst fluid with any of the following: positive cytology for mucinous epithelial cells, k-ras mutation, or carcinoembryonic antigen >200 ng/mL) are best considered for treatment. Intentional use of cyst ablation for other types of cysts has not been evaluated; however, a neuroendocrine tumor has been unexpectedly found at surgery following ablation.[40] This emphasizes the difficulty of nonoperative diagnosis of pancreatic cysts, and that careful selection of patients for this treatment is critical.

Ablation of BD-IPMNs is controversial because of the concern about injection of ablative agents into cysts that communicate with the main pancreatic duct. Mucinous cystic neoplasms rarely communicate with the main pancreatic duct and therefore may be considered safer for injection. Oh and colleagues[40] performed endoscopic retrograde cholangiopancreatography (ERCP) in all patients and excluded any cysts that communicated with the main pancreatic duct. However, Gan and colleagues[35] and DeWitt and colleagues[38] did not perform ERCP before ablation and treated BD-IPMNs on a case-by-case basis. Review of studies published to date does not demonstrate that treatment of BD-IPMNs is associated with an increased rate of complications compared with the treatment of other types of cysts. It is also unclear whether pancreatitis associated with cyst ablation is due to a ductal or parenchymal injury. Further studies comparing complication rates of different types of cysts are needed.

Patient Selection

From large surgical series and consensus statements, experts generally agree on which patients with pancreatic cysts are surgically fit to undergo an operation, and pancreatic surgery should be offered to those patients. As with any new technique, however, there is controversy about which patient may be considered for cyst ablation. There is little disagreement that patients with high-risk or symptomatic benign pancreatic cysts who either refuse or are not fit for surgery may be considered for ablation.[42] However, the use of cyst ablation in incidentally identified lesions or those that may not meet the criteria for surgical resection is more controversial.[42]

Studies to date have generally excluded patients with pancreatic cysts who have the following clinical features: active or ongoing pancreatitis, ascites, portal hypertension, and coagulopathy. Furthermore imaging of a dilated pancreatic duct (because of the concern about possible MD-IPMN) or features suggestive of malignancy (masslike lesions, suspicious liver or pulmonary lesions, and enlarged lymph nodes) should not be offered cyst ablation.

RESULTS OF PANCREATIC CYST ABLATION
Change from Baseline Cyst Size

To date, 5 published prospective studies[35–40] have evaluated the role of EUS-guided pancreas cyst ablation. However, some studies[37,40] include patients from earlier reports. Endpoints in all 5 studies include EUS or radiologic assessment of changes in baseline cyst size after ablation (**Table 2**). In the only study that uses EUS imaging 3 months after ablation to evaluate for size change, DeWitt and colleagues[38] found that a single lavage with 80% ethanol resulted in a greater mean percentage of decrease in cyst surface area compared with saline solution lavage. When size change is evaluated by cross-sectional imaging, cyst resolution (defined as no visible residual cyst) ranges from 33% to 35% for ethanol lavage alone.[35,38] Korean investigators report that the addition of paclitaxel at a concentration of 3 to 6 mg/mL numerically increases CT-defined cyst resolution (size <5% of the original cyst volume) by 60% to 79%.[36,37,40] Initial experience in the United States similarly reported cyst resolution in 50% of patients ablated with ethanol and paclitaxel (**Figs. 1–5**).[43] Treatment with 2 ethanol ablations seems to increase resolution compared with 1 ethanol ablation.[41]

If pancreatic cyst ablation is to be considered as an alternative to surgical resection, studies must examine long-term follow-up of treated cysts. Cyst resolution is durable

Table 2
Complications and resolution rates in studies on EUS-guided pancreatic cyst ablation

References	Complications	Image Resolution	% Ablated Based on Histopathology	Median Follow-Up, mo (Range)
Gan et al,[35] 2005	None	35%	Variable amount of epithelial ablation (n = 5)	At least 3 mo but not stated
Oh et al,[36] 2008	Pancreatitis (10%)	79%	None	9 (6–23)
Oh et al,[37] 2009[a]	Pancreatitis (7%) Abdominal Pain (7%)	60%	Not stated (n = 2)	8.5 (6–18)
DeWitt et al,[38] 2009	Pancreatitis (4.5%) Intracystic Bleeding (2%) Abdominal Pain at 2 h (14%) Abdominal Pain at 7 d (20%)	33%	0% (n = 1) 50%–75% (n = 2) 100% (n = 1)	At least 3 mo but not stated
Oh et al,[40] 2011[b]	Fever (2%) Pancreatitis (2%) Abdominal pain (2%)	62%	0% (n = 1) 25% (n = 1) 40% (n = 1) 100% (n = 1)	20 (12–44)

[a] Includes patients from reference.[36]
[b] Includes patients from reference.[36,37]

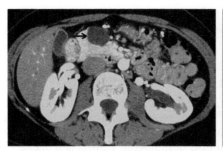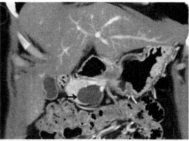

Fig. 1. Axial and coronal dual phase CT scan in a 54-year-old woman without any history of alcohol abuse or pancreatic disease who underwent CT scan during a visit to the emergency department for suspected renal stones. Multiple cystic lesions were present within the pancreas and she was referred to the authors' hospital where repeat CT was obtained and shown here. The largest cyst (*black arrows*) measured 2.8 × 2.0 × 1.9 cm and was located in the head.

in most cases with a median follow-up of approximately 2 years.[39,40] However, cyst regrowth after treatment has been observed[40] and should prompt referral when appropriate for surgical resection. Long-term studies are essential to document whether cyst ablation may be persistent in treated patients.

Complications

As with any ablative technique, safety and treatment success are important initial parameters for assessment. EUS-guided cyst ablation has generally been a very well-tolerated treatment. The initial pilot study[35] that evaluated the safety of injecting increasing concentrations of up to 80% ethanol found no treatment-related complications (see **Table 2**). However, subsequent studies reported pancreatitis in 2% to 10%, abdominal pain in 2% to 20%, fever in 2%, and intracystic bleeding in 2%. To date, no cases of severe pancreatitis, bleeding requiring transfusions, or deaths have been reported.

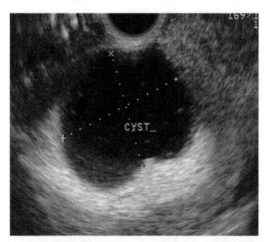

Fig. 2. Linear EUS view of the unilocular cyst measuring 2.9 × 2.0 cm. Fine-needle aspiration from the cyst fluid demonstrated no malignant cells, carcinoembryonic antigen 1200 ng/mL and amylase 175. Several other subcentimeter cysts were seen throughout the pancreas. The main pancreatic duct was normal. The clinical diagnosis was a multifocal SB-IPMN. Surgery was recommended to the patient but she declined and was treated with EUS-guided cyst ablation.

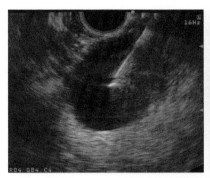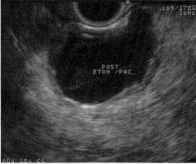

Fig. 3. The pancreatic cyst immediately before and after EUS-guided cyst ablation. Initially, 10 mL of cyst fluid was aspirated. This was followed by injection and re-aspiration of 10 mL of 100% ethanol over 5 minutes. This mixture was removed and a total of 10 mL of paclitaxel was injected and left in place. No complications from injection occurred.

Histopathology from Surgical Resection

In published series, surgery has generally been performed after cyst ablation for the following reasons: (1) persistent cyst by follow-up imaging studies, (2) cyst regrowth after successful ablation, (3) possible cyst-related symptoms, or (4) patient/provider preference for operative management. Histopathology after resection in these patients has shown variable degrees of cyst epithelial ablation ranging from 0% to 100% (see **Table 2**). Although a decrease in cyst size following ablation suggests successful treatment, epithelial ablation from histopathology provides the strongest evidence available of the potential efficacy of this therapy. The correlation of histopathology with imaging evidence of cyst resolution or size change is unknown.

There are important clinical implications from histologic evidence of remnant epithelial ablation after cyst ablation. First, the neoplastic potential of residual epithelium remains, and hence close observation of treated patients is required, even those in whom resolution is observed by cross-sectional imaging. Re-treatment of persistent cysts may be considered when appropriate. Second, cyst ablation with ethanol and/or paclitaxel is currently not an acceptable alternative to surgical resection in fit patients. Thus, patients with pancreatic cysts who meet accepted criteria for surgical resection should be offered surgery rather than cyst ablation.

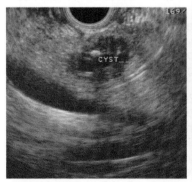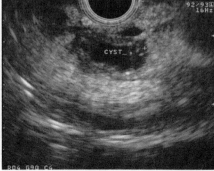

Fig. 4. Linear EUS 3 months after initial cyst ablation with the cyst now measuring 15 × 8 mm in maximal diameter. The cyst wall measures 3.5 mm in thickness and mural calcifications are visible. Repeat ablation with ethanol (2 mL) and paclitaxel (2 mL) was performed without complications.

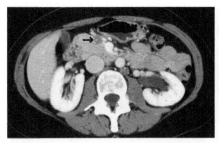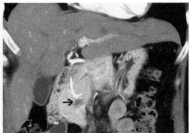

Fig. 5. Axial and coronal dual phase CT scan 6 months after the second ablation. Three-dimensional measurements showed only 1% of the original cyst volume remains (*black arrows*), which is consistent with complete ablation.

SUMMARY AND FUTURE DIRECTIONS

Pancreatic cysts represent a wide spectrum of invariably benign to precancerous and malignant neoplasms. Surgical resection, when appropriate, is curable for benign lesions such as MCNs but is associated with rare mortality and frequent morbidity. EUS-guided pancreatic cyst ablation with ethanol and/or paclitaxel offers a nonoperative treatment for patients refusing or not eligible for surgery. Studies to date have documented that cyst ablation is relatively safe and can lead to image-defined cyst resolution in up to two-thirds of patients. Histopathology after resection in these patients has shown variable degrees of cyst epithelial ablation ranging from 0% to 100%. Future research investigating the safety of this procedure, modifications of reported ablation techniques, choice and number of the lavage agents used, and the criteria to optimize selection of the appropriate pancreatic cysts for treatment is needed.

REFERENCES

1. Al-Haddad M, Schmidt MC, Sandrasegaran K, et al. Diagnosis and treatment of cystic pancreatic tumors. Clin Gastroenterol Hepatol 2011;9:635–48.
2. Reddy RP, Smyrk TC, Zapiach M, et al. Pancreatic mucinous cystic neoplasm defined by ovarian stroma: demographics, clinical features, and prevalence of cancer. Clin Gastroenterol Hepatol 2004;2:1026–31.
3. D'Angelica M, Brennan MF, Suriawinata AA, et al. Intraductal papillary mucinous neoplasms of the pancreas: an analysis of clinicopathologic features and outcome. Ann Surg 2004;239:400–8.
4. Lee KS, Sekhar A, Rofsky NM, et al. Prevalence of incidental pancreatic cysts in the adult population on MR imaging. Am J Gastroenterol 2010;105:2079–84.
5. de Jong K, Nio CY, Hermans JJ, et al. High prevalence of pancreatic cysts detected by screening magnetic resonance imaging examinations. Clin Gastroenterol Hepatol 2010;8:806–11.
6. Laffan TA, Horton KM, Klein AP, et al. Prevalence of unsuspected pancreatic cysts on MDCT. AJR Am J Roentgenol 2008;191:802–7.
7. Tanaka M, Tanaka M, Chari S, et al. International consensus guidelines for management of intraductal papillary mucinous neoplasms and mucinous cystic neoplasms of the pancreas. Pancreatology 2006;6:17–32.
8. Sugiyama M, Izumisato Y, Abe N, et al. Predictive factors for malignancy in intraductal papillary-mucinous tumours of the pancreas. Br J Surg 2003;90:1244–9.
9. Matsumoto T, Aramaki M, Yada K, et al. Optimal management of the branch duct type intraductal papillary mucinous neoplasms of the pancreas. J Clin Gastroenterol 2003;36:261–5.

10. Khalid A, Brugge W. ACG practice guidelines for the diagnosis and management of neoplastic pancreatic cysts. Am J Gastroenterol 2007;102:2339–49.
11. Allen PJ, D'Angelica M, Gonen M, et al. A selective approach to the resection of cystic lesions of the pancreas: results from 539 consecutive patients. Ann Surg 2006;244:572–82.
12. Goh BK, Tan YM, Cheow PC, et al. Cystic lesions of the pancreas: an appraisal of an aggressive resectional policy adopted at a single institution during 15 years. Am J Surg 2006;192:148–54.
13. Horvath KD, Chabot JA. An aggressive resectional approach to cystic neoplasms of the pancreas. Am J Surg 1999;178:269–74.
14. Galanis C, Zamani A, Cameron JL, et al. Resected serous cystic neoplasms of the pancreas: a review of 158 patients with recommendations for treatment. J Gastrointest Surg 2007;11:820–6.
15. Kiely JM, Nakeeb A, Komorowski RA, et al. Cystic pancreatic neoplasms: enucleate or resect? J Gastrointest Surg 2003;7:890–7.
16. Pausawasdi N, Heidt D, Kwon R, et al. Long-term follow-up of patients with incidentally discovered pancreatic cystic neoplasms evaluated by endoscopic ultrasound. Surgery 2010;147:13–20.
17. Rautou PE, Lévy P, Vullierme MP, et al. Morphologic changes in branch duct intraductal papillary mucinous neoplasms of the pancreas: a midterm follow-up study. Clin Gastroenterol Hepatol 2008;6:807–14.
18. Salvia R, Crippa S, Falconi M, et al. Branch-duct intraductal papillary mucinous neoplasms of the pancreas: to operate or not to operate? Gut 2007;56:1086–90.
19. Salvia R, Partelli S, Crippa S, et al. Intraductal papillary mucinous neoplasms of the pancreas with multifocal involvement of branch ducts. Am J Surg 2009;198: 709–14.
20. Tanno S, Nakano Y, Nishikawa T, et al. Natural history of branch duct intraductal papillary-mucinous neoplasms of the pancreas without mural nodules: long-term follow-up results. Gut 2008;57:339–43.
21. Kang MJ, Jang JY, Kim SJ, et al. Cyst growth rate predicts malignancy in patients with branch duct intraductal papillary mucinous neoplasms. Clin Gastroenterol Hepatol 2011;9:87–93.
22. Sawai Y, Yamao K, Bhatia V, et al. Development of pancreatic cancers during long-term follow-up of side-branch intraductal papillary mucinous neoplasms [erratum in Endoscopy 2011;43:79]. Endoscopy 2010;42:1077–84.
23. Gelczer RK, Charboneau JW, Hussain S, et al. Complications of percutaneous ethanol ablation. J Ultrasound Med 1998;17:531–3.
24. Xiao YY, Tian JL, Li JK, et al. CT-guided percutaneous chemical ablation of adrenal neoplasms. AJR Am J Roentgenol 2008;190:105–10.
25. Bartolozzi C, Lencioni R. Ethanol injection for the treatment of hepatic tumours. Eur Radiol 1996;6:682–96.
26. Larssen TB, Jensen DK, Viste A, et al. Single-session alcohol sclerotherapy in symptomatic benign hepatic cysts. Long-term results. Acta Radiol 1999;40: 636–8.
27. Yang CF, Liang HL, Pan HB, et al. Single-session prolonged alcohol-retention sclerotherapy for large hepatic cysts. AJR Am J Roentgenol 2006;187:940–3.
28. Hanna RM, Dahniya MH. Aspiration and sclerotherapy of symptomatic simple renal cysts: value of two injections of a sclerosing agent. AJR Am J Roentgenol 1996;167:781–3.
29. Mohsen T, Gomha MA. Treatment of symptomatic simple renal cysts by percutaneous aspiration and ethanol sclerotherapy. BJU Int 2005;96:1369–72.

30. Monzani F, Del Guerra P, Caraccio N, et al. Percutaneous ethanol injection therapy of autonomous nodule and amiodarone-induced thyrotoxicosis. Thyroidology 1994;6:99–102.
31. Fukumoto K, Kojima T, Tomonari H, et al. Ethanol injection sclerotherapy for Baker's cyst, thyroglossal duct cyst, and branchial cleft cyst. Ann Plast Surg 1994;33:615–9.
32. Kinoshita Y, Shimada T, Murakami Y, et al. Ethanol sclerosis can be a safe and useful treatment for pericardial cyst. Clin Cardiol 1996;19:833–5.
33. Akhan O, Baykan Z, Oguzkurt L, et al. Percutaneous treatment of a congenital splenic cyst with alcohol: a new therapeutic approach. Eur Radiol 1997;7:1067–70.
34. Rowinsky EK, Donehower RC. Paclitaxel (Taxol). N Engl J Med 1995;332:1004–14.
35. Gan SI, Thompson CC, Lauwers GY, et al. Ethanol lavage of pancreatic cystic lesions: initial pilot study. Gastrointest Endosc 2005;61:746–52.
36. Oh HC, Seo DW, Lee TY, et al. New treatment for cystic tumors of the pancreas: EUS guided ethanol lavage with paclitaxel injection. Gastrointest Endosc 2008;67:636–42.
37. Oh HC, Seo DW, Kim SC, et al. Septated cystic tumors of the pancreas: is it possible to treat them by endoscopic ultrasonography-guided intervention? Scand J Gastroenterol 2009;44:242–7.
38. DeWitt J, McGreevy K, Schmidt CM, et al. Endoscopic ultrasound-guided ethanol versus saline lavage for pancreatic cysts: a randomized double blinded study. Gastrointest Endosc 2009;70:710–23.
39. DeWitt J, DiMaio CJ, Brugge WR. Long-term follow-up of pancreatic cysts that resolve radiologically after EUS-guided ethanol ablation. Gastrointest Endosc 2010;72:862–6.
40. Oh HC, Seo DW, Song TJ, et al. Endoscopic ultrasonography-guided ethanol lavage with paclitaxel injection treats patients with pancreatic cysts. Gastroenterology 2011;140:172–9.
41. Dimaio CJ, Dewitt JM, Brugge WR. Ablation of pancreatic cystic lesions: the use of multiple endoscopic ultrasound-guided ethanol lavage sessions. Pancreas 2011;40:664–8.
42. Fernández-Del Castillo C. EUS treatment of pancreatic cysts: let's keep the alcohol (and the chemotherapy) locked in the cupboard. Gastroenterology 2011;140:2144–5.
43. DeWitt JM, Al-Haddad MA, Sherman S, et al. Endoscopic ultrasound guided pancreatic cyst ablation with ethanol and paclitaxel: will it also work in the Western Hemisphere? Gastrointest Endosc 2011;73:AB173.

EUS-Guided Vascular Access and Therapy

Frank Weilert, MD[a], Kenneth F. Binmoeller, MD[b],*

KEYWORDS

- Endoscopic ultrasound • Vascular access
- Gastrointestinal bleeding

INTRODUCTION

Endoscopic ultrasound (EUS) has developed since the 1980s from a niche tool to an interventional platform that intersects traditional boundaries between interventional radiology and minimally invasive surgery. It has become an essential skill for interventional endoscopists of the twenty-first century. This is exemplified in the developments of pseudocyst drainage and celiac neurolysis that are now well established as key interventions.

Vascular access and therapy are emerging as new targets for EUS-guided interventions. Most major thoracic and abdominal vessels serve as landmarks that guide routine diagnostic and therapeutic EUS procedures. The proximity of these vessels to the gastrointestinal (GI) tract could provide a preferred port of entry into the vascular tree rather than that of traditional femoral, jugular, or subclavian access performed by interventional radiologists.

EUS provides the perfect combination of real-time imaging and minimally invasive interventional endoscopy capabilities. Development of the radial scanning echoendoscope in the 1980s enabled detailed visualization of structures within and outside the GI wall. Real-time visualization of a needle as it is advanced into the target area for biopsy or injection became possible with the advent of the curved linear array (CLA) echoendoscope in the 1990s.

Vessels have been a target for therapy by interventional radiology for several decades. Refractory GI bleeding is treated by selective angiographic embolization. Transjugular intrahepatic portosystemic shunt (TIPSS) is widely used for refractory bleeding esophageal or gastroesophageal varices (GV) associated with portal hypertension.[1,2] Placement of endovascular grafts is mainstream and the first reports of transaortic valve implantation have emerged.[3] EUS offers an attractive alternative approach to vascular therapy of vessels in close proximity to the GI tract. Major

[a] Peter Stokes Endoscopy Unit, Waikato District Health Board, Waikato Hospital, Pembroke Street, Hamilton 3200, New Zealand; [b] Paul May and Frank Stein Interventional Endoscopy Services, California Pacific Medical Center, Suite 600, Stanford Building, San Francisco, CA 94115, USA
* Corresponding author.
E-mail address: binmoek@sutterhealth.org

Gastrointest Endoscopy Clin N Am 22 (2012) 303–314
doi:10.1016/j.giec.2012.04.019
1052-5157/12/$ – see front matter © 2012 Elsevier Inc. All rights reserved.

vascular structures, including the heart, aorta, celiac axis, portal vein (PV), hepatic veins (HVs), and mesenteric vessels, and aberrant vascular shunts, such as spenorenal shunts associated with portal hypertension, are easily identified. Even smaller vascular structures, such as the gastroduodenal artery, splenic vessels, hepatic artery, and PV branches, can be confidently traced and identified.

NONVARICEAL GASTROINTESTINAL BLEEDING

Endoscopic techniques for nonvariceal GI bleeding effectively treat the majority of the more than 400,000 hospitalizations per year[4,5] with well-established therapeutic interventions, such as injection of epinephrine,[6–8] thermal contact therapy,[9–12] and mechanical hemostasis with clip[13] and band ligation.[14] EUS-guided vascular therapy was first reported in a case series of 5 patients with refractory bleeding from hemosuccus pancreaticus, a Dieulafoy lesion, duodenal ulceration, and GI stromal tumor.[15] These patients had presented with at least 3 bleeding episodes and required multiple units of packed red blood cells and repeated endoscopic and vascular therapies, which were ineffective. EUS-guided injection therapy of absolute alcohol and/or cyanoacrylate (CYA) was delivered directly into the bleeding vessels. Real-time monitoring by Doppler ultrasound was used to conclude the injection therapy when no visible flow could be seen in the bleeding vessel. Control of the bleeding source was achieved in all of these refractory cases without any complications.

ESOPHAGEAL VARICEAL BLEEDING

Endoscopic band ligation is well established as the preferred technique for primary and secondary therapy of esophageal varices.[16–18] Injection of sclerosants[19] has been used as rescue therapy. Recurrence is seen in 15% to 65%[20,21] and thought to be secondary to failure to treat perforating veins and collateral vessels that feed esophageal varices.[22,23] Krige and colleagues[24] found a correlation between the number of endoscopic sclerotherapy sessions required to achieve eradication and the presence of collaterals. EUS enables the visualization and targeting of perforating veins and collaterals for sclerotherapy.[23,25,26] Lahoti and colleagues[27] first reported the use of EUS-guided endoscopic sclerotherapy to achieve variceal obliteration. The sclerosant was injected into the esophageal varices, directed at the perforating vessels until flow was completely impeded. All 5 treated patients achieved variceal obliteration after an average of 2.2 sessions. No recurrent bleeding was reported after a mean follow-up period of 15 months. De Paulo and colleagues[28] reported a randomized controlled trial of 50 patients comparing endoscopic sclerotherapy and EUS-guided sclerotherapy of esophageal collateral veins. They found similar numbers of sessions to achieve obliteration and similar rebleeding rates, but rebleeding was significantly associated with the presence of collateral vessels. A larger randomized trial is needed to determine the potential benefit of EUS-guided sclerotherapy of esophageal varices.

GASTRIC VARICEAL BLEEDING

Vascular anatomy of GV is classified into 2 types: type 1 (localized type) consists of a single varicose vessel with almost the same diameter as the inflow/outflow vein, and type 2 (diffuse type) consists of multiple varicose vessels with complex connecting ramifications.[29] GV exist in connection with esophageal varices as 2 types: gastroesophageal varices type 1 (GOV1) are found along the lesser curvature, and gastroesophageal varices type 2 (GOV2) are found at the cardia. Isolated GV (IGV) exist as 2 types: IGV1 are located in the fundus, and IGV2 are sporadic. These distinctions are important in predicting the frequency of bleeding and the response to treatment.[30]

GV are less common than esophageal varices but may be present in up to 20% of patients with portal hypertension. As many as 65% of GV bleed over 2 years.[30] Variceal ligation has performed well in esophageal varices; however, results with GV have not been favorable.[31] Sclerosants have had less success in the treatment of GV, because they are associated with a high incidence of complications, including gastric ulcerations and perforation and recurrent bleeding rates of 37% to 53%.[30,31]

Direct endoscopic CYA injection of bleeding GV, first described by Soehendra in the 1980s,[32] is widely considered first-line therapy.[33] N-butyl-2-CYA has been used in multiple case series and randomized trials with hemostasis rates of 58% to 100% and rebleeding rates of 0% to 40%.[16] Rengstorff and Binmoeller[34] reported on the use of 2-octyl-CYA in 25 patients with GV with similar hemostasis rates and a 4% rebleeding rate over 11 months.

The major and most serious complication of CYA therapy is systemic embolization. This is well described in individual case reports, including fatal cerebral infarct (**Table 1**).[35] Entrapment of the needle in the varix by glue[36,37] and damage to scope have also been reported. The injection technique, including the injection volume and the ratio of the Histoacryl/Lipiodol mixture, was standardized by Soehendra and colleagues[32,38] based on vitro studies and clinical experience collected in 50 initial cases treated under fluoroscopy.

Table 1 Major complications reported with CYA injection	
See et al, 1986	Cerebral embolism
Gallet et al, 1995	Cardiac embolism
D'Imperio et al, 1996	Needle stuck in varix, embolism
Shim et al, 1996	PV and splenic vein thrombosis
Naga and Foda, 1997	Pulmonary embolism
Cheng et al, 1998	Splenic vein thrombosis
Tsokos et al, 1998	Pulmonary embolism
Rösch, 1998	Pulmonary, cerebral, coronary embolism
Battaglia et al, 2000	Visceral fistula formation
Irisawa et al, 2000	Left renal vein thrombosis
Lo et al, 2000	Bleeding ulcer, sepsis
Hwang et al, 2001	Pulmonary embolism
Türler et al, 2001	Pulmonary embolism, sepsis
Iwase et al, 2002	Bleeding ulcer
Dhiman et al, 2002	Embolism, needle stuck in varix
Tan et al, 2002	Embolism, sepsis
Greenwald et al, 2003	Pulmonary embolism
Sato et al, 2004	Splenic vein occlusion
Wahl et al, 2004	Recurrent bacteraemia
Kok et al, 2004	Bleeding ulcer, pulmonary embolism
Yu et al, 2005	Splenic artery embolism, splenic infarct

Data from Soehendra N, Nam V, Grimm H. Endoscopic obliteration of large esophagogastric varices with bucrylate. Endoscopy 1986;18:25–6.

EUS-GUIDED CYANOACRYLATE INJECTION

Delivery of CYA under EUS guidance has been previously reported[39] and has the advantage of enabling precise delivery of glue into the varix lumen. EUS also enables assessment of vessel obliteration after treatment with Doppler. This may have prognostic significance, because rebleeding risk after CYA injection has been linked to residual patency of treated varices.[40]

EUS can display the main feeding vein system, which derives from the left gastric vein trunk, posterior gastric vein, short gastric vein, or outflowing vein system[40,41] with gastrorenal shunts.[42] Romero-Castro and colleagues[43] described a small case series targeting the feeder vessel rather than the varix lumen proper, under EUS guidance. The rationale for targeting the perforating vessel was to minimize the amount of CYA needed to achieve obliteration of GV and thereby reduce the risk of embolization. The investigators targeted the perforating vein using a 1:1 mixture of N-butyl-2-CYA plus lipiodol. The lipiodol enabled fluoroscopic visualization of the injected vessel and confirmation that the feeder vessel had been accurately targeted. There was no rebleeding or complications observed. The limitation of this approach is that identification of the perforating vessel with EUS can be difficult and time consuming, as acknowledged by the investigators. Furthermore, because the perforating vessel may be afferent or efferent, contrast should be injected before treatment to determine directional flow relative to the varix.

An advantage of EUS-guided treatment is the lack of dependency on direct varix visualization. Even in the presence of retained food or blood that may obstruct the endoscopic view, the varix lumen can be accurately targeted for glue injection.

EUS-GUIDED COILING

To avoid issues with glue embolization, 2 small cases series have described deployment of commercially available stainless steel coils. Levy and colleagues[44] used a 22-gauge needle loaded with a microcoil. The stylet was used to advance the constrained coil to the tip of the needle. Once the needle was inserted into the largest (1.4-cm) varix, the stylet was further advanced to deliver the coil. Two additional coils were each placed into separate varices. Rebleeding occurred and repeat EUS therapy was recommended. At EUS, the previously treated varices were thrombosed. Two additional coils were placed into untreated varices. Romero-Castro and colleagues[45] used coils of 0.035 in diameter, 50 mm to 150 mm in length, and with diameters of 8 mm to 15 mm, deployed through a 19-gauge needle. In one patient with a large gastrorenal shunt, the investigators failed to achieve obliteration of GV despite deployment of 13 coils. The investigators subsequently delivered 9 additional coils into the perforating feeding vein. Cost becomes a consideration when using such large numbers of coils to achieve varix obliteration.

COMBINED CYANOACRYLATE INJECTION AND COILING

In an ex vivo study, the authors deployed a coil in a container of heparinized blood, followed by injection of 1 mL of CYA glue. The glue immediately adhered to the synthetic fibers on the coil and both coil and adherent glue were removed in one piece from the container. Outside the container, the glue was firmly adherent to the coil and no residual glue was identified in the container. The authors hypothesized that the deployment of a coil before CYA injection may serve as a scaffold to retain CYA at the site of injection and serve 2 potential benefits: (1) concentrating the glue at the site of coil deployment and (2) reducing (and possibly eliminating) the risk of glue embolization. Furthermore, the coil itself may contribute to varix obliteration and hemostasis.

The authors reported their first use of coil and CYA as rescue treatment after standard endoscopy-guided CYA treatment failed in a patient with massive gastric fundal variceal (GFV) bleeding.[46] They recently reported experience using a combined approach of CYA injection after deployment of a single coil in a series of 30 patients with GFV.[47] The procedure was successful in all patients, with immediate hemostasis achieved for active bleeding. The average volume of CYA (2-octyl-CYA) injected was 1.4 mL per patient after coil deployment. This was 1 mL less than the average amount injected per patient in a previous study using the same CYA injected alone.[38] There was no damage to the echoendoscope related to glue injections and no procedure-related complications. Of 24 patients with follow-up endoscopy, 23 (95.8%) had complete GFV obliteration after a single treatment session, with no intravariceal flow on EUS color Doppler imaging (**Figs. 1** and **2**). Recurrent bleeding from GFV developed in 1 patient at 21 days. This patient underwent a second successful treatment with EUS-guided coil and CYA. No patients required surgical or percutaneous shunt procedures.

A limitation of the echoendoscope is the difficulty maneuvering into retroflexion to visualize and access GFV. The gastric fundus can be well visualized, however, on EUS with the transducer positioned in the distal esophagus. The authors, therefore, elected to treat GFV from the esophagus with the echoendoscope in an orthograde position. Apart from enabling EUS-guided access to GFV, this transesophageal approach is not hindered by gastric contents, such as blood and food, which tend to accumulate in the fundus. There is also no disruption of the gastric mucosa overlying the varix, which is usually thinned and at high risk of back bleeding after varix puncture. The transesophageal approach also allows visualization of the diaphragmatic crus muscle, which is sandwiched between the esophageal and gastric fundic walls (**Fig. 3**). The crus muscle was intentionally included in the path of access to GFV (transcrural puncture), hypothesizing that the crus muscle—a thick fibromuscular bundle approximately 1 cm in thickness—acts as a stabilizing backboard to GFV.

The authors used both conventional and a prototype forward view (FV) CLA echoendoscopes for EUS-guided treatment. They found the FV-CLA instrument to have several technical advantages: (1) more perpendicular needle orientation to the target lesion; (2) uniaxis instrumentation imparting an increased forward transfer of force to the tip of the needle; (3) front-view optics that improve endoscopic visualization; and (4) accessory water jet channel for water filling and irrigation. These advantages have been previously described in other clinical applications of the FV-CLA

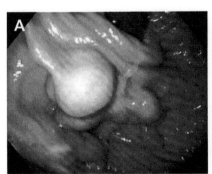 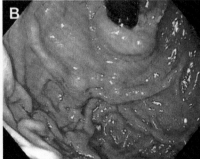

Fig. 1. Endoscopic views showing (A) large gastric fundal varices before treatment and (B) fundal varices eradicated 3 months after treatment.

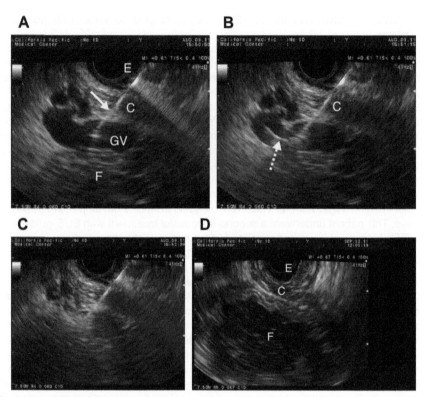

Fig. 2. Transesophageal EUS view showing (*A*) fundal varix targeted with a 19-gauge needle (*arrow*), (*B*) deployment of coil (*broken arrows*) through the 19-gauge needle, (*C*) injection of 1 mL of CYA glue through the 19-gauge needle to obliterate the varix lumen, and (*D*) eradication of fundal varices. C, crus muscle; E, esophagus; F, fundus.

echoendoscope.[48,49] The injection and deployment technique are summarized in **Box 1**. Comparative studies are needed to determine the benefit of combined CYA and coil treatment of GV over CYA alone as well as the advantages of EUS guidance over endoscopy guidance.

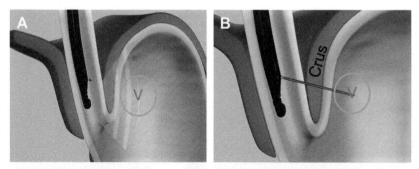

Fig. 3. Anatomic cartoon illustrating transesophageal imaging (*A*) and injector needle access (*B*) to a gastric fundal varix (V) from the distal esophagus. The CLA echoendoscope is positioned in the distal esophagus.

Box 1

Technique of EUS-guided coil and CYA treatment of GFV

1. Gastric fundus is filled with water

2. The echoendoscope is retracted to the distal esophagus to sonographically visualize the gastric fundus

3. The GFV is punctured with a fine-needle aspiration (FNA) needle using a transesophageal-transcrural approach (see **Fig. 2A**)

4. A single coil is delivered into the varix through an FNA needle using the stylet as a pusher (see **Fig. 2B**)

5. After coil deployment, 1 mL of CYA is immediately injected through the same needle, using normal saline solution to flush the glue through the catheter (see **Fig. 2C**)

6. Absence of flow in the varix is confirmed with color Doppler

7. If the varix has persistent flow, an additional 1 mL of CYA is injected.

PORTAL VEIN ANGIOGRAPHY AND PRESSURE MEASUREMENTS

PV angiography and pressure measurements can add important clinical information for the management of patients with chronic liver disease and portal hypertension. Direct transcutaneous transhepatic portal pressure measurements are not used in clinical practice, however, because of technical difficulties and the high rate of complications.[50] EUS may permit PV access, contrast injection, and monitoring the PV pressure. Magno and colleagues[51] demonstrated the feasibility and safety of EUS-guided PV puncture and angiography. Direct measurements of the PV pressure under EUS guidance was first reported by Lai and colleagues,[52] who inserted a 22-gauge FNA needle, under EUS guidance, into the extrahepatic PV and obtained pressure measurements . The investigators were not able to attain the PV pressure measurement in 15% of their animals. Such a high rate of failure was probably related to the small caliber of the FNA needle used and the difficulties in holding the needle's position inside the PV to obtain reliable continuous pressure readings. These experiments were also complicated by intraperitoneal bleeding and hematoma formation at the sites of the PV puncture.[52]

Giday and colleagues[53] performed transhepatic PV catheterization with a modified endoscopic retrograde cholangiopancreatography catheter, which allowed them to perform good-quality portal angiography and obtain continuous portal pressure readings over 1 h, with consistent results and minimal variability within each animal. The position of the catheter inside the PV was stable and was not influenced by the animal's respiratory motions or movements of the operator or endoscope. To prevent complications, the investigators performed a transhepatic puncture of the PV with the FNA needle to create a transhepatic route for catheter placement into the PV. Hepatic parenchyma surrounded the catheter was thought to tamponade the track after catheter removal to prevent postprocedural bleeding.[53]

TRANSJUGULAR INTRAHEPATIC PORTOSYSTEMIC SHUNT

Decompression of the portal system by placement of a TIPSS is frequently used for the treatment of portal hypertension and its complications.[1] The effectiveness of TIPSS has been well documented in the treatment of acute variceal bleeding,[2,33] the prevention of recurrent variceal bleeding,[54] and the management of refractory ascites.[55] TIPSS is a widely used technique, predominantly performed by interventional radiologists, and limited to tertiary-referral centers.

Buscaglia and colleagues[56] first described EUS-guided creation of an intrahepatic portosystemic shunt (IPSS) in a live porcine model. The technique of IPSS placement was simple and straightforward: under direct EUS observation, the HV and the PV were sequentially punctured with a 19-gauge FNA needle, a guide wire was advanced through the needle into the PV, and a stent was inserted over the guide wire and deployed with its distal end inside the PV and the proximal end inside the HV. All steps of the procedure were clearly seen by EUS.

The authors' group[57] recently reported the use of a lumen-apposing stent in the endoscopic management of this disease through the creation of a transgastric IPSS. The AXIOS (Xlumena, Mountain View, CA, USA) is a fully coated, dual-flanged metal stent constrained in a 10.5F delivery catheter. When expanded, the flange and body diameters measure 10 mm and 4 mm, respectively. The length of the AXIOS is 8 mm. A therapeutic 3.7-mm working channel echoendoscope was advanced into the stomach of 5 healthy animals and used to locate the PV and inferior vena cava (IVC). A 0.035 guide wire was advanced and placed into the PV. The needle was then exchanged for the AXIOS delivery catheter. The distal anchor flange (lower arrow) of the AXIOS was deployed in the PV and the proximal anchor flange (upper arrow) was deployed in the IVC (**Fig. 4**A). Gross necropsy on all animals confirmed stent placement between the PV and IVC and no evidence of tissue injury or hematoma (see **Fig. 4**B).

MICROCOIL EMBOLIZATION

Interventional radiologists have performed selective embolization of the right branch of the PV to produce compensatory hypertrophy of the left hepatic lobe in patients undergoing right hepatectomy. Preliminary results in an animal model[58] suggest EUS-guided coil embolization of the right PV can produce the intended hypertrophy of the left hepatic lobe. Matthes and colleagues[59] reported on the injection of the polymer (Enteryx) into the main PV, to occlude the vessel. These anecdotal reports in the animal model support a role for EUS-guided delivery of different devices or compounds to occlude small and large vessels. Further studies are needed to determine the potential benefit over percutaneous approaches.

ACCESS TO THE HEART

The proximity of the heart to the esophagus lends itself to EUS-guided intervention. Fritscher-Ravens and colleagues[60] described EUS-guided puncture of the heart. In porcine studies, an FNA needle could be introduced repeatedly into the left atrium, followed by the injection of saline. Reaching the aortic valve was thought to be more

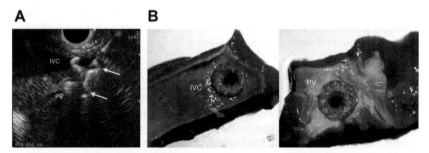

Fig. 4. (A) EUS view showing placement of dual-flanged metal stent (arrows) across IVC and PV and (B) necropsy specimen confirming lumen apposing stent positioning across IVC and PV.

difficult because of the moving target, but ablation therapy was thought technically possible. The coronary artery was successfully punctured in several of the animals. No significant injury was observed in 2 acute and 6 survival animals. The investigators also reported EUS-guided pericardial fluid aspiration in 3 patients and puncture of a left atrial mass in a third patient.

HURDLES TO DISSEMINATION OF EUS-GUIDED VASCULAR THERAPY

EUS is becoming increasingly available throughout the United States, Europe, and Asia. Specific training programs are still limited in number, however, and variable in content. Some endoscopic societies are setting specific training requirements for EUS training (Conjoint Committee for Endoscopy Training in Australia and New Zealand) whereas others leave these to specific training institutions.[61] Competency in interventional EUS will continue to require training and mentorship in a high-volume tertiary interventional endoscopy unit. The generation of high-quality data in a research environment is necessary to validate and standardize procedures.

SUMMARY

The GI tract provides a unique window to access vascular structures in the mediastinum and abdomen. The advent of interventional EUS has enabled access to these structures with a standard FNA needle. Sclerosants, CYA, and, more recently, coils can be delivered through the lumen of an FNA needle. EUS-guided treatment of varices has been largely reserved as rescue therapy for refractory bleeding but has theoretic advantages over conventional endoscopy-guided treatment. Controlled studies are needed to determine the role of EUS-guided treatment for primary and secondary prevention of variceal bleeding. There is a growing list of novel indications for EUS-guided vascular therapy that require further study. Data are still limited and multicenter, prospective controlled trials are needed to show clinical effectiveness and safety in humans. The development of new tools designed for EUS-guided vascular therapy is needed.

REFERENCES

1. Colombato L. The role of transjugular intrahepatic portosystemic shunt (TIPS) in the management of portal hypertension. J Clin Gastroenterol 2007;41:S344–51.
2. Boyer T, Haskal Z, AASLD practice guideline. The role of transjugular intrahepatic portosystemic shunt in the management of portal hypertension. Hepatology 2005;41:1–15.
3. Webb J, Cribier A. Percutaneous transarterial aortic valve implantation. Eur Heart J 2011;32:140–7.
4. Longstreth G. Epidemiology and outcome of patients hospitalized with acute lower gastrointestinal hemorrhage: a population-based study. Am J Gastroenterol 1997;92:419–24.
5. Longstreth G. Epidemiology of hospitalization for acute upper gastrointestinal hemorrhage: a population-based study. Am J Gastroenterol 1995;90:206–10.
6. Lin H, Hsieh Y, Tseng G. A prospective, randomized trial of large-versus small-volume endoscopic injection of epinephrine for peptic ulcer bleeding. Gastrointest Endosc 2002;55:615–9.
7. Song S, Chung J, Moon YM. Comparison of the hemostatic effect of endoscopic injection with fibrin glue and hypertonic saline-epinephrine for peptic ulcer bleeding: a prospective randomized trial. Endoscopy 1997;29:827–33.

8. Kubba A, Murphy W, Palmer KR. Endoscopic injection for bleeding peptic ulcer: a comparison of adrenaline alone with adrenaline plus human thrombin. Gastroenterology 1996;111:623–8.
9. Kanai M, Hamada A, Endo Y. Efficacy of argon plasma coagulation in nonvariceal upper gastrointestinal bleeding. Endoscopy 2004;36:1085–8.
10. Chau C, Siu W, Law B. Randomized controlled trial comparing epinephrine injection plus heat probe coagulation versus epinephrine injection plus argon plasma coagulation for bleeding peptic ulcers. Gastrointest Endosc 2003;57:455–61.
11. Jensen D, Kovacs T, Jutabha R. Randomized trial of medical or endoscopic therapy to prevent recurrent ulcer hemorrhage in patients with adherent clots. Gastroenterology 2002;123:407–13.
12. Laine L, Estrada R. Randomized trial of normal saline solution injection versus bipolar electrocoagulation for treatment of patients with high-risk bleeding ulcers: is local tamponade enough? Gastrointest Endosc 2002;55:6–10.
13. Chou Y, Hsu P, Lai K. A prospective, randomized trial of endoscopic hemoclip placement and distilled water injection for treattment of high-risk bleeding ulcers. Gastrointest Endosc 2003;57:324–8.
14. Mumtaz R, Shaukat M, Ramirez F. Outcomes of endoscopic treatment of gastroduodenal Dieulafoy's lesion with rubber band ligation and thermal/injection therapy. J Clin Gastroenterol 2003;36:310–4.
15. Levy M, Wong Kee Song L, Farnell M. Endoscopic ultrasound (EUS)-guided angiotherapy of refractory gastrointestinal bleeding. Am J Gastroenterol 2008;103: 352–9.
16. De Franchis R, Primignani M. Endoscopic treatments for portal hypertension. Semin Liver Dis 1999;19:439–55.
17. Helmy A, Hayes P. Review article: current endoscopic therapeutic options in the management of variceal bleeding. Aliment Pharmacol Ther 2001;15:575–94.
18. Marrero J, Scheiman J. Prevention of recurrent variceal bleeding: as easy as A.P.C.? Gastrointest Endosc 2002;56:600–3.
19. Asaki S. Efficacy of endoscopic pure ethanol injection method for gastrointestinal ulcer bleeding. World J Surg 2000;24:294–8.
20. Sarin S, Govil A, Jain A. Prospective randomized trial of endoscopic sclerotherapy versus variceal band ligation for esophageal varices: influence on gastropathy, gastric varices and variceal recurrence. J Hepatol 1997;26:826–32.
21. Hou M, Lin H, Lee FY, et al. Recurrence of esophageal varices following endoscopic treatment and its impact on rebleeding: comparison of sclerotherapy and ligation. J Hepatol 2000;32:202–8.
22. Irisawa A, Obara K, Bhutani M. Role of para-esophageal collateral veins in patients with portal hypertension based on the results of endoscopic ultrasonography and liver scintigraphy analysis. J Gastroenterol Hepatol 2003;18:309–14.
23. Irisawa A, Saito A, Obara K. Endoscopic recurrence of esophageal varices is associated with the specific EUS abnormalities: severe peri-esophageal collateral veins and large perforating veins. Gastrointest Endosc 2001;53:77–84.
24. Krige J, Bornman P, Goldberg P, et al. Variceal rebleeding and recurrence after endoscopic injection sclerotherapy: a prospective evaluation in 204 patients. Arch Surg 2000;135:1315–22.
25. Toyonaga A, Iwao T. Paraesophageal collaterals in endoscopic therapies for esophageal varices: good or bad? J Gastroenterol Hepatol 2001;16:489–90.
26. Konishi Y, Nakamura T, Kida H, et al. Catheter US probe EUS evaluation of gastric cardia and perigastric vascular structures to predict esophageal variceal recurrence. Gastrointest Endosc 2002;55:197–203.

27. Lahoti S, Catalano M, Alcocer E, et al. Obliteration of esophageal varices using EUS-guided sclerotherapy with color Doppler. Gastrointest Endosc 2000;51:331–3.
28. De Paulo G, Ardengh J, Nakao F, et al. Treatment of esophageal varices: a randomized controlled trial comparing endoscopic sclerotherapy and EUS-guided sclerotherapy of esophageal collateral veins. Gastrointest Endosc 2006;63:396–402.
29. Arakawa M, Masuzaki T, Okuda K. Pathomorphology of esophageal and gastric varices. Semin Liver Dis 2002;22:73–82.
30. Sarin S, Lahoti D, Saxena S. Prevalence, classification and natural history of gastric varices: a long-term follow-up study in 568 portal hypertension patients. Hepatology 1992;16:1343–9.
31. Trudeau W, Prindiville T. Endoscopic injection sclerosis in bleeding gastric varices. Gastrointest Endosc 1986;32:264–8.
32. Soehendra N, Nam V, Grimm H. Endoscopic obliteration of large esophagogastric varices with bucrylate. Endoscopy 1986;18:25–6.
33. De Franchis R. Evolving consensus in portal hypertension. Report of the Baveno IV consensus workshop on methodology of diagnosis and therapy in portal hypertension. J Hepatol 2005;43:167–76.
34. Rengstorff D, Binmoeller K. A pilot study of 2-octyl cyanoacrylate injection for treatment of gastric fundal varices in humans. Gastrointest Endosc 2004;59:553–8.
35. Seewald S, Leong T, Imazu H, et al. A standardized injection technique and regimen ensures success and safety of N-butyl-2-cyanoacrylate injection for the treatment of gastric fundal varices. Gastrointest Endosc 2008;68:447–54.
36. Dhiman R, Chawla Y, Taneja S. Endoscopic sclerotherapy of gastric variceal bleeding with N-butyl-2-cyanoacrylate. J Clin Gastroenterol 2002;35:222–7.
37. Bhasin D, Sharma B, Prasad H. Endoscopic removal of sclerotherapy needle from gastric varix after N-butyl-2-cyanoacrylate injection. Gastrointest Endosc 2000;51:497–8.
38. Soehendra N, Grimm H, Nam V. [10 years experience with endoscopic sclerotherapy of esophagogastric varices]. Chirurgie 1989;60:594–8 [in German].
39. Lee Y, Chan F, Ng E, et al. EUS-guided injection of cyanoacrylate for bleeding gastric varices. Gastrointest Endosc 2000;52:168–74.
40. Iwase H, Suga S, Morise K. Color Doppler endoscopic ultrasonography for the evaluation of gastric varices and endoscopic obliteration with cyanoacrylate glue. Gastrointest Endosc 1995;41:150–4.
41. Hino S, Kakutani H, Ikeda H. Hemodynamic analysis of esophageal varices using color Doppler endoscopic ultrasonography to predict recurrence after endoscopic treatment. Endoscopy 2001;33:869–72.
42. Kakutani H, Hino S, Ikeda K. Use of the curved linear-array echo endoscope to identify gastrorenal shunts in patients with gastric fundal varices. Endoscopy 2004;36:710–4.
43. Romero-Castro R, Pellicer-Bautista F, Jimenez-Saenz M. EUS-guided injection of cyanoacrylate in perforating feeding veins in gastric varices: results in 5 cases. Gastrointest Endosc 2007;66:402–7.
44. Levy M, Wong Kee Song L, Kendrick M. EUS-guided coil embolization for refractory ectopic variceal bleeding. Gastrointest Endosc 2008;67:572.
45. Romero-Castro R, Pellicer-Bautista F, Giovannini M. Endoscopic ultrasound (EUS)-guided coil embolization therapy in gastric varices. Endoscopy 2010; 42(Suppl 2):E35–6.
46. Sanchez-Yague A, Shah J, Nguyen-Tang T. EUS-guided coil embolization of gastric varices after unsuccessful endoscopic glue injection. Gastrointest Endosc 2009;69:AB6.

47. Binmoeller K, Weilert F, Shah J, et al. EUS-guided transesophageal treatment of gastric fundal varices with combined coiling and cyanoacrylate glue injection. Gastrointest Endosc 2011;74(5):1019–25.
48. Nguyen-Tang T, Shah J, Sanchez-Yague A. Use of the front-view forward-array echoendoscope to evaluate right colonic subepithelial lesions. Gastrointest Endosc 2010;72:606–10.
49. Binmoeller K. Optimizing interventional EUS: the echoendoscope in evolution. Gastrointest Endosc 2007;66:917–9.
50. Armonis A, Patch D, Burroughs A. Hepatic venous pressure measurement: an old test as a new prognostic marker in cirrhosis? Hepatology 1997;25:245–8.
51. Magno P, Ko C, Buscaglia J. EUS-guided angiography: a novel approach to diagnostic and therapeutic interventions in the vascular system. Gastrointest Endosc 2007;66:587–91.
52. Lai L, Poneros J, Santilli J. EUS-guided portal vein catheterization and pressure measurement in an animal model: a pilot study of feasibility. Gastrointest Endosc 2004;59:280–3.
53. Giday S, Clarke J, Buscaglia J, et al. EUS-guided portal vein catheterization: a promising novel approach for portal angiography and portal vein pressure measurements. Gastrointest Endosc 2008;67:338–42.
54. D'Amico G, Pagliaro L, Bosch J. The treatment of portal hypertension: a meta-analytic view. Hepatology 1995;22:332–53.
55. Gines P, Uriz J, Calahorra B. Transjugular intrahepatic portosystemic shunt versus repeated paracentesis plus intravenous albumin for refractory ascites in cirrhosis. A multicenter randomized comparative study. Gastroenterology 2002; 123:1839–47.
56. Buscaglia J, Dray X, Shin E, et al. A new alternative for a transjugular intrahepatic portosystemic shunt: EUS-guided creation of an intrahepatic portosystemic shunt (with video). Gastrointest Endosc 2009;69:941–7.
57. Binmoeller K, Shah J. EUS-guided transgastric intrahepatic portosystemic shunt using the axios stent. Gastrointest Endosc 2011;73:AB167.
58. Vazquez-Sequeiros E, Foruny Olcina J. Endoscopic ultrasound guided vascular access and therapy: a promising indication. World J Gastrointest Endosc 2010; 2(6):198–202.
59. Matthes K, Sahani D, Holalkere N, et al. Feasibility of endoscopic ultrasound-guided portal vein embolization with Enteryx. Acta Gastroenterol Belg 2005;68: 412–5.
60. Fritscher-Ravens A, Ganbari A, Mosse C. Transesophageal endoscopic ultrasound-guided access to the heart. Endoscopy 2007;39:385–9.
61. Conjoint Committee for the Recognition of Training in GastroIntestinal Endoscopy (CCRTGE). Available at: http://conjoint.gesa.org.au/information.html. Accessed May 1, 2012.

Endoscopic Ultrasound-Guided Antitumor Agents

Yousuke Nakai, MD, PhD[a,b], Kenneth J. Chang, MD[a],*

KEYWORDS

- Drug delivery • Endoscopic ultrasound • Fine needle aspiration
- Pancreatic cancer

RATIONALE

The development of linear-array endoscopic ultrasound (EUS) scan, with its real-time guidance of needle advancement, changed EUS from a diagnostic procedure to an interventional procedure. EUS-guided fine needle aspiration has been established as a tissue acquisition method[1–3] and application of this technique to variable interventional procedures is increasingly reported, such as drainage of pseudocyst[4–7] or biliary tract[8–10] and injection of drugs. Celiac plexus or ganglion neurolysis for pain control in pancreatic diseases[11,12] and botulinum toxin injection in achalasia[13] are the 2 major current EUS-guided fine-needle injection (EUS-FNI) procedures. Because EUS-FNI has demonstrated its feasibility and safety in the delivery of medication, this procedure has attracted attention as a method of antitumor-agent delivery as well as radioactive seeds[14–16] and fiducial markers.[17,18] This strategy can be applied to any organ within the reach of EUS. However, EUS-FNI greatly affects pancreatic cancer for 2 reasons: its anatomic location and the dismal prognosis of this cancer. Various organs and major vessels surrounding the pancreas make access to the pancreas difficult, but EUS provides better access than other modalities such as computed tomography (CT). Despite extensive basic and clinical research, the prognosis of pancreatic cancer is still dismal, and surgical resection still represents the only possibility of cure. In patients with advanced pancreatic cancer with distant metastasis, systemic chemotherapy or palliation is the standard of care (SOC). In patients with locally advanced or borderline resectable pancreatic cancer, aggressive downstaging of the tumor with neoadjuvant chemoradiation therapy can lead to a better chance of R0 resection and better survival. However, the response to antitumor agents in pancreatic cancer is limited because of

[a] Division of Gastroenterology and Hepatology, H.H. Chao Comprehensive Digestive Disease Center, University of California, Irvine, 101 The City Drive, Orange, CA 92868, USA; [b] Department of Gastroenterology, Graduate School of Medicine, The University of Tokyo, 7-3-1 Hongo Bunkyo-ku, Tokyo 113-8655, Japan
* Corresponding author.
E-mail address: kchang@uci.edu

Gastrointest Endoscopy Clin N Am 22 (2012) 315–324
doi:10.1016/j.giec.2012.04.014
1052-5157/12/$ – see front matter © 2012 Elsevier Inc. All rights reserved.

poor drug delivery resulting from abundant desmoplasia and the hypovascular nature of the tumor. By injecting the antitumor agent directly into the tumor under EUS guidance, these hurdles can be overcome less invasively.

Another target for EUS-guided antitumor delivery is neuroendocrine tumor (NET). Pancreatic NET is less aggressive and can be cured by surgery, but some patients who are not eligible for pancreatic surgery because of their age or comorbidity can benefit from local therapy with EUS-FNI using alcohol as well as placement of radioactive seeds for brachytherapy and placement of fiducial marker for image-guided radiation therapy.

The following is a literature review of EUS-guided antitumor agents.

CURRENT LITERATURE
Cytoimplant

The authors reported their first phase I trial of EUS-guided injection of allogenic mixed lymphocyte culture (cytoimplant) in patients with advanced pancreatic cancer.[19] The strategy of cytoimplant is that cytokine production directly within a tumor can induce its regression by host antitumor effector mechanisms, and it is a well-established fact that mixed lymphocyte culture results in the release of cytokines and the activation of immune effector cells.

Eight patients with unresectable adenocarcinoma of the pancreas were enrolled to evaluate the safety and feasibility: 4 patients in stage II, 3 in stage III, and 1 in stage IV. EUS-guided single injection of cytoimplants was performed in escalating doses of 3, 6, or 9 billion cells, using a 22-guage FNA needle. After localizing the tumor on EUS, the needle was advanced through the bulk of the tumor by real-time EUS guidance. After a well was created with the needle, the needle was slowly withdrawn while the cytoimplant was simultaneously injected in a slow steady fashion. There were no procedure-related complications. There were no bone marrow, hemorrhagic, infectious, renal, cardiac, and pulmonary toxicities. There were 3 transient grade 3 gastrointestinal toxicities, and 3 patients had transient episodes of hyperbilirubinemia that were reversed by the replacement of biliary stents. Seven of 8 patients (86%) experienced low-grade fever that responded to acetaminophen, and fever was resolved within the first 4 weeks. No patient had procedure-induced pancreatitis, and toxicities were not dose related. Of the 8 patients enrolled, there were 2 patients with partial responses and 1 patient with minor response, with a median survival of 13.2 months. There was no obvious correlation between tumor response and survival. With the injection of cytoimplant and the proposed immunologic reaction, the tumor volume on imaging studies may hypothetically remain unchanged or increase despite the reduction of malignant cells. Although this was a study with a small sample size and a subsequent multicenter randomized trial of EUS-guided cytoimplant injection versus conventional chemotherapy was terminated because of negative results in the interim analysis, this phase I study first demonstrated the feasibility of EUS-FNI as a delivery method of antitumor agent.

GENE THERAPY
ONYX-015

ONYX-015 (dl1520) is an E1B-55kD gene-deleted replication-selective adenovirus that preferentially replicates in and kills malignant cells. A phase I trial of injection of ONYX-015 into locally advanced pancreatic cancer was performed under CT guidance (n = 22). The treatment was well tolerated without significant virus-related toxicity.[20] Although objective responses were not demonstrated, 6 minor responses of injected tumors were reported. However, repeated intratumoral injection of ONYX-015 under CT guidance is cumbersome. In addition, a single needle pass is insufficient for the spread of adenovirus throughout the pancreatic cancer with significant amounts of fibrosis. Subsequently, a phase I/II trial was performed under EUS guidance.[21] The feasibility, tolerability, and efficacy of EUS injection of ONYX-015 into unresectable pancreatic carcinomas were evaluated in 21 patients. Patients underwent 8 sessions of ONYX-015 delivered by EUS injection into the primary pancreatic tumor over 8 weeks. The final 4 treatments were given in combination with gemcitabine (intravenous [IV], 1000 mg/m^2). Patients received 2×10^{10} (n = 3) or 2×10^{11} (n = 18) virus particles/treatment. No objective responses were demonstrated on day 35 after 4 injections of ONYX-015 as a single agent. After combination treatment with virus plus gemcitabine, objective partial regressions of 50% were seen in 2 patients (10%). There was no clinical pancreatitis despite mild, transient elevations in lipase levels in a minority of patients, but 2 patients had sepsis before the institution of prophylactic oral antibiotics. Two patients had duodenal perforations from the endoscope tip. No perforations occurred after the protocol was changed to transgastric injections.

TNFerade

TNFerade was constructed as a second-generation adenovector, which expresses the complementary DNA (cDNA) encoding human tumor necrosis factor (TNF). To further optimize local effectiveness and minimize systemic toxicity, the radiation-inducible immediate response early growth response (Egr) -1 promoter was placed upstream of the transcriptional start site of the human TNF cDNA. This vector was engineered to ensure that maximal gene expression and subsequent TNF secretion are constrained in space and time by radiation therapy. Human clinical trials have been performed in pancreatic, esophageal, and rectal cancers.

In patients with pancreatic cancer, long-term results of phase I/II study of EUS or percutaneous transabdominal delivery of TNFerade with chemoradiation were reported in patients with locally advanced pancreatic cancer.[22] Five-week treatment consisted of weekly injections of 4×10^9, 4×10^{10}, 4×10^{11}, and 1×10^{12} particle units (PU) TNFerade, continuous infusion 5-FU (200 mg/m^2/d, 5 d/wk) and 50.4 Gy radiation (1.8 Gy fractions). TNFerade was delivered with a single-needle pass by percutaneous transabdominal approach whereas up to 4 injections were given by EUS (**Figs. 1–3**).

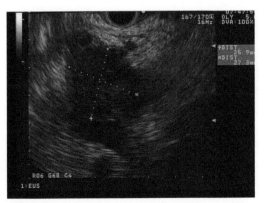

Fig. 1. A 71-year-old man with T4 cancer in the neck of pancreas. Pretreatment tumor size was 27.3 × 25.9 mm on EUS.

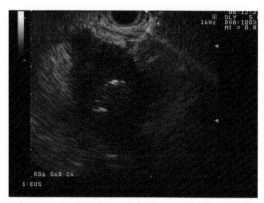

Fig. 2. EUS-FNI of TNFerade. The TNFerade was injected under real-time EUS guidance.

Fifty patients completed this dose-escalation study (n = 27 for EUS, n = 23 for PTA). Dose-limiting toxicities (DLTs) occurred in 3 EUS patients at 1×10^{12} PU (2 patients with pancreatitis, and 1 patient with cholangitis). Major grade 3 to 4 adverse events were gastrointestinal bleeding, deep vein thrombosis (DVT), pulmonary emboli, pancreatitis, and cholangitis. The median time to tumor progression was 108 days (95% confidence interval [CI], 67–198 days) and the median overall survival (OS) was 297 days (95% CI, 201–316 days). The best median survival was seen in the 4 $\times 10^{11}$ PU cohort of 332 days (95% CI, 154–316 days). Seven patients underwent surgical resection some time after treatment, and 6 had negative surgical margins. One patient had a complete pathologic response. Given the high rate of pathologically negative surgical resection after downstaging, this treatment seemed to be promising.

Subsequently, a phase II/III randomized controlled trial of SOC (chemoradiation therapy) with and without TNFerade was conducted. The authors' single center experience of this trial demonstrated longer OS in 20 patients treated by SOC with TNFerade compared with 9 patients treated by SOC alone (14.7 vs 11.1 months, P = .022).[23] However, the final results of this phase II/III study did not show superiority by addition of TNFerade (abstract submitted to ASCO annual meeting 2012). Median OS for TNFerade was 10.1 (95% CI, 9.1–11.7) months, compared with 10.0 (95% CI,

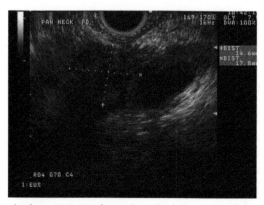

Fig. 3. EUS at 4 weeks from EUS-FNI showed marked decrease of the tumor size (17.8 × 14.6 mm).

7.6–11.2) months for SOC. However, a subgroup analysis showed patients with T1 to T3 tumors and cancer antigen (CA) 19-9 U/mL levels less than 1000 had a longer survival with the addition of TNFerade (10.9 vs 9.0 months; $P = .04$). Thus, patient selection is especially important with this therapy. The most appropriate patients seem to be those with borderline resectable, locally advanced tumors.

In locally advanced esophageal cancer, a multicenter phase I dose-escalating trial of intratumoral injection of TNFerade with chemoradiotherapy was performed.[24] Five weekly injections of TNFerade, dose-escalated logarithmically from 4×10^8 to 4×10^{11} PU, were given in combination with cisplatin 75 mg/m^2 and 5-FU 1000 mg/m^2/day IV for 96 hours on days 1 and 29, and concurrent radiotherapy (RT) to 45Gy. Surgery was performed 9 to 15 weeks after treatment. Six patients (29%) had pathologic complete response, observed among 21 patients. Dose-limiting toxicities were not observed. The most frequent potentially related adverse events were fatigue (54%), fever (38%), nausea (29%), vomiting (21%), esophagitis (21%), and chills (21%). At the top dose of 4×10^{11} PU, 5 out of 8 patients developed thromboembolic events. The median OS was 47.8 months. The 3- and 5-year OS and disease-free survival were 54% and 41%, and 38% and 38%, respectively. These results, especially the long-term prognosis, are encouraging and warrant further study (randomized control trial).

A pilot study of TNFerade with capecitabine and radiation therapy as neoadjuvant chemoradiation therapy[25] was performed in 9 patients with T3, T4, or N1 rectal cancer. Patients received RT to a total dose of 50.4 to 54 Gy in combination with capecitabine 937.5 mg/m^2 orally twice a day. TNFerade at a dose of 4×10^{10} PU was injected into the rectal tumor on the first day of RT and weekly for a total of 5 injections. Surgery was performed 5 to 10 weeks after the completion of chemoradiation. Grade 3 hematologic toxicity was observed in 2 patients. Eight patients completed all treatments. Discontinuation of treatment was necessary in 1 patient with grade 3 hematologic toxicity concurrent with ileitis. One grade 2 catheter-associated thrombosis was observed, but there were no other thrombotic events. There was no toxicity directly attributable to FNI procedure. A complete pathologic response was observed in 2 of 9 patients. This study confirmed the feasibility of EUS-FNI of antitumor agents in rectal cancer.

ONCOGEL

OncoGel[26] is a combination of the chemotherapeutic drug paclitaxel and ReGel (MacroMed Inc, Salt Lake City, UT, USA), a thermosensitive, controlled-release delivery system. ReGel is a triblock copolymer comprising poly(D,L lactide-co-glycolide) (PLGA) and polyethylene glycol (PEG) with the basic structure of PLGA–PEG–PLGA. ReGel is transformed from a water-soluble polymer to a water-insoluble biodegradable hydrogel at body temperature. Paclitaxel was selected as an ideal drug for local anticancer therapy based on its compatibility with ReGel. After intratumoral injection, Oncogel releases paclitaxel continuously into the adjacent tissue for up to 6 weeks.

EUS-guided FNI of Oncogel into the pancreas was reported in animal studies. In the first study,[27] OncoGel was injected under EUS guidance into the tail of the pancreas of 3 pigs, using a 22-gauge needle. The animals were monitored for 4 to 5 days after the injection, and no signs of pancreatitis were observed clinically. A depot of OncoGel was observed both grossly and histologically. There was no evidence of extravasation of OncoGel out of the pancreas, and cross–sectional histologic studies demonstrated the depot but no evidence of pancreatitis. In the second study,[28] tissue paclitaxel concentrations were evaluated after EUS-guided OncoGel injection in the pancreas of 8 pigs. Eight pigs underwent injection of 1, 2, 3, or 4 mL (n = 2 per group). After

14 days, clinically significant tissue concentrations of paclitaxel were detected at a distance of 30 to 50 mm from the depot in the animals that underwent an injection of 3 and 4 mL of the agent. These results demonstrated the safety and feasibility of EUS-guided OncoGel injection as a potential, minimally invasive local treatment option for unresectable pancreatic tumors.

In clinical settings, OncoGel was first evaluated in a phase 1 dose escalation study of superficially accessible solid tumors.[29] Subsequently, EUS-guided OncoGel injection was evaluated in esophageal cancer as a phase 2 trial.[30] EUS can provide easy access, measurement of tumor response, and visualization of OncoGel injection in esophageal cancer. Single EUS-guided OncoGel injection was evaluated in 11 patients with inoperable esophageal cancer who were candidates for palliative external-beam RT. Three cohorts of patients received approximately one-third of the tumor volume with increasing paclitaxel concentrations to achieve 0.48, 1.0, and 2.0 mg paclitaxel/cm^3 tumor volume. After injection, RT was initiated (50.4 Gy in 1.8 Gy fractions). Tumor response by EUS performed at week 11, approximately 5.5 weeks after completion of RT, showed 2 partial response (18%), 6 stable disease (55%), and 2 progressive disease (18%). EUS was unable to pass through the esophagus in 1 patient because of tumor invasion of the lumen. Biopsy results were negative for cancer in 4 patients. Systemic exposure after OncoGel administration was minimal. Peak paclitaxel plasma concentrations were low (0.53–2.73 ng/mL, less than 0.3% of the lowest C_{max} reported after IV paclitaxel infusions) and directly related to the absolute amount of paclitaxel administered. The addition of EUS-guided OncoGel injection to RT in esophageal cancer seemed to be safe and feasible. The combination of EUS-guided antitumor agent injection with conventional anticancer treatment is one of the new directions to be explored.

GEMCITABINE

Levy and colleagues.[31] reported EUS-FNI of gemcitabine in 36 patients with unresectable pancreatic cancer. Systemic chemotherapy with gemcitabine has long been the standard treatment of metastatic pancreatic cancer since a randomized controlled trial showed superiority over 5-fluorouracil. Hence the idea of direct injection of gemcitabine would emerge as a treatment option for pancreatic cancer. The investigators hypothesized that direct intratumoral injection of chemotherapy would enhance the direct drug specific effects as well as boost local radiation effect within the tumor bed. Patients underwent EUS-FNI with gemcitabine (40 mg/mL) and at 4 to 14 days after EUS-FNI, and before initiating standard chemoradiotherapy, toxicities were assessed. A mean of 2.7 needle passes (range 1–4) and mean total volume of 2.5 mL (range 0.7–7.0) was injected per patient, corresponding to an intratumoral injection of 90 mg (range 28–280 mg) of gemcitabine. There were no procedure-related complications or grade 3 or higher adverse events associated with intratumoral therapy. Survival at 6 months and 1 year was 76% and 46%, respectively. Three patients initially deemed unresectable have been downstaged and undergone R0 resection. This study suggests the feasibility and safety of intratumoral EUS-FNI of gemcitabine for pancreatic cancer. These data again offer promise in terms of tumor downstaging and impact on survival by EUS-FNI of antitumor agents.

EUS-GUIDED IMMUNOTHERAPY

Immunotherapy is a theoretically attractive option, especially in patients with pancreatic cancer, which is usually refractory to conventional chemotherapy or radiation therapy. Tumor antigen–loaded dendritic cells (DCs) have been considered as a therapeutic vaccine for inducing tumor specific immunity because DCs are the most potent antigen-presenting cells. To optimize a sufficient immune response, the strategy of first inducing apoptosis (RT or chemotherapy) followed by in vivo provocation of immunity by direct intratumor injection of DCs has been used.

Irisawa and colleagues[32] reported a pilot trial of EUS-FNI of unpulsed immature DCs in 7 patients with unresectable pancreatic cancer refractory to gemcitabine. Five of 7 patients received irradiation before initial EUS-FNI of DCs to induce apoptosis and necrosis. Patients received intratumoral injection of 10 billion or more immature DCs at 2 to 3 sites on days 1, 8, and 15. The cycles were repeated every 28 days. No complication associated with EUS-FNI was noted. CA19-9 level decreased in 3 patients; 3 had mixed response (a regression of main pancreatic tumors, whereas other lesions remained stable or progressed).

Subsequently, Hirooka and colleagues[33] performed a pilot trial of combination therapy of gemcitabine with immunotherapy using OK432-pulsed DCs in 5 patients with inoperable locally advanced pancreatic cancer. OK432 is a widely used maturation stimulus for DCs. Patients received GEM IV administration at 1000 mg/m^2 (day 1) and EUS-FNI of OK432-pulsed DCs into a tumor, followed by IV infusion of lymphokine-activated killer cells stimulated with anti-CD3 monoclonal antibody (CD3-LAKs) (day 4), at 2-week intervals. No serious treatment-related adverse events were observed. One patient had partial response and 2 had sustained stable disease for more than 6 months. DC-based vaccination combined with GEM administration.

These 2 studies, despite being small study populations, suggested that immunotherapy via intratumoral injection of DCs under EUS guidance can be potential treatment options in the future.

EUS-GUIDED ALCOHOL ABLATION OF AN INSULINOMA

Alcohol ablation of tumor was most reported in the treatment of hepatocellular carcinoma via percutaneous route under transabdominal ultrasound guidance.[34] EUS-FNI of alcohol was used in pain control of pancreatic cancer as celiac plexus or ganglion neurolysis.[11,12] Jurgensen and colleagues[35] reported a patient with pancreatic NET who refused surgical resection and was successfully treated by ethanol injection. A total of 8 mL of 95% alcohol was injected into a 13-mm symptomatic insulinoma under EUS guidance with complete resolution based on clinical, morphologic, and biochemical data. Levy and colleagues[36] reported 6 cases with symptomatic insulinoma who underwent EUS-FNI or intraoperative ultrasound (IOUS)-guided FNI of 99% ethanol. Surgery was not performed because of comorbidities (n = 2), recent incomplete resection (n = 1), or tumor location requiring pancreaticoduodenectomy (n = 3). Tumor locations were head (n = 4), body (n = 1), or tail (n = 1) and the tumor size was 16.6 mm (range 11–21). For 2 patients undergoing IOUS-guided FNI, 1 treatment session was performed, whereas for 4 patients undergoing EUS-FNI, a mean of 2.3 (range 1–3) treatment sessions was performed with 3 (range 2–5) injections per session. An ethanol injection volume per session was 0.75 mL (0.12–3.0) and 1.2 mL (0.8–1.5) in EUS-FNI and IOUS-guided FNI, respectively. No complication developed in 4 patients treated with EUS-FNI, but 1 patient had minor bleeding and the other developed a 1.7 cm fluid collection in the ablative bed and an 8 cm pseudocyst, which did not require intervention, with IOUS-guided FNI. The similar technique of EUS-guided alcohol injection was also reported in a patient with left adrenal metastasis of non–small cell lung cancer for palliation of cancer-related pain.[37] EUS-guided alcohol injection seems to have its role in patients with insulinoma who are poor candidates for surgical resection. However, there are no prospective trials with a large sample size yet. The appropriate needle type or size and amount of alcohol still remain to be elucidated, and the risk of pancreatitis should always be considered as a possible complication of this procedure.

TECHNICAL HURDLES AND FUTURE DIRECTIONS

Most of the clinical studies mentioned previously are still experimental with a small study population. Prospective randomized controlled trials with a large study population are necessary to confirm the role of EUS-FNI in cancer treatment. As opposed to systemic chemotherapy, EUS-FNI of antitumor agent only exerts antitumor effects locally. Therefore, appropriate patient selection with truly local disease is important to use EUS-FNI treatment. EUS-FNI antitumor treatment of most cancers cannot be offered as monotherapy, but as part of combination multidisciplinary treatment including chemotherapy or chemoradiation therapy. Because the development of new anticancer drugs has been in progresses, the best combination of local antitumor agents along with biologics and conventional chemotherapy or chemoradiation therapy should be pursued.

The best delivery method of antitumor agents is also unclear. Theoretically, EUS can provide a better and safer access and can enable the effective delivery of antitumor agents even into multiple sites in 1 session. The superiority of EUS-FNI over percutaneous approach, however, has not been proven. The other concern is that EUS is not uniformly available, even among cancer centers.

Development of specific devices including FNA needles suited for the administration of antitumor agents is another issue to be solved. A needle that is specific for antitumor agent delivery should have sufficient caliber and be able to deliver the drug into the tumor in a uniform, sterile, and diffuse manner. To plan, monitor, and diffuse appropriate drug delivery throughout the tumor, a new EUS system such as three-dimensional ultrasound-CT dual imaging[38] should be developed.

In conclusion, although EUS-FNI of antitumor agents has not yet been established as a standard option in cancer treatment, its feasibility and safety has been proven in both animal and human trials. We are merely waiting for a potent and effective agent to deliver. Once the agent is identified, large prospective randomized controlled trials are needed to prove it's efficacy (in combination) over standard therapy. Unlike the development of endoscopy, the life cycle of these antitumor agents are considerably longer, yet we remain optimistic that they will play an important role in cancer therapy.

REFERENCES

1. Vilmann P, Jacobsen GK, Henriksen FW, et al. Endoscopic ultrasonography with guided fine needle aspiration biopsy in pancreatic disease. Gastrointest Endosc 1992;38:172–3.
2. Chang KJ, Katz KD, Durbin TE, et al. Endoscopic ultrasound-guided fine-needle aspiration. Gastrointest Endosc 1994;40:694–9.
3. Giovannini M, Seitz JF, Monges G, et al. Fine-needle aspiration cytology guided by endoscopic ultrasonography: results in 141 patients. Endoscopy 1995;27: 171–7.
4. Grimm H, Binmoeller KF, Soehendra N. Endosonography-guided drainage of a pancreatic pseudocyst. Gastrointest Endosc 1992;38:170–1.
5. Varadarajulu S, Christein JD, Tamhane A, et al. Prospective randomized trial comparing EUS and EGD for transmural drainage of pancreatic pseudocysts (with videos). Gastrointest Endosc 2008;68:1102–11.

6. Varadarajulu S, Lopes TL, Wilcox CM, et al. EUS versus surgical cyst-gastrostomy for management of pancreatic pseudocysts. Gastrointest Endosc 2008;68:649–55.
7. Park DH, Lee SS, Moon SH, et al. Endoscopic ultrasound-guided versus conventional transmural drainage for pancreatic pseudocysts: a prospective randomized trial. Endoscopy 2009;41:842–8.
8. Giovannini M, Moutardier V, Pesenti C, et al. Endoscopic ultrasound-guided bilioduodenal anastomosis: a new technique for biliary drainage. Endoscopy 2001; 33:898–900.
9. Yamao K, Bhatia V, Mizuno N, et al. EUS-guided choledochoduodenostomy for palliative biliary drainage in patients with malignant biliary obstruction: results of long-term follow-up. Endoscopy 2008;40:340–2.
10. Hara K, Yamao K, Niwa Y, et al. Prospective clinical study of EUS-guided choledochoduodenostomy for malignant lower biliary tract obstruction. Am J Gastroenterol 2011;106:1239–45.
11. Gunaratnam NT, Sarma AV, Norton ID, et al. A prospective study of EUS-guided celiac plexus neurolysis for pancreatic cancer pain. Gastrointest Endosc 2001; 54:316–24.
12. Levy MJ, Topazian MD, Wiersema MJ, et al. Initial evaluation of the efficacy and safety of endoscopic ultrasound-guided direct Ganglia neurolysis and block. Am J Gastroenterol 2008;103:98–103.
13. Hoffmanm BJ, Knapple W, Bhutani MS, et al. EUS-guided injection of botulinum toxin (Botox) for achalasia: final report of an open study. Gastrointest Endosc 1997;45:AB174.
14. Sun S, Qingjie L, Qiyong G, et al. EUS-guided interstitial brachytherapy of the pancreas: a feasibility study. Gastrointest Endosc 2005;62:775–9.
15. Sun S, Xu H, Xin J, et al. Endoscopic ultrasound-guided interstitial brachytherapy of unresectable pancreatic cancer: results of a pilot trial. Endoscopy 2006;38: 399–403.
16. Jin Z, Du Y, Li Z, et al. Endoscopic ultrasonography-guided interstitial implantation of iodine 125-seeds combined with chemotherapy in the treatment of unresectable pancreatic carcinoma: a prospective pilot study. Endoscopy 2008;40:314–20.
17. Park WG, Yan BM, Schellenberg D, et al. EUS-guided gold fiducial insertion for image-guided radiation therapy of pancreatic cancer: 50 successful cases without fluoroscopy. Gastrointest Endosc 2010;71:513–8.
18. Varadarajulu S, Trevino JM, Shen S, et al. The use of endoscopic ultrasound-guided gold markers in image-guided radiation therapy of pancreatic cancers: a case series. Endoscopy 2010;42:423–5.
19. Chang KJ, Nguyen PT, Thompson JA, et al. Phase I clinical trial of allogeneic mixed lymphocyte culture (cytoimplant) delivered by endoscopic ultrasound-guided fine-needle injection in patients with advanced pancreatic carcinoma. Cancer 2000;88:1325–35.
20. Mulvihill S, Warren R, Venook A, et al. Safety and feasibility of injection with an E1B-55 kDa gene-deleted, replication-selective adenovirus (ONYX-015) into primary carcinomas of the pancreas: a phase I trial. Gene Ther 2001;8:308–15.
21. Hecht JR, Bedford R, Abbruzzese JL, et al. A phase I/II trial of intratumoral endoscopic ultrasound injection of ONYX-015 with intravenous gemcitabine in unresectable pancreatic carcinoma. Clin Cancer Res 2003;9:555–61.
22. Hecht JR, Farrell JJ, Senzer N, et al. EUS or percutaneously guided intratumoral TNFerade biologic with 5-fluorouracil and radiotherapy for first-line treatment of locally advanced pancreatic cancer: a phase I/II study. Gastrointest Endosc 2012;75:332–8.

23. Chang KJ, Ashida R, Muthusamy R, et al. Overall survival in locally advanced pancreatic cancer patients treated with a biologic using endoscopic ultrasound (EUS) FNI or CT-Guided Injection: a single institution experience. Gastrointest Endosc 2009;69:AB132–3.

24. Chang KJ, Reid T, Senzer N, et al. Phase I evaluation of TNFeradeTM biologic plus chemoradiotherapy prior to esophagectomy for locally advanced resectable esophageal cancer. Gastrointest Endosc 2012. [Epub ahead of print].

25. Citrin D, Camphausen K, Wood BJ, et al. A pilot feasibility study of TNFerade biologic with capecitabine and radiation therapy followed by surgical resection for the treatment of rectal cancer. Oncology 2010;79:382–8.

26. Elstad NL, Fowers KD. OncoGel (ReGel/paclitaxel)–clinical applications for a novel paclitaxel delivery system. Adv Drug Deliv Rev 2009;61:785–94.

27. Linghu E, Matthes K, Mino-Kenudson M, et al. Feasibility of endoscopic ultrasound-guided OncoGel (ReGel/paclitaxel) injection into the pancreas in pigs. Endoscopy 2005;37:1140–2.

28. Matthes K, Mino-Kenudson M, Sahani DV, et al. EUS-guided injection of paclitaxel (OncoGel) provides therapeutic drug concentrations in the porcine pancreas (with video). Gastrointest Endosc 2007;65:448–53.

29. Vukelja SJ, Anthony SP, Arseneau JC, et al. Phase 1 study of escalating-dose OncoGel (ReGel/paclitaxel) depot injection, a controlled-release formulation of paclitaxel, for local management of superficial solid tumor lesions. Anticancer Drugs 2007;18:283–9.

30. DuVall GA, Tarabar D, Seidel RH, et al. Phase 2: a dose-escalation study of OncoGel (ReGel/paclitaxel), a controlled-release formulation of paclitaxel, as adjunctive local therapy to external-beam radiation in patients with inoperable esophageal cancer. Anticancer Drugs 2009;20:89–95.

31. Levy MJ, Alberts SR, Chari ST, et al. EUS guided intra-tumoral gemcitabine therapy for locally advanced and metastatic pancreatic cancer. Gastrointest Endosc 2011;73:AB144–5.

32. Irisawa A, Takagi T, Kanazawa M, et al. Endoscopic ultrasound-guided fine-needle injection of immature dendritic cells into advanced pancreatic cancer refractory to gemcitabine: a pilot study. Pancreas 2007;35:189–90.

33. Hirooka Y, Itoh A, Kawashima H, et al. A combination therapy of gemcitabine with immunotherapy for patients with inoperable locally advanced pancreatic cancer. Pancreas 2009;38:e69–74.

34. Shiina S, Teratani T, Obi S, et al. Percutaneous ethanol injection therapy for liver tumors. Eur J Ultrasound 2001;13:95–106.

35. Jurgensen C, Schuppan D, Neser F, et al. EUS-guided alcohol ablation of an insulinoma. Gastrointest Endosc 2006;63:1059–62.

36. Levy M, Topazian M. Ultrasound guided ethanol ablation of insulinomas: a new treatment option. Gastrointest Endosc 2011;73:AB102.

37. Artifon EL, Lucon AM, Sakai P, et al. EUS-guided alcohol ablation of left adrenal metastasis from non-small-cell lung carcinoma. Gastrointest Endosc 2007;66: 1201–5.

38. Minami Y, Chung H, Kudo M, et al. Radiofrequency ablation of hepatocellular carcinoma: value of virtual CT sonography with magnetic navigation. AJR Am J Roentgenol 2008;190:W335–41.

Endoscopic Ultrasound-Guided Fiducial Markers and Brachytherapy

Zhendong Jin, MD[a], Kenneth J. Chang, MD[b],*

KEYWORDS

- Endoscopic ultrasound • Fiducial markers • Brachytherapy
- Pancreatic cancer • Radioactive seeds

The value of endoscopic ultrasound (EUS) has been expanded from diagnosis to treatment. Because the local resolution of EUS in anatomy is high and the puncture path has many advantages, EUS-guided implant treatment has been performed and is demonstrated with broad application.

EUS-GUIDED FIDUCIAL MARKERS

The linear echo-endoscope facilitates EUS-guided interventions such as fiducial placement. Fiducial markers are radiopaque spheres, coils, or seeds that are implanted in or near the tumor. The objective is to demarcate the extent of tumors to facilitate image-guided radiation therapy (IGRT).[1–11]

Stereotactic body radiation therapy (SBRT) techniques rely on IGRT to permit escalation of radiation dose to tumors while simultaneously minimizing dose to normal tissues. Implantation of fiducials into the region of interest facilitates quantification of respiratory-associated tumor motion as well as delineation of the local extent of malignant disease. In addition, fiducial markers enable reproducible daily treatment delivery.

There are several studies on the feasibility of EUS-guided fiducial placement for a variety of tumors.[2–11] Two publications discuss the feasibility of EUS-guided fiducial placement for locally advanced and recurrent pancreatic cancer.[2,7] SBRT has been introduced into the locally advanced pancreatic cancer armamentarium by investigators at Stanford University.[12] Recent evidence has also suggested the feasibility of five high dose fractions of radiation before pancreatic cancer resection.[13]

[a] Department of Gastroenterology, Changhai Hospital of Second Military Medical University, 168 Changhai Road, Shanghai 200433, China; [b] Division of Gastroenterology and Hepatology, H.H. Chao Comprehensive Digestive Disease Center, University of California, Irvine, 101 The City Drive, Orange, CA 92868, USA
* Corresponding author.
E-mail address: kchang@uci.edu

Gastrointest Endoscopy Clin N Am 22 (2012) 325–331
doi:10.1016/j.giec.2012.04.012
1052-5157/12/$ – see front matter © 2012 Elsevier Inc. All rights reserved.

However, there is no published evidence regarding the utility of EUS-implanted markers for SBRT as part of a neoadjuvant regimen for the subset of patients specifically designated to have "borderline resectable" pancreatic cancer.[14,15]

The previous positioning of radiation required CT-guided percutaneous placement of some location markers. The process was often difficult because it was necessary to pass through some abdominal organs, important ducts and vessels, and so forth. Under the guidance of EUS, these small particles are implanted in the pancreas and liver tumors with a 19-gauge fine needle. EUS-guided implantation of gold particles is a more convenient and effective way of localizing these tumors and can be done during the same session as EUS or FNA for diagnosis and local staging. Most recently, a new fiducial marker delivery needle has been developed which is a smaller 22-gauge needle with four seeds preloaded into the needle for sequential deployment (**Figs. 1** and **2**).

EUS-GUIDED IODINE-125 IMPLANTATION IN PANCREATIC CANCER
Rationale

The radioactive seeds recommended in brachytherapy are iodine-125, iridium-192, or palladium-103. Compared with the latter two sources, iodine-125 has a longer half-time of 59.7 days, which is appropriate in targeting rapidly growing tumors, such as with pancreatic cancer. Iridium-192 is always introduced in brachytherapy for gynecologic malignancies, such as endometrial cancer, with a similar survival rate as external beam radiotherapy.[16] Palladium-103 has been widely accepted as a standard particle in brachytherapy for prostate and breast cancers.[17,18] Iodine-125 source is sodium iodide-125 and the package is a titanium alloy tube sealed by laser. Each seed source is 4.5 mm in length and 0.8 mm in diameter, with a mean photon energy of 27 to 35 keV gamma ray, an initial dose rate of 7 centigray per hour and a mean radioactivity of 0.694 plus or minus 0.021 MCi (25.6 megabecquerel). The spillover of radiation

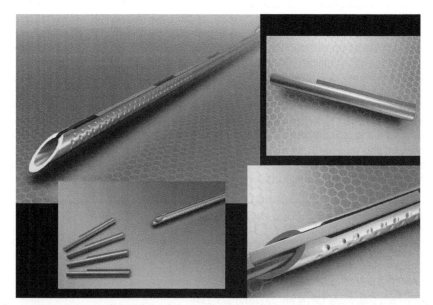

Fig. 1. New 22-gauge fiducial marker needle device that preloads four markers into the needle for sequential deployment (Cook Medical, Winston-Salem, NC, USA).

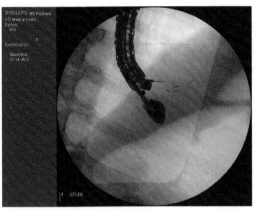

Fig. 2. Fluoroscopic image of four markers placed into the target tissue in the pancreas using new 22-gauge needle device (Cook Medical).

beyond the region of interest is certainly a potential concern. However, the penetration distance in human tissue for each seed is only 1.7 cm, which allows for precise localization of the energy inside the tumor instead of irradiating the surrounding organs. For the same reason, the implanted seeds are harmless to the patient's close contacts. The potential harm to the operators can be minimized by adequate shielding.

The most notable feature of radioactive seeds is the low dose rate. The low dose rate can maintain enough radiation dosage in the target while minimizing damage to surrounding normal tissue. Currently, the most common radioactive seed used clinically is iodine-125. When the doubling time of pancreatic cancer cells is short, it may be difficult to reach the adequate treatment dose in a relatively short interval after implantation. The effects of treatment of radioactive particles may also be less than ideal. At this time, external beam radiotherapy (XRT) or XRT combined with brachytherapy should still be considered standard of care, unless maximal dosage has already been reached or access to conventional XRT is difficult.

Current Literature

The first reported cases of EUS-guided brachytherapy were applied to head and neck cancer[19] and recurrent esophageal cancer in a mediastinal lymph node.[20] By searching PubMed with the strategy of "brachytherapy," "seeds," "endoscopy," and "pancreatic cancer" from January 2000 to July 2010, a list of nine reports were summarized. Before EUS-guided radioactive seeds implantation could be applied in human tumor treatment, animal studies were necessary to confirm the safety and to simulate the protocol. Owing to the resemblance of anatomy and physiology to humans, the pig represents a suitable animal model. Sun and colleagues[21] pioneered the EUS-mediated implantation, with four iodine-125 seeds in each pig. All the six pigs tested tolerated the trial; the median diameter of the lesion around the seed was 3.8 cm after sacrifice. The surrounding pancreas was sonographically normal and no seed migration occurred. Most important, localized tissue necrosis and fibrosis were only achieved in seed-containing pancreas, without significant complications. The usage of 18 or 19 gauge needles was shown to be safe puncturing through the gastric wall. The study firstly confirmed that EUS-guided implantation of radioactive seeds was a safe and minimally invasive technique for interstitial brachytherapy.

Under EUS, the maximal diameter of the tumor is measured by real-time sector ultrasound and the relationship between the surrounding vasculature and the tumor is then identified. The puncture points should be determined by color Doppler technology to prevent the injury to the pancreatic duct or the vessels.

The only available two clinical trials on EUS-guided brachytherapy of the pancreas come from China.[22,23] The number of patients enrolled in these two studies was 15 and 22, respectively, with stage III or IV pancreatic cancer in most of the cases. The study conducted by Sun and colleagues[22] reported an estimated median survival time of 10.6 months and 27% of the patients reached partial tumor response toward a mean 22 seeds load per patient. Procedure-related pancreatitis or pseudocyst was only found in three patients, which was considered mild and easily managed. With the combination of gemcitabine, Jin and colleagues[23] further evaluated the clinical efficacy and safety of EUS-guided interstitial implantation of radioactive iodine-125 seeds in advanced pancreatic cancer. Although the novel technique did not significantly improve the overall survival rate, it showed an estimated median survival time of 9.0 months, with a partial remission rate of 13.6%, and an estimated 1-year survival rate at 27.3%. Moreover, the visual analog scale pain score significantly dropped from 5.07 to 1.73 1 week after brachytherapy and maintained for 1 month. Therefore, these two reports show promising preliminary data that pancreatic cancer can be treated safely with EUS-brachytherapy. Additional larger studies are needed to establish this as an acceptable option for inoperable pancreatic cancer. Compared with brachytherapy monotherapy as reported by Sun and colleagues,[22] the brachytherapy-chemotherapy combination treatment did not seem to show a better tumor response or long-term outcome.[23] Single gemcitabine chemotherapy provides a median 1-year survival rate of 21% (11.0%–37.2%).[24] Having shown initial safety and feasibility in these preliminary clinical trials, the next step is to conduct randomized controlled trials with long-term follow-up to evaluate the efficacy between single EUS-guided implantation and single standardized chemotherapy. It would also be of interest to compare the efficacy and tolerability between EUS-guided brachytherapy and conventional external beam radiation.

EUS-GUIDED CELIAC GANGLION RADIATION FOR PAIN RELIEF

Ameliorating pain is a critical component of therapy in patients with unresectable pancreatic cancer, with studies showing improved quality of life and survival with optimal pain management. Partial pain relief can be achieved with effective intratumoral brachytherapy. Celiac plexus neurolysis (CPN) and celiac plexus block (CPB) have been considered the first-line adjuvant therapies for the treatment of pain in pancreatic patients with cancer.[25] Gunaratnam and colleagues[26] reported that EUS-guided CPN reduced pain in 78% pancreatic of patients with cancer. However, CPN can only relieve the pain to a limited degree, with short duration, and the analgesic effect is inversely correlated with the extent of invasion of celiac ganglia.[27–29] EUS-guided brachytherapy with the implantation of iodine-125 seeds beside the celiac ganglion seems to be another option for pain relief. Recently, Wang and colleagues[30] performed a pilot trial in a porcine model. Four pigs in each group were implanted with one 0.4 MCi or 0.8 MCi iodine-125 seed in either side of the celiac ganglion area with the help of EUS. Pigs implanted with nonradioactive seeds were used as controls. All animals were sacrificed and the celiac ganglia were checked on days 14 and 60. Compared with the control group, neuronal apoptosis in the ganglion was seen in both brachytherapy groups, and the intensity of necrosis increased with the radiation dose increasing. More apoptotic cells (index as 0.53

and 0.94, respectively) were seen on day 60 of irradiation than on day 14 (0.27 and 0.76, respectively) in both the 0.4 MCi and 0.8 MCi groups. There were no significant complications during the experiment. This is the first preliminary evidence for the feasibility and safety of EUS-guided celiac neuron brachytherapy. This new technique may introduce an alternative treatment for pain-accompanied pancreatic diseases in humans. However, iodine-125 seeds, which have a long decay period, may have a slower onset but longer durability of analgesia compared with CPN or CPB. More animal and clinical trials are needed to determine whether celiac ganglion radiation is superior to classic CPN, and whether the technique can be eventually applied in clinical practice.

Jin reported iodine-125 seeds under EUS guidance were implanted beside the celiac ganglion in 15 patients with the 0.7 MCi (group 1) and 15 were treated with pharmacologic therapy (group 2) (Jin Z, personal communication, 2012). Immediate and long-term efficacy, mean analgesic consumption, mortality, and morbidity were evaluated. A mean number of four radioactive seeds per patient were implanted into the celiac ganglia. Immediately after the procedure, pain relief and analgesic consumption did not differ between the two groups. On the contrary, three patients reported pain exacerbation. However, 10 days later, patients in group 1 reported significant pain relief compared with those in group 2. Mean analgesic consumption was lower in group 1. There were no deaths. No complications such as transient diarrhea, hypotension, or infection occurred. Drug-related adverse effects were constipation (6 of 15 patients in group 1 vs 13 of 15 in group 2), nausea and/or vomiting (4 of 15 patients in group 1 vs 12 of 15 in group 2).

SUMMARY

The currently commercially available radioactive seeds have a fixed length that is too long for certain situations. For example, it may be difficult to advance seeds into the pancreatic head and uncinate process, where the echoendoscope and needle device are in a severe angle. However, the delivery is relatively easy when the scope and needle are in a straight position, as with tumors in the pancreatic neck, body, or tail. The development of new radioactive particles with smaller size, or even in liquid form, would help overcome these limitations.

Although the exact seed number needed for brachytherapy can be calculated by three-dimensional computer software, the exact model for EUS-guided implantation has not been established. For instance, the goal of precise and evenly spaced placement of radioactive seeds in three-dimensional space is very difficult if not impossible. Therefore, future development must incorporate a sophisticated treatment planning system based on EUS imaging.

REFERENCES

1. Vignesh S, Jamidar P. EUS-guided pancreatogastrostomy and pancreatobulbostomy in patients with pancreatic-duct obstruction inaccessible to transpapillary endoscopic therapy: working our way to NOTES. Gastrointest Endosc 2007;65: 242–6.
2. Sanders MK, Moser AJ, Khalid A, et al. EUS-guided fiducial placement for stereotactic body radiotherapy in locally advanced and recurrent pancreatic cancer. Gastrointest Endosc 2010;71:1178–84.
3. DiMaio CJ, Nagula S, Goodman KA, et al. EUS-guided fiducial placement for image-guided radiation therapy in GI malignancies by using a 22-gauge needle (with videos). Gastrointest Endosc 2010;71:1204–10.

4. Ammar T, Coté GA, Creach KM, et al. Fiducial placement for stereotactic radiation by using EUS: feasibility when using a marker compatible with a standard 22-gauge needle. Gastrointest Endosc 2010;71:630–3.

5. Owens DJ, Savides TJ. Backloaded fiducial placement using a bone wax seal to facilitate EUS-guided fiducial placement. Gastrointest Endosc 2009;69(2 Suppl 1): S253.

6. Pishvaian AC, Collins B, Gagnon G, et al. EUS-guided fiducial placement for CyberKnife radiotherapy of mediastinal and abdominal malignancies. Gastrointest Endosc 2006;64:412–7.

7. Park WG, Yan BM, Schellenberg D, et al. EUS-guided gold fiducial insertion for image-guided radiation therapy of pancreatic cancer: 50 successful cases without fluoroscopy. Gastrointest Endosc 2010;71:513–8.

8. Van Dam J, Varadarajulu S, Jin Z, EUS 2008 Working Group. EUS 2008 Working Group document: evaluation of EUS-guided implantation therapy (with video). Gastrointest Endosc 2009;69(Suppl 2):S49–53.

9. Berzin TM, Majumder S, Mahadevan A, et al. Comparison of EUS vs. surgery for placement of fiducials in patients with pancreatic cancer. Gastrointest Endosc 2010;71:AB285.

10. Owens DJ, Savides TJ. EUS placement of metal fiducials by using a backloaded technique with bone wax seal. Gastrointest Endosc 2009;69:972–3.

11. Ghassemi S, Faigel DO. EUS-guided placement of fiducial markers using a 22-gauge needle. Gastrointest Endosc 2009;69:AB337–8.

12. Koong AC, Le QT, Ho A, et al. Phase I study of stereotactic radiosurgery in patients with locally advanced pancreatic cancer. Int J Radiat Oncol Biol Phys 2004;58:1017–21.

13. Hong TS, Ryan DP, Blaszkowsky LS, et al. Phase I study of preoperative short-course chemoradiation with proton beam therapy and capecitabine for resectable pancreatic ductal adenocarcinoma of the head. Int J Radiat Oncol Biol Phys 2011;79:151–7.

14. Evans DB, Erickson BA, Ritch P. Borderline resectable pancreatic cancer: definitions and the importance of multimodality therapy. Ann Surg Oncol 2010;17: 2803–5.

15. Chun YS, Milestone BN, Watson JC, et al. Defining venous involvement in borderline resectable pancreatic cancer. Ann Surg Oncol 2010;17:2832–8.

16. Hampton T. Clinical trials probe new therapies for some difficult-to-treat cancers. JAMA 2008;300:384–5.

17. Herstein A, Wallner K, Merrick G, et al. There is a wide range of predictive dosimetric factors for I-125 and pd-103 prostate brachytherapy. Am J Clin Oncol 2008;31:6–10.

18. Ravi A, Caldwell CB, Keller BM, et al. Online gamma-camera imaging of 103Pd seeds (OGIPS) for permanent breast seed implantation. Phys Med Biol 2007; 52:5921–32.

19. Maier W, Henne K, Krebs A, et al. Endoscopic ultrasound-guided brachytherapy of head and neck tumours. A new procedure for controlled application. J Laryngol Otol 1999;113(1):41–8.

20. Lah JJ, Kuo JV, Chang KJ, et al. EUS-guided brachytherapy. Gastrointest Endosc 2005;62(5):805–8.

21. Sun S, Qingjie L, Qiyong G, et al. EUS-guided interstitial brachytherapy of the pancreas: a feasibility study. Gastrointest Endosc 2005;62:775–9.

22. Sun S, Xu H, Xin J, et al. Endoscopic ultrasound-guided interstitial brachytherapy of unresectable pancreatic cancer: results of a pilot trial. Endoscopy 2006;38:399–403.

23. Jin Z, Du Y, Li Z, et al. EUS-guided interstitial implantation of iodine 125 seeds combined with chemotherapy in the treatment of unresectable pancreatic carcinoma: a prospective pilot study. Endoscopy 2008;40:314–20.
24. Xie DR, Liang HL, Wang Y, et al. Meta-analysis on inoperable pancreatic cancer: a comparison between gemcitabine-based combination therapy and gemcitabine alone. World J Gastroenterol 2006;12:6973–81.
25. Michaels AJ, Draganov PV. Endoscopic ultrasonography guided celiac plexus neurolysis and celiac plexus block in the management of pain due to pancreatic cancer and chronic pancreatitis. World J Gastroenterol 2007;13:3575–80.
26. Gunaratnam NT, Sarma AV, Norton ID, et al. A prospective study of EUS-guided celiac plexus neurolysis for pancreatic cancer pain. Gastrointest Endosc 2001; 54:316–24.
27. Yan BM, Myers RP. Neurolytic celiac plexus block for pain control in unresectable pancreatic cancer. Am J Gastroenterol 2007;102:430–8.
28. Wiersema MJ, Wiersema LM. Endosonography-guided celiac plexus neurolysis. Gastrointest Endosc 1996;44:656–62.
29. Akhan O, Ozmen MN, Basgun N, et al. Long-term results of celiac Ganglia block: correlation of grade of tumoral invasion and pain relief. AJR Am J Roentgenol 2004;182:891–6.
30. Wang K, Jin Z, Du Y, et al. Evaluation of endoscopic ultrasound guided celiac ganglion radiation with iodine 125 seeds: a pilot study in porcine model. Endoscopy 2009;41:346–51.

Endoscopic Ultrasound Image Enhancement Elastography

Julio Iglesias-Garcia, MD, PhD*,
J. Enrique Domínguez-Muñoz, MD, PhD

KEYWORDS

- Endoscopic ultrasound • Elastography • Pancreatic tumors
- Lymph nodes

INTRODUCTION

Endoscopic ultrasound (EUS) has evolved in recent years into a technique with a major clinical impact in digestive and mediastinal diseases.[1–3] In fact, EUS has represented a major advance in the diagnosis and staging of several tumors, and can determine a change in diagnosis and management in 25% to 50% of cases.[4–7] However, EUS is not only useful providing excellent images for detection and staging of several malignancies, it also provides guidance for fine-needle aspiration (FNA) and biopsies of almost all lesions detected during a standard procedure. Overall accuracy of EUS-guided FNA can be considered excellent, with sensitivities between 80% and 85%, and specificities close to 100%.[8–14]

However, differential diagnosis of certain lesions, based only on B-mode image can be challenging and EUS-guided FNA and/or biopsy is technically demanding and multiple punctures of the lesions can be necessary to obtain sufficient tissue for cyto-histologic assessment.[15,16] EUS-guided FNA can also be associated with false-negative results, mainly in patients with solid pancreatic masses with the underlying diagnosis of chronic pancreatitis.[17] Another limitation is related to the evaluation of lymph nodes. When several lymph nodes appear suspicious, the choice of which one to puncture is not always clear.[18] Finally, EUS and EUS-guided FNA are associated with a small, but not insignificant, morbidity.[19,20]

Disclosures: Dr Julio Iglesias-Garcia is International Advisor of Cook-Medical.
Gastroenterology Department, Foundation for Research in Digestive Diseases (FIENAD), University Hospital of Santiago de Compostela, c/Choupana s/n, 15706 Santiago de Compostela, Spain
* Corresponding author.
E-mail address: julio.iglesias.garcia@sergas.es

Gastrointest Endoscopy Clin N Am 22 (2012) 333–348
doi:10.1016/j.giec.2012.04.011
1052-5157/12/$ – see front matter © 2012 Elsevier Inc. All rights reserved.

giendo.theclinics.com

With this background, new methods allowing better characterization of lesions evaluated by EUS are essential to avoid the realization of unnecessary FNA and/or biopsies, to allow more accurate characterization of lesions before the puncture, and possibly to reduce complication rates. One of these new available methods is elastography.

It is well known that certain diseases, such as cancer, may induce changes in tissue stiffness. Elastography is a method for the real-time evaluation of tissue stiffness. This technique has been previously used for the analysis of superficial organ lesions, such as those of the breast and prostate.[21,22] Elastographic images are an index of tissue elasticity, which may be related to histopathologic features. It has been considered virtual biopsy.[23,24] Now, elastographic evaluation can be performed by EUS. Several studies have demonstrated that EUS-elastography is a promising technique with a high accuracy for the differential diagnosis of solid pancreatic tumors and lymph nodes.

This article analyzes the theoretical aspects and methodology of elastography, and reviews the actual indications and further development of this relatively novel method.

THEORY AND TECHNICAL ASPECTS OF ELASTOGRAPHY

Elastography is based on the knowledge that some diseases (among them cancer) lead to a change in tissue hardness (elasticity modulus) and is an outgrowth of the well-known breast ultrasound fremitus technique, during which the patient is asked to hum while color or power Doppler is used to examine the breast.[25–27] Softer portions of the breast vibrate more in response to the humming, whereas cancers and other solid lesions present a lower vibration rate and thus are seen as areas of decreased color, even if they are isoechoic on the ordinary B-mode ultrasound. Elastography examines the elastic properties of tissues by applying a slight compression to the tissue and comparing an image obtained before and after this compression. Both data obtained are compared by using a cross-correlation technique to determine the amount of displacement each small portion of tissue presented in response to the compression applied by the ultrasound transducer.[28,29] The tissue elasticity distribution is calculated from the strain and the stress of the examined structures. Although the strain field can be estimated from the radio frequency signals returned from tissue structures before and after compression, it is impossible to measure the stress field directly within the tissue. Another problem is that the compression of harder tissue structures is often followed by a lateral displacement of these structures. It is nearly impossible to represent the volume of this sideslip with conventional two-dimensional methods, but its calculation is indispensable for an accurate determination of the tissue elasticity of the examined structures. To overcome these problems, the extended combined autocorrelation method has been developed, allowing the reconstruction of the tissue elasticity of the examined structures based on the three-dimensional finite element model. The new technique enables highly accurate estimation of the tissue elasticity distribution and adequate compensation of sideslips. The elasticity imaging can be performed in real time with the elastography module, which can be integrated into different HITACHI platforms (Hitachi Medical Systems Europe, Zug, Switzerland).[30] Features of the elastographic patterns shown with the first generation of elastography, in terms of homogeneity or heterogeneity and predominant color, closely correlate with the histologic features of the lesion. New generations of elastography can also provide a quantitative elastographic evaluation.

PROCEDURE TECHNIQUE AND CRITERIA

As with traditional color Doppler imaging, EUS tissue-elasticity imaging is performed with conventional EUS probes. The vibrations and compressions are provided physiologically by vascular pulsation and respiratory motion. The elastography module available for use with EUS scopes today provides two generations of this technique. The first generation allows a qualitative evaluation and the second generation allows a quantitative evaluation of tissue stiffness.

Qualitative EUS-Elastography

Elastography modules provided in the ultrasound devices enables real-time elastographic evaluation and recording. The technology is based on the detection of small structure deformations within the B-mode image caused by compression, so that the strain is smaller in hard tissue than in soft tissue.[21] The degree of deformation is used as an indicator of the stiffness of the tissue.[31] Different elasticity values (on a scale of 1–255) are marked with different colors resulting in different tissue elasticity patterns, represented in color superimposed over the conventional B-mode. The system is set-up to use a hue color map (red-green-blue), where hard tissue areas are shown in dark blue, medium-hard tissue areas in cyan, intermediate tissue areas in green, medium-soft tissue areas in yellow, and soft tissue areas in red. During the procedure, two-panel images are shown, with the usual conventional grayscale B-mode image on the right side and the elastographic image on the left side (**Fig. 1**). To perform a correct elastographic evaluation, the probe needs to be attached to the wall just exerting the pressure needed for an optimal and stable B-mode image at 7.5 MHz. The region of interest (ROI) for the elastographic evaluation is manually selected and, when possible, the whole targeted lesion as well as surrounding tissues needs to be included. Maximal sensitivity for elastographic registration should be used to give the final elastographic evaluation and, because elastographic images tend to show rapid changing colors, a stable image for at least 5 s is required for the final color pattern definition.[32]

Initial clinical research involving elastography was focused on the evaluation of breast masses and initial patterns were described in these lesions. Three different patterns have been identified in elastograms of breast cancers: a well-defined, very hard (dark) mass or nodule; a moderately hard mass or nodule containing much harder (darker) foci within it; and a very dark or hard central core surrounded by a somewhat

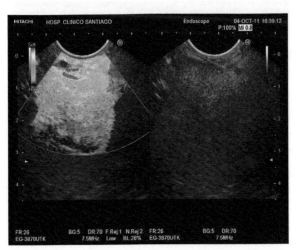

Fig. 1. Qualitative EUS-elastography of a normal pancreas showing a specific color distribution.

softer or less dark peripheral component.[26] Although with conventional ultrasound or EUS fibrosis generally appears as hyperechogenic regions with posterior acoustic shadowing (an appearance also seen in cancers), with elastography it generally appears as a uniform, moderately hard region with no distinct foci of increased hardness. Preliminary work in breast tissue elastography has shown that it can correctly classify most benign and malignant masses.[24] For EUS-elastography, different patterns have been described (see later discussion).[32,33]

Quantitative EUS-Elastography

There are two options to perform a quantitative elastographic evaluation: using the calculation of hue-histogram with specific software or using the new elastography module allowing the strain ratio calculation.

Hue histogram

Possibly one of the most useful tools available in digital medical images is the histogram—a graphical representation of the colors (hues) distribution. Specific software is freely available that allows performing this evaluation (ImageJ software, NIH, Bethesda, MD, USA).[34]

Calculation of hue-histograms is based on the qualitative EUS elastographic image obtained during the standard procedure. Once the optimal elastographic image is selected, the lesion to study for the hue-histogram is manually selected. For the hue-histogram analysis, on the x-axis of the histogram the numeric values of the elasticity are displayed on a scale from 0 (softest) to 255 (hardest). On the y-axis, the height of the spikes displayed indicates the number of pixels of each elasticity level found in the ROI. In the new HITACHI machines, software is included that allows the calculation of the hue-histogram. However, there is a slight difference compared with the ImageJ software in which the scale is from 0 to 250, but 0 is the hardest and 255 the softest (**Fig. 2**). Consequently, the mean value of the histogram corresponds to the global hardness or elasticity of the tumors.[35]

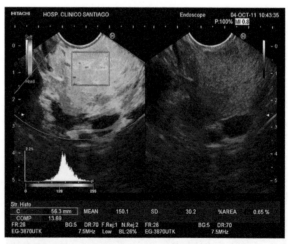

Fig. 2. Quantitative EUS-elastography based on hue-histogram analysis of normal pancreas. The histogram analysis is performed from an area selected at the ROI. The mean value of this evaluation is shown at the bottom of the image (150.1).

Strain ratio

Strain ratio was developed to add quantitative diagnostic information to pattern recognition. Strain ratio is based on the assumption that the hardness of connective or fat tissue does not vary between individuals. Taking into account that colors obtained during the elastographic evaluation are relative to each ROI, the relationship between the color patterns of lesions and the surrounding tissue sometimes provides the most meaningful data. The software extracts various features from real-time images. It converts the color values inside of the ROI into a relative strain value and calculates other features of the elastographic image, such as the mean of the relative strain value, the standard deviation of the relative strain value, and the proportion of the blue region in the region analyzed. This software also allows evaluation of the uniformity of the target area and quantifies the number of objective parameters of the distribution of hardness.[36]

Calculation of strain ratio is based on the qualitative EUS elastographic image obtained during the standard procedure. Two areas (A and B) from the ROI are selected for quantitative elastographic analysis. Area A represents the area of the target lesion, including the biggest possible area of the lesion. Area B refers to a soft (red) reference area outside the area under investigation, with the gut wall being the best option to select. The quotient B/A (strain ratio) is the measure of the quantitative elastographic evaluation (**Fig. 3**).[37]

CLINICAL APPLICATIONS OF EUS-ELASTOGRAPHY

This article focuses on the accepted and potential indications of EUS-elastography. First, the usefulness of this new technique in the diagnosis and management of pancreatic diseases is reviewed. Second, the focus is on the management of lymph nodes. Finally, the future and theoretical indications of EUS-elastography are commented on.

Evaluation of Pancreatic Diseases

As previously noted, EUS provides high-resolution images of the pancreas and it is considered one of the most accurate methods for the diagnosis and staging of chronic inflammatory, cystic, and neoplastic pancreatic diseases.[4,38,39] However,

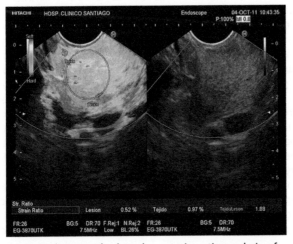

Fig. 3. Quantitative EUS-elastography based on strain ratio analysis of normal pancreas. Area A is representative of pancreatic parenchyma and area B corresponds to a soft area from the gut wall. The quotient B/A is display at the bottom of the image (1.88).

differentiation between pancreatic cancer and focal pancreatitis remains a challenge based only on B-mode imaging, particularly in cases of advanced chronic pancreatitis.[4] Several studies have attempted to establish EUS-imaging criteria for the discrimination between benign inflammatory lesions and malignant tumors. However, despite the high resolution of EUS, overall accuracy in this setting is not higher than 75%.[40] EUS-elastography seems to be a useful tool in the evaluation of pancreatic diseases.

Differential diagnosis of solid pancreatic lesions

Giovannini and colleagues[41] published the first experience with elastography in pancreatic solid lesions. They analyzed 24 pancreatic masses using a subjective scoring system based on different color patterns of the images. Lesions appearing mostly blue (harder) were classified as malignant. Based on this classification, sensitivity and specificity for detecting malignancy was 100% and 67%, respectively. The investigators performed a more refined classification. Score 1 (normal pancreatic tissue) was given to a homogeneous low elastographic area (soft or green). Score 2 (fibrosis) was given to images with heterogeneity of the elastographic area in the soft-tissue range (green, yellow, and red). Score 3 (early pancreatic adenocarcinoma) was given to an elastographic image that was largely blue (hard) with minimal heterogeneity. Score 4 (hypervascular lesion, such as neuroendocrine tumor or small pancreatic metastasis) was given to an image with a hypoechoic region in the center of the tumor, with appearance of a small green area surrounded by blue or harder tissue. Finally, score 5 (advanced pancreatic adenocarcinoma) was assigned to lesions that were largely blue on elastography images but with heterogeneity of softer tissue colors representing necrosis. Subsequently, Giovannini and colleagues[42] published the results from a multicenter study, including 121 pancreatic masses. Elastography showed a malignant aspect (blue color) for all pancreatic adenocarcinomas, endocrine tumors, pancreatic metastases, and pancreatic sarcomas. All inflammatory masses presented a benign aspect (mixed green and low intensity of blue). Using the previous classification, considering score 1 and 2 as benign and 3 to 5 as malignant, sensitivity, specificity, positive predictive value, and negative predictive value in the differentiation between benign and malignant pancreatic masses were 92.3%, 80.6%, 93.3%, and 78.1%, with an overall accuracy of 89.2%. An interobserver agreement evaluation on 30 cases showed a kappa score of 0.785 for determination of malignancy. Iglesias-Garcia and colleagues[32] have published their experience with qualitative EUS-elastography in 130 patients with solid pancreatic masses and 20 controls. The investigators detected four different patterns, similar to those described by Giovannini and colleagues. These include a homogeneous green pattern present only in normal pancreas; a heterogeneous, green-predominant pattern, with slight yellow and red lines, present only in inflammatory pancreatic masses; a heterogeneous, blue-predominant pattern, with slight green areas and red lines and a geographic appearance, present mainly in pancreatic malignant tumors (among them pancreatic adenocarcinoma); and a homogeneous blue pattern, present only in pancreatic neuroendocrine malignant lesions. By using this classification, sensitivity, specificity, positive and negative predictive values, and overall accuracy of EUS-elastography for malignancy were 100%, 85.5%, 90.7%, 100%, and 94.0%, respectively. An interobserver agreement analysis was also conducted in which both endosonographers agreed in 121 cases and the 20 controls, with a kappa value of 0.772. **Fig. 4** shows the different patterns previously described for solid pancreatic lesions.

However, not all studies have shown the same level of accuracy. Janssen and colleagues[43] analyzed 20 patients with normal pancreas, 20 with chronic pancreatitis,

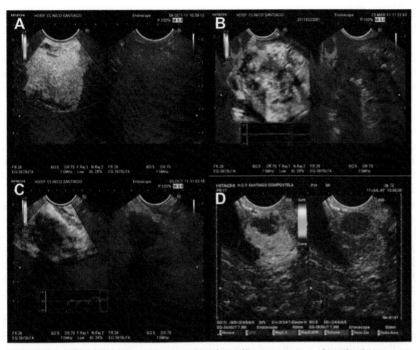

Fig. 4. Qualitative EUS-elastography, showing the different patterns described in pancreatic solid lesions. (*A*) Homogeneous green pattern from normal pancreas. (*B*) Heterogeneous green predominant pattern from chronic pancreatitis. (*C*) Heterogeneous blue predominant pattern from a pancreatic adenocarcinoma. (*D*) Homogeneous blue predominant patter from a neuroendocrine pancreatic tumor.

and 33 with focal pancreatic lesions, with less optimistic results. They performed a subanalysis of the patients with focal pancreatic lesions, describing that all tumors presented a similar pattern that was a heterogeneous, mixed green and blue, with irregular distribution—except neuroendocrine tumor, which presented a more homogeneous pattern. However, the investigators only included one inflammatory mass, so most of the lesions included were noninflammatory. Hirche and colleagues[44] presented their results on 70 patients with unclassified solid pancreatic lesions and 10 controls. They could only perform an adequate elastographic evaluation in 56% of patients, related to difficulty with including the whole lesion and enough surrounding tissue in the ROI, especially with lesions larger than 35 mm or those far away from the transducer. Overall, EUS-elastography predicted the nature of pancreatic lesions with poor diagnostic sensitivity (41%), specificity (53%), and accuracy (45%).

More recent studies have analyzed the usefulness of the quantitative EUS-elastography. Iglesias-Garcia and colleagues[37] have published data on 86 consecutive patients and 20 controls, using the calculation of the strain ratio, based on HITACHI software. The mean size of the pancreatic masses was 31.4 plus or minus 12.3 mm. The final diagnoses were pancreatic adenocarcinoma (n = 49), inflammatory mass (n = 27), malignant neuroendocrine tumor (n = 6), metastatic oat-cell lung cancer (n = 2), pancreatic lymphoma (n = 1), and pancreatic solid pseudopapillary tumor (n = 1). The strain ratio was significantly higher among patients with pancreatic malignant tumors compared with those with inflammatory masses. Healthy pancreas showed a mean strain ratio of 1.68 (95%, CI 1.59–1.78). Inflammatory masses had a higher strain ratio (mean 3.28, 95%, CI 2.61–3.96) than healthy pancreas (P<.001), but lower than pancreatic adenocarcinoma (mean 18.12, 95%, CI 16.03–20.21; P<.001). As a group, endocrine tumors presented the highest strain ratio (mean 52.34, 95%, CI 33.96–70.71). **Fig. 5** shows the strain ratio evaluation of different solid pancreatic lesions. Sensitivity and specificity of strain ratio for detecting pancreatic malignancies for a cut-off point of 6.04 were 100% and 92.9%, respectively (area under the receiver operating characteristic [ROC] curve = 0.983). This was higher than the accuracy obtained with the qualitative elastography. Another recent study retrospectively evaluated 109 patients with solid pancreatic masses using the same methodology. The final diagnosis was chronic pancreatitis in 20 patients (6 without focal masses, 7 with an inflammatory mass, and 7 with autoimmune pancreatitis), pancreatic cancer in 72 patients, pancreatic neuroendocrine tumor in 9 patients, and normal pancreas in 8 patients. In the qualitative evaluation, all pancreatic cancer showed intense blue coloration; however, inflammatory masses presented a mixed coloration pattern of green, yellow, and low-intensity blue. Regarding the quantitative evaluation, mean strain ratio was 23.66 plus or minus 12.65 for inflammatory masses and 39.08 plus or minus 20.54 for pancreatic cancer (P<.05).[45]

Săftoiu and colleagues[35] have evaluated the usefulness of hue-histograms for quantitative EUS-elastography. In this study, including 22 controls, 11 chronic pancreatitis patients, 32 pancreatic adenocarcinomas, and 3 neuroendocrine tumors, for a cutoff of 175 for the mean hue histogram values, the sensitivity, specificity, and accuracy of differentiation of benign and malignant masses were 91.4%, 87.9%, and 89.7%, respectively. The positive and negative predictive values were 88.9% and 90.6%, respectively. Recently, a multicenter study was published using the same methodology

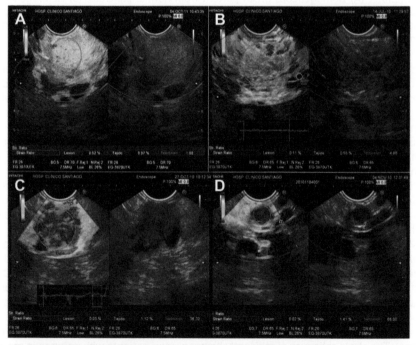

Fig. 5. Quantitative EUS-elastography, showing the different strain ratio values from pancreatic solid lesions. (*A*) Normal pancreas. (*B*) Inflammatory mass in chronic pancreatitis. (*C*) Pancreatic adenocarcinoma. (*D*) Neuroendocrine pancreatic tumor.

and, after analyzing 258 patients (211 with pancreatic adenocarcinoma and 47 with chronic pancreatitis), the average-hue histogram analysis of the data indicated a sensitivity of 93.4%, a specificity of 66.0%, a positive predictive value of 92.5%, a negative predictive value of 68.9%, and an overall accuracy of 85.4%, based on a cut-off value of 175. The area under the ROC curve was 0.854.[46] The investigators have conducted a recent study comparing both modalities of quantitative EUS-elastography, strain ratio, and hue histogram, finding no differences in accuracy for the differentiation between benign and malignant pancreatic masses (**Fig. 6**).

Table 1 summarizes the published results of EUS-elastography in the differential diagnosis of solid pancreatic masses.

Diagnosis of chronic pancreatitis

There are few data available on the usefulness of EUS-elastography for the diagnosis of chronic pancreatitis. Only the study published by Janssen and colleagues[43] showed objective data on the usefulness of elastography in this field. In this study, the subgroup of patients with chronic pancreatitis presented patterns with irregular color, mixing green areas with the presence of heterogenic strands, predominantly hard (blue). These changes were clearly different from those observed in the control group (patients without pancreatic diseases), who presented homogeneous patterns, predominantly green and yellow. In the authors' experience, a normal pancreas presents a homogeneous green predominant pattern and a pancreas with chronic pancreatitis presents an irregular and heterogeneous green predominant pattern with isolated mixed areas (yellow and blue) associated. On the other hand, a recent study

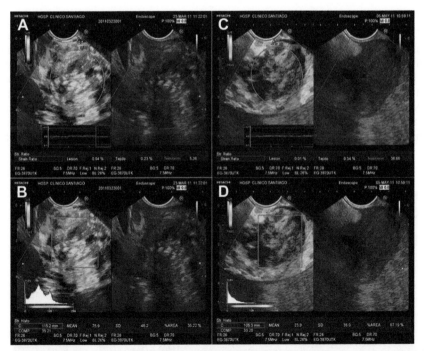

Fig. 6. Quantitative EUS elastographic evaluation of an inflammatory mass in a chronic pancreatitis (A, B) and a pancreatic adenocarcinoma (C, D); both with strain ratio and hue-histogram analysis.

Table 1
Accuracy of EUS-elastography in the differential diagnosis of solid pancreatic lesions

	Author	Year	Sensitivity (%)	Specificity (%)
Qualitative EUS-Elastography	Giovannini et al[41]	2006	100	67
	Giovannini et al[42]	2009	92.3	80
	Janssen et al[43]	2007	93.8	65.4
	Săftoiu et al[50]	2006	91.7	94.4
	Iglesias-Garcia et al[32]	2009	100	85.5
Quantitative EUS-Elastography	Săftoiu et al[35]	2008	91.4	87.9
	Iglesias-Garcia et al[32]	2010	100	92.9
	Săftoiu et al[46]	2011	93.4	66

conducted at the authors' department, evaluating the usefulness of quantitative EUS-elastography (based on the calculation of the strain ratio) in chronic pancreatitis demonstrated favorable results. The study included 178 patients, who were classified according to the number of EUS criteria for chronic pancreatitis and followed the Rosemont classification. The strain ratio obtained was significantly different between the different Rosemont groups: 1.80 (95%, CI 1.73–1.80) in a normal pancreas, 2.40 (95%, CI 2.21–2.56) in the indeterminate group, 2.85 (95%, CI 2.69–3.02) in the group suggestive of chronic pancreatitis, and 3.62 (95%, CI 3.24–3.99) in the group consistent with chronic pancreatitis ($P<.001$). The investigators also detected an excellent correlation between the total number of EUS criteria for chronic pancreatitis and the strain ratio ($r = 0.801$; $P<.0001$) (**Fig. 7**).[47]

Differential Diagnosis of Lymph Nodes

EUS provides highly accurate images of lymph nodes. However, the differential diagnosis of pathologic lymph nodes remains a challenge. Current EUS criteria for malignant lymph nodes (round, hypoechogenicity, diameter >1 cm, and distinct margins) are helpful in targeting lesions, but problems exist with specificity and overlap of these features with benign lymph nodes.[18] EUS-guided FNA has increased the overall accuracy in this setting. However, as previously noted, it is technically demanding and can be associated with complications.[48] Another important point is that, in certain situations, several lymph nodes can be detected in the same patient and making the

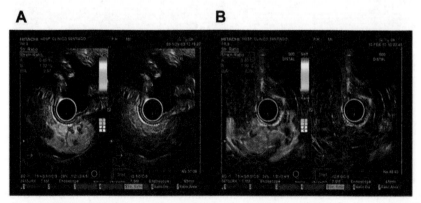

Fig. 7. Quantitative EUS elastographic evaluation in a patient with EUS findings suggestive of chronic pancreatitis (*A*) and consistent with chronic pancreatitis (*B*).

decision of which lymph node to biopsy to obtain a diagnosis challenging. The assessment of the risk of malignancy is a key point for clinical decision-making and subsequent invasive staging procedures and the development of a noninvasive imaging procedure is essential. The application of EUS-elastography for the exclusion of malignancy or preferential targeting of the most suspicion lymph nodes may be useful in this setting.

Giovannini and colleagues[41] published the first experience with elastography in the evaluation of lymph nodes. They analyzed 25 patients with 31 lymph nodes, 3 located at the cervical area, 17 in the mediastinum, 5 at the celiac arterial trunk region, and 6 at the aortocaval region. EUS elastographic images were interpreted as showing malignancy in 22 cases, benign lesions in 7 cases, and indeterminate in 2 cases, based on the predominant color (blue was considered malignant and green benign). There were no false-negative findings, but there were five false-positive findings. Indeterminate cases were associated with heterogeneity of images and, finally, were classified as benign lesions. Sensitivity and specificity for determining malignancy was 100% and 50%, respectively. The investigators performed a classification of EUS elastographic images into five different scores, including the evaluation of solid pancreatic masses, in the manner previously defined. The same investigators conducted a multicenter study, including 101 lymph nodes. These lymph nodes were classified as malignant in 57 cases and benign in 44 cases. Elastographic images were interpreted as benign in (score 1 + 2) in 38 cases, indeterminate (score 3) in 10 cases, and malignant (score 4 + 5) in 53 cases. Considering a score of 1 or 2 as benign and 3 to 5 as malignant, the sensitivity, specificity, positive predictive value, and negative predictive value in the differentiation between benign and malignant lymph nodes were 91.8%, 82.5%, 88.8%, and 86.8%, respectively, with an overall accuracy of 88.1%. An interobserver agreement evaluation on 30 cases showed a kappa score of 0.657 for determining malignancy of lymph nodes.[42] Janssen and colleagues[49] evaluated the feasibility of qualitative EUS-elastography of the dorsal mediastinum; comparing the elastographic patterns of lymph nodes to the gold standard (EUS-guided FNA). Sixty-six lymph nodes were examined (37 benign and 29 malignant at the histologic evaluation). Of the 37 benign lymph nodes, 31 showed a homogeneous pattern of intermediate elasticity, whereas a dominance of hard tissue with variable patterns was found in 23 of 29 malignant lymph nodes. Applying these criteria, the accuracy range among the three examiners was between 81.8% and 87.9% for benign lymph nodes and between 84.6% and 86.4% for malignant ones. The interobserver agreement was excellent (kappa = 0.84).

Lariño-Noia and colleagues[33] also evaluated the usefulness of qualitative EUS-elastography in the evaluation of lymph nodes. This study included 57 patients with 63 lymph nodes (54 mediastinal and 9 abdominal). The investigators defined three different elastographic patterns: a predominant blue pattern, a predominant green pattern and a mixed pattern (blue and green without predominance). Final histologic diagnosis was 31 malignant lymph nodes and 32 benign. From the 31 patients with malignant lymph nodes 24 showed a predominant blue pattern and 7 showed a mixed pattern. From the 32 patients with benign lymph nodes, 23 cases demonstrated a predominant green pattern, 2 showed a blue predominant pattern, and 7 showed a mixed pattern. With these findings the probability of having benign lymph nodes with a predominant green pattern was 100%. The probability of having malignant lymph nodes with a predominant blue pattern was 92.3%. The probability of having benign and/or malignant lymph nodes with a mixed pattern was 50% (**Fig. 8**).

Săftoiu and colleagues[50] published their first experience of patients diagnosed by EUS with cervical, mediastinal, or abdominal lymph nodes. The investigators included

A   B

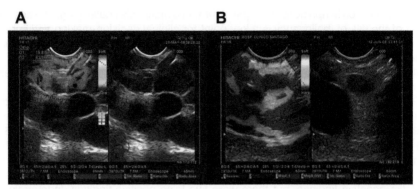

Fig. 8. Qualitative EUS-elastography of lymph nodes, showing different patterns. (*A*) Predominant green pattern in a patient with sarcoidosis and (*B*) a predominant blue pattern in a patient with malignant lymph nodes, metastasis from oat-cell lung cancer.

a total number of 42 lymph nodes. By using a qualitative analysis, based on the five predefined patterns, sensitivity, specificity, and accuracy for the differentiation between benign and malignant lymph nodes were 91.7%, 94.4%, and 92.86%, respectively.

There are few data on the usefulness of quantitative EUS-elastography for the evaluation of lymph nodes. Săftiou and colleagues also analyzed in their previous study[50] the usefulness if the quantitative analysis based on separate red, green and blue (RGB) channel histogram values of the EUS-elastography images. This method allowed an excellent discrimination between benign and malignant lymph nodes. Sensitivity, specificity, and accuracy for the differential diagnosis of 95.8%, 94.4%, and 95.2%, respectively were based on a cut-off level of 0.84. Săftoiu and colleagues[51] subsequently published their experience on quantitative EUS-elastography, based on the evaluation of hue histogram for the evaluation of lymph nodes. The investigators included patients diagnosed by EUS with cervical, mediastinal, or abdominal lymph nodes, with a total number of 85 lymph nodes examined in 54 patients, with a final diagnosis confirmed in 78 cases (37 were considered as benign and 41 as malignant). By using a mean hue value cutoff of 166 (middle of green-blue rainbow scale), the sensitivity, specificity, and accuracy for malignant lymph nodes were 85.4%, 91.9%, and 88.5%, respectively, based on a cutoff level of 166, with an area under the curve of 0.928.

Table 2 summarizes the published results of EUS-elastography in the differential diagnosis of lymph nodes.

Table 2				
Accuracy of EUS-elastography in the differential diagnosis of lymph nodes				
	Author	**Year**	**Sensitivity (%)**	**Specificity (%)**
Qualitative EUS-Elastography	Giovannini et al[41]	2006	100	50
	Giovannini et al[42]	2009	91.8	82.5
	Janssen et al[49]	2007	86.8	87.9
	Săftoiu et al[50]	2006	91.7	94.4
Quantitative EUS-Elastography	Săftoiu et al[50]	2006	95.8	94.4
	Săftoiu et al[51]	2007	85.4	91.9

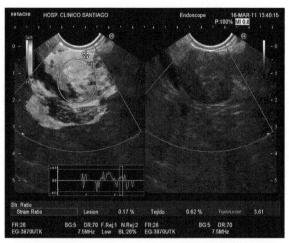

Fig. 9. Quantitative EUS-elastography of a left suprarenal gland mass, with a strain ratio of 3.61, corresponding to an adenoma.

Other Indications

There are no data about new applications of EUS-elastography. However, we can consider some future developments of this technique. Considering all accepted indications of EUS, it seems that EUS-elastography might be of help in the differentiation of solid lesions of the left suprarenal gland, to distinguish between adenoma and metastasis (in the authors' short experience in this field, we have found that EUS-elastography is helpful in this context) (**Fig. 9**). Owing to the proximity of the liver, it can also be helpful for determining malignancy of solid liver lesions (**Fig. 10**).[52] There are also some ongoing studies that are trying to evaluate the utility of elastography in the staging of gastric and esophageal cancer, by defining the infiltration of surrounding organs based on the elastographic patterns. Another proposed indication is for the evaluation of rectal wall involvement in patients with inflammatory bowel disease.

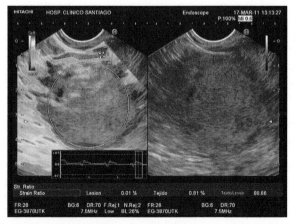

Fig. 10. Quantitative EUS-elastography of a solid liver mass, with a strain ratio of 88.66, finally corresponding to a hepatocellular carcinoma.

With this background of new possible indications, EUS-elastography will have many new clinical applications in the near future.

SUMMARY

EUS-elastography, both qualitative and quantitative, is an emerging technique, with the capability to differentiate fibrotic or inflammatory tissue from malignant lesions. This new methodology has proven to be useful in the differential diagnosis of solid pancreatic masses and lymph nodes, but also in the evaluation of patients with suspected chronic pancreatitis. However, further research is needed to completely define the place of this technique in routine clinical work and also to determine future indications.

REFERENCES

1. Dye CE, Waxman I. Endoscopic ultrasound. Gastroenterol Clin North Am 2002; 31(3):863–79.
2. Tamerisa R, Irisawa A, Bhutani MS. Endoscopic ultrasound in the diagnosis, staging, and management of gastrointestinal and adjacent malignancies. Med Clin North Am 2005;89:139–58.
3. Byrne MF, Jowell PS. Gastrointestinal imaging: endoscopic ultrasound. Gastroenterology 2002;122:1631–48.
4. Iglesias-García J, Lariño Noia J, Domínguez Muñoz JE. Endoscopic ultrasound in the diagnosis and staging of pancreatic cancer. Rev Esp Enferm Dig 2009; 101(9):631–8.
5. Giovannini M. The place of endoscopic ultrasound in bilio-pancreatic pathology. Gastroenterol Clin Biol 2010;34(8-9):436–45.
6. Gill KR, Wallace MB. Endoscopic ultrasound and staging of non-small cell lung cancer. Minerva Med 2007;98(4):323–30.
7. De Luca L, Di Bella S, D'Amore E. Mediastinal and gastric EUS: indications and technique examination. Minerva Med 2007;98(4):423–9.
8. Erickson RA. EUS-guided FNA. Gastrointest Endosc 2004;60(2):267–79.
9. Dumonceau JM, Polkowski M, Larghi A, et al. Indications, results, and clinical impact of endoscopic ultrasound (EUS)-guided sampling in gastroenterology: European Society of Gastrointestinal Endoscopy (ESGE) Clinical Guideline. Endoscopy 2011;43(10):897–912.
10. Turner BG, Cizinger S, Agarwal D, et al. Diagnosis of pancreatic neoplasia with EUS and FNA: a report of accuracy. Gastrointest Endosc 2010;71(1):91–8.
11. Iglesias-García J, Dominguez-Muñoz JE, Lozano-Leon A, et al. Impact of endoscopic-ultrasound fine needle biopsy for diagnosis of pancreatic masses. World J Gastroenterol 2007;13:289–93.
12. Chang KJ, Nguyen P, Erickson RA, et al. The clinical utility of endoscopic ultrasound-guided fine-needle aspiration in the diagnosis and staging of pancreatic carcinoma. Gastrointest Endosc 1997;45:387–93.
13. Vilmann P, Annema J, Clementsen P. Endosonography in bronchopulmonary disease. Best Pract Res Clin Gastroenterol 2009;23(5):711–28.
14. Nguyen TQ, Kalade A, Prasad S, et al. Endoscopic ultrasound guided fine needle aspiration (EUS-FNA) of mediastinal lesions. ANZ J Surg 2011;81(1-2):75–8.
15. Erickson RA, Sayage-Rabie L, Beisner RS. Factors' predicting the number of EUS-guided fine-needle passes for diagnosis of pancreatic malignancies. Gastrointest Endosc 2000;51:184–90.

16. Binmoeller KF, Rathod VD. Difficult pancreatic mass FNA: tips for success. Gastrointest Endosc 2002;56:S86–93.

17. Varadarajulu S, Tamhane A, Eloubeidi MA. Yield of EUS-guided FNA of pancreatic masses in the presence or the absence of chronic pancreatitis. Gastrointest Endosc 2005;62:728–36.

18. Bhutani MS, Hawes RH, Hoffman BJ. A comparison of the accuracy of echo features during endoscopic ultrasound (EUS) and EUS-guided fine needle aspiration for diagnosis of malignant lymph node invasion. Gastrointest Endosc 1997; 45:474–9.

19. Micames C, Jowell PS, White R, et al. Lower frequency of peritoneal carcinomatosis in patients with pancreatic cancer diagnosed by EUS-guided FNA vs. percutaneous FNA. Gastrointest Endosc 2003;58:690–5.

20. Eloubeidi MA, Tamhane A, Varadajulu S. Frequency of major complications after EUS-guided FNA of solid pancreatic masses: a prospective evaluation. Gastrointest Endosc 2006;63:622–9.

21. Itoh A, Ueno E, Tohno E, et al. Breast disease: clinical application of US elastography for diagnosis. Radiology 2006;239:341–50.

22. Cochlin DL, Ganatra RH, Griffiths DF. Elastography in the detection of prostatic cancer. Clin Radiol 2002;57:1014–20.

23. Krouskop TA, Wheeler TM, Kallel F, et al. Elastic moduli of breast and prostate tissues under compression. Ultrason Imaging 1998;20:260–74.

24. Giovannini M. Contrast-enhanced endoscopic ultrasound and elastosonoendoscopy. Best Pract Res Clin Gastroenterol 2009;23:767–79.

25. Chaudhari MH, Forsberg F, Voodarla A, et al. Breast tumor vascularity identified by contrast enhanced ultrasound and pathology: initial results. Ultrasonics 2000; 38:105–9.

26. Fornage BD. Recent advances in breast sonography. JBR-BTR 2000;83:75–80.

27. Garra BS, Cespedes EI, Ophir J, et al. Elastography of breast lesions: initial clinical results. Radiology 1997;202:79–86.

28. Gao L, Parker KJ, Lerner RM, et al. Imaging of the elastic properties of tissue—a review. Ultrasound Med Biol 1996;22:959–97.

29. Ophir J, Cespedes EI, Garra BS, et al. Elastography: ultrasound imaging of tissue strain and elastic modulus in vivo. Eur J Ultrasound 1996;3:49–70.

30. Giovannini M. Endoscopic ultrasound elastography. Pancreatology 2011; 11(Suppl 2):34–9.

31. Frey H. Real-time elastography. A new ultrasound procedure for the reconstruction of tissue elasticity. Radiologie 2003;43:850–5.

32. Iglesias-Garcia J, Lariño-Noia J, Abdulkader I, et al. Endoscopic ultrasound elastography for the characterization of solid pancreatic masses. Gastrointest Endosc 2009;70:1101–8.

33. Lariño-Noia J, Iglesias-García J, Álvarez-Castro A, et al. Usefulness of endoscopic ultrasound (EUS) elastography for the detection of malignant infiltration of mediastinal and abdominal lymph nodes [abstract]. Gastroenterology 2009.

34. Ferreira T, Rasband W. The ImageJ user guide—Version 1.44. Available at: http://imagej.nih.gov/ij/docs/user-guide.pdf. Accessed April 4, 2012.

35. Săftoiu A, Vilmann P, Gorunescu F, et al. Neural network analysis of dynamic sequences of EUS elastography used for the differential diagnosis of chronic pancreatitis and pancreatic cancer. Gastrointest Endosc 2008;68:1086–94.

36. Hirooka Y, Itoh A, Kawashima H, et al. Diagnosis of pancreatic disorders using contrast-enhanced endoscopic ultrasonography and endoscopic elastography. Clin Gastroenterol Hepatol 2009;7:S63–7.

37. Iglesias-Garcia J, Lariño-Noia J, Abdulkader I, et al. Quantitative endoscopic ultrasound elastography: an accurate method for the differentiation of solid pancreatic masses. Gastroenterol 2010;139:1172–80.
38. Seicean A. Endoscopic ultrasound in chronic pancreatitis: where are we now? World J Gastroenterol 2010;16(34):4253–63.
39. Brugge WR. Evaluation of pancreatic cystic lesions with EUS. Gastrointest Endosc 2004;59:698–707.
40. Galasso D, Carnuccio A, Larghi A. Pancreatic cancer: diagnosis and endoscopic staging. Eur Rev Med Pharmacol Sci 2010;14(4):375–85.
41. Giovannini M, Hookey LC, Bories E, et al. Endoscopic ultrasound elastography: the first step towards virtual biopsy? Preliminary results in 49 patients. Endoscopy 2006;38:344–8.
42. Giovannini M, Botelberge T, Bories E, et al. Endoscopic ultrasound elastography for evaluation of lymph nodes and pancreatic masses: a multicenter study. World J Gastroenterol 2009;15:1587–93.
43. Janssen J, Schlörer E, Greiner L. EUS elastography of the pancreas: feasibility and pattern description of the normal pancreas, chronic pancreatitis, and focal pancreatic lesions. Gastrointest Endosc 2007;65:971–8.
44. Hirche TO, Ignee A, Barreiros AP, et al. Indications and limitations of endoscopic ultrasound elastography for evaluation of focal pancreatic lesions. Endoscopy 2008;40:910–7.
45. Itokawa F, Itoi T, Sofuni A, et al. EUS elastography combined with the strain ratio of tissue elasticity for diagnosis of solid pancreatic masses. J Gastroenterol 2011; 46(6):843–53.
46. Săftoiu A, Vilmann P, Gorunescu F, et al. Accuracy of endoscopic ultrasound elastography used for differential diagnosis of focal pancreatic masses: a multicenter study. Endoscopy 2011;43:596–603.
47. Iglesias-Garcia J, Lariño-Noia J, Dominguez-Muñoz JE. [Elastography in the evaluation of chronic pancreatitis]. Gastroenterol Hepatol 2011;34(9):629–34 [in Spanish].
48. Micames CG, McCrory DC, Pavey DA, et al. Endoscopic ultrasound-guided fine-needle aspiration for non-small cell lung cancer staging: A systematic review and metaanalysis. Chest 2007;131(2):539–48.
49. Janssen J, Dietrich CF, Will U, et al. Endosonographic elastography in the diagnosis of mediastinal lymph nodes. Endoscopy 2007;39(11):952–7.
50. Săftoiu A, Vilmann P, Hassan H, et al. Analysis of endoscopic ultrasound elastography used for characterisation and differentiation of benign and malignant lymph nodes. Ultraschall Med 2006;27(6):535–42.
51. Săftoiu A, Vilmann P, Ciurea T, et al. Dynamic analysis of EUS used for the differentiation of benign and malignant lymph nodes. Gastrointest Endosc 2007;66(2): 291–300.
52. Iglesias-García J, Lariño-Noia J, Souto R, et al. Endoscopic ultrasound (EUS) elastography of the liver. Rev Esp Enferm Dig 2009;101(10):717–9.

Endoscopic Ultrasound: Contrast Enhancement

Masayuki Kitano, MD, PhD*, Hiroki Sakamoto, MD, PhD,
Masatoshi Kudo, MD, PhD

KEYWORDS

- Endoscopic ultrasonography • Contrast enhancement
- Contrast-enhanced harmonic EUS
- Ultrasound contrast agents • Sonazoid • SonoVue
- Definity • Microbubbles

ULTRASOUND CONTRAST AGENTS

Intra-arterial infusion of carbon dioxide (CO_2) gas was the first technology used for contrast-enhanced ultrasonography.[1-3] In this method, CO_2 is infused into the regional artery through a catheter during angiography. Fundamental B-mode ultrasonography sufficiently depicts signals from CO_2 microbubbles in a real-time manner.[1-3] Although intra-arterial CO_2 infusion combined with ultrasonography allows imaging with very high spatial and time resolutions, it has the limitation that ultrasonographic scanning must be performed during angiography.[1-3]

Intravenous ultrasound contrast agents are more convenient for contrast-enhanced ultrasonography because their use requires only a bolus infusion of the agent from a peripheral vein.[4,5] There are several ultrasound contrast agents commercially available.[4,5] Most of them are microbubbles consisting of gas covered with a lipid or phospholipid membrane. A certain range of acoustic power induces microbubble oscillation or breakage.[6,7] When microbubbles are oscillated or broken, signals are emitted that have different frequencies from the transmitted signals.[6,7] These signals can then be depicted by contrast-enhanced ultrasonography.[6,7]

The first-generation ultrasound contrast agents included Levovist (Schering AG, Berlin, Germany), which is composed of microbubbles of room air covered with a palmitic acid membrane.[4-7] Levovist required high acoustic power to oscillate or break its microbubbles. To overcome this disadvantage, second-generation ultrasound contrast agents, including SonoVue (Bracco Imaging, Milan, Italy), Sonazoid (Daiichi-Sankyo, Tokyo, Japan; GE Health care Milwaukee, WI, USA), and Definity (Lantheus Medical

Department of Gastroenterology and Hepatology, Kinki University School of Medicine, 377-2 Ohnohigashi, Osakasayama, 589-8511 Japan
* Corresponding author.
E-mail address: m-kitano@med.kindai.ac.jp

Gastrointest Endoscopy Clin N Am 22 (2012) 349–358
doi:10.1016/j.giec.2012.04.013
1052-5157/12/$ – see front matter © 2012 Elsevier Inc. All rights reserved.

Imaging, North Billerica MA, USA), were created.[4-6] These agents are composed of gasses different from room air, and microbubbles of these agents can be oscillated or broken by lower acoustic powers.[4-6] These second-generation agents are more suitable for endoscopic ultrasonography (EUS) because the small transducer of EUS produces limited acoustic power.[8]

VASCULAR ASSESSMENT BY EUS

In the early days of EUS development, it was difficult to enhance vessels by mechanical radial EUS.[9] The first reports about contrast-enhanced EUS used fundamental B-mode EUS with an intravenous ultrasound contrast agent composed of sonicated albumin.[10,11] Although this method slightly enhanced the signals from lesions with rich vessels such as neuroendocrine tumors and cystic tumors in the pancreas, it did not enhance signals of other diseases and has a limitation in selective depiction of the contrast agent.[10,11] Electronic EUS equipped with color and power Doppler modes first enabled the identification of large vessels with colored images.[12] In particular, this method allowed the visualization of large vessels behind the gastrointestinal wall and improved the avoidance of intervening vessels during needle puncture. However, those modes only detect large vessels with fast flow because they depict the phase shift of signals from quickly moving substances.

Ultrasound contrast agents located in vessels emit phase shift (pseudo-Doppler) signals and enhance Doppler signals from vessels.[13] Contrast-enhanced Doppler EUS (CD-EUS) is used to evaluate not only large vessels but also tumor vascularity, by enhancing the intratumoral vessels (**Fig. 1**).[14-20] However, even the use of ultrasound contrast agents cannot depict fine vessels with slow flow because Doppler ultrasonography has low sensitivity to low flow.[7,8,15] Moreover, contrast-enhanced Doppler ultrasonography suffers from poor spatial resolution as well as motion and blooming artifacts, which can make it difficult to evaluate tumor vascularity.[7,8,15] Motion artifacts refer to the low signal intensity of flowing blood compared with that of tissue movement.[7] Blooming refers to the widened appearance of a blood vessel with power Doppler compared with the results with fundamental B-mode imaging (see **Fig. 1**).[7]

Contrast-enhanced harmonic imaging was developed to allow for more specific imaging of ultrasound contrast agents.[6-8] The main purpose of contrast-enhanced harmonic ultrasonography is the selective sensitive depiction of signals from

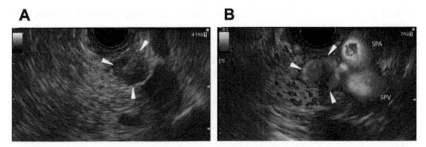

Fig. 1. Typical conventional EUS and contrast-enhanced power Doppler EUS images of a small endocrine tumor in the pancreas. (A) The conventional EUS image shows a small hypoechoic nodule (*arrowheads*) of 10 mm in diameter in the body of the pancreas. (B) The contrast-enhanced power Doppler EUS image shows abundant vessels in the nodule (*arrowheads*), although blooming artifact is observed at vessels in the nodule. Blooming artifact is also observed in the splenic artery (SPA) and splenic vein (SPV).

microbubbles in situ by filtrating signals from the tissue. The most important advantage of contrast-enhanced harmonic ultrasonography over contrast-enhanced Doppler ultrasonography is that it can depict microbubbles even though they do not flow.[6–8] By depicting microbubbles located in microvasculature, contrast-enhanced harmonic ultrasonography allowed imaging of parenchymal perfusion. In addition, it can depict vessels with very high resolution without Doppler-related artifacts.

Contrast-enhanced harmonic EUS (CH-EUS) was impossible with Levovist because the transducer of the echoendoscope was too small to oscillate and break the microbubbles, necessitating the use of CD-EUS.[9,15] Because second-generation ultrasound contrast agents can be oscillated or broken by lower acoustic powers,[4–6,9] CH-EUS can be used with these agents.

CONTRAST-ENHANCED DOPPLER EUS

Intravenous ultrasound contrast agents improve the Doppler detection of flow in vessels. CD-EUS is significantly more sensitive and accurate than power Doppler EUS in detecting the relatively hypovascular ductal adenocarcinomas of the pancreas.[14–16] Hypovascularity as a sign of ductal carcinomas in CD-EUS obtained a sensitivity of 85% to 94% and a specificity of 71% to 100%.[14–18] EUS is also a highly sensitive method for detection of pancreatic ductal carcinomas, particularly small ones.[9,21,22] In a study comparing the abilities of CD-EUS and contrast-enhanced multidetector-row computed tomography (MDCT) to diagnose small pancreatic tumors, the sensitivities for detecting pancreatic carcinomas sized 2 cm or less by EUS and MDCT were 94% and 50%, respectively, and CD-EUS diagnosed small pancreatic carcinomas sized 2 cm or less as tumors with hypoenhancement significantly better than MDCT.[15] EUS is also useful to detect small neuroendocrine tumors.[19,23,24] Detection rate of EUS for neuroendocrine tumors (92%–95%) is significantly higher than that of MDCT (63%–81%).[19,24] Ishikawa and colleagues[19] reported on the usefulness of EUS combined with contrast enhancement in the preoperative localization of pancreatic endocrine tumors. In their report, CD-EUS indicated that hyperenhancement was observed in 98% of neuroendocrine tumors.[19] In those previous reports about CD-EUS, ductal carcinomas and neuroendocrine tumors are characterized by CD-EUS as solid lesions with hypoenhancement and hyperenhancement, respectively. Taking into consideration the superiority of EUS in the detection rates, CD-EUS is a promising tool to characterize small pancreatic tumors that cannot be detected by other imaging methods.

In discrimination between benign and malignant mediastinal and abdominal lymph nodes, 2 groups reported the usefulness of CD-EUS.[20,25] Kanamori and colleagues[20] found that all malignant lymph nodes showed a defect of enhancement (sensitivity 100%), whereas diffuse enhancement was observed in 86% of benign lymph nodes (specificity 86%). Hocke and colleagues[25] used the following criteria for malignant lymph nodes: irregular appearance of the vessels and only arterial vessels visible. Using these criteria, the sensitivity and specificity in differentiating malignant from benign lymph nodes were 60% and 91%, respectively. If malignant lymphoma were excluded, the sensitivity of the CD-EUS for malignant lymph nodes increased to 73%.[25] Even though those reports differ in criteria and diagnostic accuracy for malignancy, CD-EUS is useful for characterization of enlarged lymph nodes.

PRINCIPLE OF CONTRAST HARMONIC IMAGING

When exposed to a certain range of ultrasonic beams, the microbubbles of ultrasound contrast agents are disrupted or resonated, which releases a large amount of harmonic signals (**Fig. 2**).[6–8] When the tissues and microbubbles receive transmitted ultrasound waves, both produce harmonic components that are integer multiples of the fundamental frequency; however, the harmonic content from the microbubbles is higher than that from the tissues (see **Fig. 2**).[6–8] Selective depiction of the second harmonic component visualizes the signals from the microbubbles more strongly than those from the tissues.

When ultrasound pulses are transmitted multiple times in succession, the signals from the contrast agents vary greatly in phase (see **Fig. 2**), with no relation to its motion.[9,26,27] The signals in the part without contrast agents are hardly changed between multiple transmissions. This specific feature of the contrast agents (phase shifts) is also used for contrast-enhanced harmonic imaging.[9,26,27] Extended pure harmonic detection (ExPHD) is a mode for EUS systems that is specific for contrast harmonic imaging, which receives not only the second harmonic components but also signals with the relative phase shifts (see **Fig. 2**).[9,26,27] This processing enhances the imaging of signals from microbubbles in vessels with very slow flow without Doppler-related artifacts.

CONTRAST-ENHANCED HARMONIC EUS

Dietrich and colleagues[28] first reported the use of contrast-enhanced, low–mechanical index, real-time EUS using adapted dynamic-contrast harmonic wide-band pulsed inversion software. Using this method, they identified the celiac trunk, common hepatic artery, splenic artery, and portal vein and its branches and collaterals in patients with portal vein thrombosis.[28]

The development of another EUS system, equipped with an echoendoscope with a broadband transducer and ExPHD mode, enabled the authors to obtain images of the microcirculation and parenchymal perfusion in digestive organs (**Fig. 3**).[26,27] In contrast, CD-EUS cannot provide images of parenchymal perfusion or of branching vessels because blooming artifacts of large vessels are observed.[27,29]

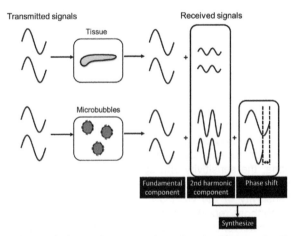

Fig. 2. Principle of extended pure harmonic detection (ExPHD) mode. The microbubbles produce stronger second harmonic signals as well as greater phase shifts than does the tissue. Contrast harmonic imaging based on the ExPHD mode selectively depicts signals from microbubbles by synthesizing the phase shift signals with the second harmonic components.

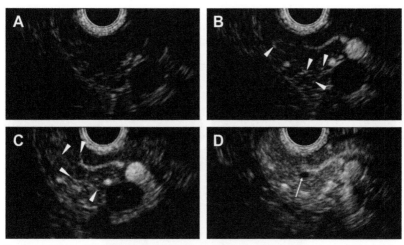

Fig. 3. Time course of CH-EUS images in a normal pancreas. (*A*) The CH-EUS image before infusion of the contrast agent. Neither signals from the tissue nor microbubbles can be observed. (*B*) The CH-EUS image 13 seconds after infusion of the contrast agent. Spotty signals from microbubbles (*arrowheads*) appear in the pancreas. (*C*) The CH-EUS image 15 seconds after infusion of the contrast agent. Fine branching vessels (*arrowheads*) are observed. (*D*) The CH-EUS image 22 seconds after infusion of the contrast agent. Diffuse parenchymal perfusion of microbubbles can be imaged. The pancreatic duct (*arrow*) is depicted as an avascular structure with strong contrast to the surrounding tissue.

The new EUS system depicts pancreatic ductal carcinomas as hypovascular nodules that mostly have irregular network-like vessels. In contrast, CH-EUS depicts most neuroendocrine tumors as a hypervascular pattern (**Fig. 4**).[27,29–31] This new CH-EUS system allowed diagnosis of pancreatic carcinomas with a high sensitivity (89%–96%) and specificity (64%–89%).[29–31] Particularly, CH-EUS was significantly more accurate than MDCT in diagnosing small ductal carcinomas (*P* = .034).[31]

Although EUS has a high spatial resolution, it misses some ductal carcinomas. Some factors, including chronic pancreatitis, a diffusely infiltrating and a recent episode of acute pancreatitis, increase the likelihood of a false-negative EUS examination.[32] CH-EUS improves the depiction of pancreatic tumors, compared with conventional EUS.[30,31] CH-EUS allowed detection of the outline of all ductal carcinomas with uncertain conventional EUS findings.[30,31] Similarly, when Imazu and colleagues[33] compared the abilities of conventional EUS and CH-EUS in terms of preoperative T staging of pancreatobiliary tumors, they found that CH-EUS correctly diagnosed T staging in 24 of 26 pancreatobiliary tumors, 6 of which were misdiagnosed by conventional EUS. In particular, CH-EUS depicted the wall of the portal vein more clearly, which means that it is superior in diagnosing portal invasion by pancreatic and bile duct cancers.[33]

CH-EUS is also used for evaluation of vascularity in organs other than the pancreas. In a study evaluating the microvasculature of benign and malignant intra-abdominal lesions of undetermined origin by CH-EUS, 96.3% of malignant lesions exhibited heterogeneous enhancement (**Fig. 5**), whereas benign lesions did not show heterogeneous enhancement.[34] This result suggests that heterogeneous enhancement on CH-EUS is a feature of malignant lesions. When CH-EUS was used for assessment of tumor vascularity of gastrointestinal stromal tumors (GISTs), CH-EUS identified

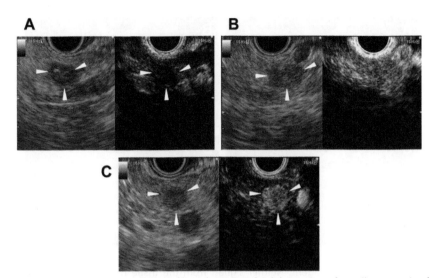

Fig. 4. Typical conventional EUS (*left*) and CH-EUS (*right*) images of small tumors in the pancreas. (*A*) A ductal carcinoma with hypoenhancement. Conventional EUS (*left*) shows a hypoechoic area (*arrowheads*) of 10 mm in diameter at the pancreas tail. CH-EUS (right) indicates that the area is hypovascular (*arrowheads*) compared with the surrounding tissue. (*B*) An inflammatory pseudotumor with isoenhancement. Conventional EUS (*left*) shows a hypoechoic area (*arrowheads*) of 11 mm at the pancreas tail. CH-EUS (*right*) indicates enhancement in this area similar to the surrounding tissue; a margin is not observed. (*C*) A neuroendocrine tumor with hyperenhancement. Conventional EUS (*left*) shows a hypoechoic mass (*arrowheads*) of 9 mm in diameter at the pancreas body. CH-EUS (*right*) indicates that enhancement (*arrowheads*) in the mass is higher than in the surrounding tissue.

irregular vessels in GISTs with high-grade malignancy (**Fig. 6**) with a sensitivity, specificity, and accuracy of 100%, 63%, and 83%, respectively, suggesting CH-EUS may play an important role in predicting the malignancy risk of GISTs.[35]

CONTRAST-ENHANCED EUS FOR EUS-GUIDED FINE-NEEDLE ASPIRATION

EUS-guided fine-needle aspiration (EUS-FNA) is a useful tool for characterizing a solid mass detected by conventional EUS.[36] If the EUS-FNA diagnosis is a malignant tumor,

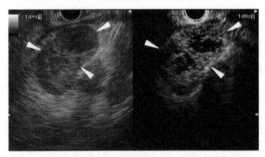

Fig. 5. Typical conventional EUS (*left*) and CH-EUS (*right*) images of a metastatic lymphadenopathy. Conventional EUS (*left*) shows a swollen lymph node (*arrowheads*) of 41 mm in diameter adjacent to the stomach. CH-EUS (*right*) indicates that enhancement in the lymph node is heterogeneous.

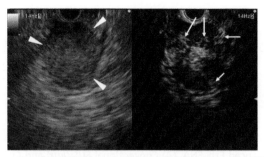

Fig. 6. Typical conventional EUS (*left*) and CH-EUS (*right*) images of a GIST with high-grade malignancy. Conventional EUS (*left*) shows a tumor (*arrowheads*) of 38 mm in diameter located in the fourth layer of the gastric wall. CH-EUS (*right*) depicts irregular vessels (*arrows*) in the tumor.

then patients should be recommended to undergo surgery, because EUS-FNA is highly specific for the identification of pancreatic carcinomas. However, deciding between surgery and follow-up in patients whose EUS-FNA findings are negative is sometimes difficult, because false-negative EUS-FNA results cannot be excluded. When Napoleon and colleagues[29] compared CH-EUS and EUS-FNA for the identification of pancreatic carcinomas, the sensitivity of CH-EUS for carcinoma identification was higher than that of EUS-FNA. Moreover, 4 of the 5 carcinomas with false-negative EUS-FNA findings had hypoenhancement. In the authors' recent study, CH-EUS was not superior to EUS-FNA for the identification of pancreatic carcinomas.[31] However, CH-EUS revealed that all ductal carcinomas with false-negative EUS-FNA findings had hypoenhancement. When the ductal carcinomas were regarded as tumors with a positive EUS-FNA finding and/or hypoenhancement on CH-EUS, combining CH-EUS with EUS-FNA improved the sensitivity of identifying ductal carcinomas from 92.2% to 100%.[31] Therefore, CH-EUS before EUS-FNA complements EUS-FNA in identifying ductal carcinomas and helps in making decisions about the next treatment approach. When CH-EUS reveals a hypovascular pattern in a pancreatic tumor, even if the EUS-FNA findings are negative, surgical resection or pathologic reevaluation by EUS-FNA of the tumor should be recommended.

As described earlier, CH-EUS is better than conventional EUS in clearly depicting the outline of some pancreatic carcinomas.[30,31] These results suggest that contrast harmonic imaging might be useful for the identification of some lesions that are not clearly defined by conventional EUS (**Fig. 7**). Consequently, it is likely that CH-EUS facilitates EUS-FNA of lesions by helping to identify the target for EUS-FNA (see **Fig. 7**). In addition, information from CH-EUS can potentially change the diagnosis and management of the lesions depicted by EUS. Romagnuolo and colleagues[37] reported 2 cases in which the management changed significantly after CH-EUS. EUS-FNA was avoided because CH-EUS revealed that a liver tumor was a hemangioma. EUS-FNA was performed in a mediastinal cystic lesion after CH-EUS confirmed it as solid.

FUTURE PERSPECTIVE OF CONTRAST-ENHANCED EUS

So far, the technique of contrast-enhanced EUS has largely been used for evaluation of vascularity. However, recent studies have revealed that this technique can also be applied for molecular imaging of vascular endothelial growth factor (VEGF) receptor.[38,39] Affinity of microbubbles for VEGF receptor may facilitate molecular profiling of angiogenesis and early assessment of antiangiogenic therapy effects.

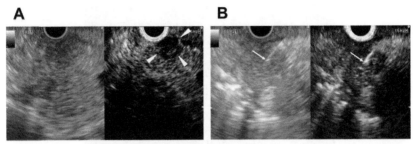

Fig. 7. Contrast-enhanced EUS-FNA. (*A*) Conventional EUS (*left*) and CH-EUS (*right*) images of a ductal carcinoma. Conventional EUS (*left*) shows a slightly hypoechoic area without a clear margin at the pancreas head. CH-EUS (*right*) depicts a tumor with hypoenhancement with a clear margin relative to the surrounding tissue. (*B*) Conventional EUS (*left*) and CH-EUS (*right*) images during needle puncture. The tumor with hypoenhancement is punctured by a needle (*arrow*) guided by CH-EUS (*right*). The targeted EUS-FNA of the hypovascular tumor detected malignant cells.

Recently, there has been a focus on EUS-guided ablation therapy for the treatment of focal pancreatic lesions. Experiments in pigs showed that contrast-enhanced EUS improved visualization of altered pancreatic vascular perfusion after local injection of ethanol, indicating that contrast-enhanced EUS can be used for follow-up of the ablated lesion.[40] Moreover, the development of contrast-enhanced EUS will be beneficial for targeted drug delivery applications in pancreatic tumors.[4,41] Drug substances, including plasmid DNA, can be delivered within the microbubbles. Strong ultrasound beams can potentially destroy microbubbles to release the drug "payload" only in the pancreas. Thus, the targeted drug delivery treatment should enhance drug action and reduce undesirable adverse effects. In the near future, the technology of contrast-enhanced EUS would expand to these promising applications.

REFERENCES

1. Matsuda Y, Yabuuchi I. Hepatic tumors: US contrast enhancement with CO_2 microbubbles. Radiology 1986;161:701–5.
2. Kudo M, Tomita S, Tochio H, et al. Small hepatocellular carcinoma: diagnosis with US angiography with intraarterial CO_2 micorbubbles. Radiology 1992;182:155–60.
3. Kato T, Tsukamoto Y, Naitoh Y, et al. Ultrasonographic and endoscopic ultrasonographic angiography in pancreatic mass lesions. Acta Radiol 1995;36:381–7.
4. Sanchez MV, Varadarajulu S, Napoleon B. EUS contrast agents: what is available, how do they work, and are they effective? Gastrointest Endosc 2009;69:571–7.
5. Reddy NK, Ioncică AM, Săftoiu A, et al. Contrast-enhanced endoscopic ultrasonography. World J Gastroenterol 2011;17:42–8.
6. Whittingham TA. Contrast-specific imaging techniques; technical perspective. In: Quaia E, editor. Contrast media in ultrasonography. Basic principles and clinical applications. Berlin: Springer; 2005. p. 43–84.
7. Kudo M. Various contrast-enhanced imaging modes after administration of Levovist. In: Kudo M, editor. Contrast harmonic imaging in the diagnosis and treatment of hepatic tumors. Tokyo: Springer; 2003. p. 22–30.
8. Kitano M, Kudo M, Maekawa K, et al. Dynamic imaging of pancreatic diseases by contrast enhanced coded phase inversion harmonic ultrasonography. Gut 2004; 53:854–9.

9. Kitano M, Kudo M, Sakamoto H, et al. Endoscopic ultrasonography and contrast-enhanced endoscopic ultrasonography. Pancreatology 2011;11(Suppl 2): 28–33.

10. Hirooka Y, Goto H, Ito A, et al. Contrast-enhanced endoscopic ultrasonography in pancreatic diseases: a preliminary study. Am J Gastroenterol 1998;93: 632–5.

11. Hirooka Y, Naitoh Y, Goto H, et al. Usefulness of contrast-enhanced endoscopic ultrasonography with intravenous injection of sonicated serum albumin. Gastrointest Endosc 1997;46:166–9.

12. Wiersema MJ, Chak A, Kopecky KK, et al. Duplex Doppler endosonography in the diagnosis of splenic vein, portal vein, and portosystemic shunt thrombosis. Gastrointest Endosc 1995;42:19–26.

13. Bhutani MS, Hoffman BJ, van Velse A, et al. Contrast-enhanced endoscopic ultrasonography with galactose microparticles: SHU508A (Levovist). Endoscopy 1997;29:635–9.

14. Hocke M, Schulze E, Gottschalk P, et al. Contrast-enhanced endoscopic ultrasound in discrimination between focal pancreatitis and pancreatic cancer. World J Gastroenterol 2006;12:246–50.

15. Sakamoto H, Kitano M, Suetomi Y, et al. Utility of contrast-enhanced endoscopic ultrasonography for diagnosis of small pancreatic carcinomas. Ultrasound Med Biol 2008;34:525–32.

16. Săftoiu A, Iordache SA, Gheonea DI, et al. Combined contrast-enhanced power Doppler and real-time sonoelastography performed during EUS, used in the differential diagnosis of focal pancreatic masses (with videos). Gastrointest Endosc 2010;72:739–47.

17. Becker D, Strobel D, Bernatik T, et al. Echo-enhanced color- and power-Doppler EUS for the discrimination between focal pancreatitis and pancreatic carcinoma. Gastrointest Endosc 2001;53:784–9.

18. Dietrich CF, Ignee A, Braden B, et al. Improved differentiation of pancreatic tumors using contrast-enhanced endoscopic ultrasound. Clin Gastroenterol Hepatol 2008;6:590–7.

19. Ishikawa T, Itoh A, Kawashima H, et al. Usefulness of EUS combined with contrast-enhancement in the differential diagnosis of malignant versus benign and preoperative localization of pancreatic endocrine tumors. Gastrointest Endosc 2010;71:951–9.

20. Kanamori A, Hirooka Y, Itoh A, et al. Usefulness of contrast-enhanced endoscopic ultrasonography in the differentiation between malignant and benign lymphadenopathy. Am J Gastroenterol 2006;101:45–51.

21. DeWitt J, Devereaux B, Chriswell M, et al. Comparison of endoscopic ultrasonography and multidetector computed tomography for detecting and staging pancreatic cancer. Ann Intern Med 2004;141:753–63.

22. Săftoiu A, Vilmann P. Role of endoscopic ultrasound in the diagnosis and staging of pancreatic cancer. J Clin Ultraound 2009;37:1–17.

23. Rösch T, Lightdale CJ, Botet JF, et al. Localization of pancreatic endocrine tumors by endoscopic ultrasonography. N Engl J Med 1992;326:1721–6.

24. Khashab MA, Yong E, Lennon AM, et al. EUS is still superior to multidetector computed tomography for detection of pancreatic neuroendocrine tumors. Gastrointest Endosc 2011;73:691–6.

25. Hocke M, Menges M, Topalidis T, et al. Contrast-enhanced endoscopic ultrasound in discrimination between benign and malignant mediastinal and abdominal lymph nodes. J Cancer Res Clin Oncol 2008;134:473–80.

26. Kitano M, Kudo M, Sakamoto H, et al. Preliminary study of contrast-enhanced harmonic endosonography with second-generation contrast agents. J Med Ultrasonics 2008;35:11–8.
27. Kitano M, Sakamoto H, Matsui U, et al. A novel perfusion imaging technique of the pancreas: contrast-enhanced harmonic EUS (with video). Gastrointest Endosc 2008;67:141–50.
28. Dietrich CF, Ignee A, Frey H. Contrast-enhanced endoscopic ultrasound with low mechanical index: a new technique. Z Gastroenterol 2005;43:1219–23.
29. Napoleon B, Alvarez-Sanchez MV, Gincoul R, et al. Contrast-enhanced harmonic endoscopic ultrasound in solid lesions of the pancreas: results of a pilot study. Endoscopy 2010;42:564–70.
30. Fusaroli P, Spada A, Mancino MG, et al. Contrast harmonic echo-endoscopic ultrasound improves accuracy in diagnosis of solid pancreatic masses. Clin Gastroenterol Hepatol 2010;8:629–34.
31. Kitano M, Kudo M, Yamao K, et al. Characterization of small solid tumors in the pancreas: contrast: the value of contrast-enhanced harmonic endoscopic ultrasonography. Am J Gastroenterol 2012;107:303–10.
32. Bhutani MS, Gress FG, Giovannini M, et al. The no endosonographic detection of tumor (NEST) study: a case series of pancreatic cancers missed on endoscopic ultrasonography. Endoscopy 2004;36:385–9.
33. Imazu H, Uchiyama Y, Matsunaga K, et al. Contrast-enhanced harmonic EUS with novel ultrasonographic contrast (Sonazoid) in the preoperative T-staging for pancreaticobiliary malignancies. Scand J Gastroenterol 2010;45:732–8.
34. Xia Y, Kitano M, Kudo M, et al. Characterization of intra-abdominal lesions of undetermined origin by contrast-enhanced harmonic EUS (with video). Gastrointest Endosc 2010;72:637–42.
35. Sakamoto H, Kitano M, Matsui S, et al. Estimation of malignant potential of GI stromal tumors by contrast-enhanced harmonic EUS (with videos). Gastrointest Endosc 2011;73:227–37.
36. DeWitt J. EUS in pancreatic neoplasms. In: Hawes RH, Fockens P, editors. Endosonography. Philadelphia: Saunders Elsevier; 2006. p. 177–203.
37. Romagnuolo J, Hoffman B, Vela S, et al. Accuracy of contrast-enhanced harmonic EUS with a second-generation perflutren lipid microsphere contrast agent (with video). Gastrointest Endosc 2011;73:52–63.
38. Willmann JK, Lutz AM, Paulmurugan R, et al. Dual-targeted contrast agent for US assessment of tumor angiogenesis in vivo. Radiology 2008;248:936–44.
39. Palmowski M, Huppert J, Ladewig G, et al. Molecular profiling of angiogenesis with targeted ultrasound imaging: early assessment of antiangiogenic therapy effects. Mol Cancer Ther 2008;7:101–9.
40. Giday SA, Magno P, Gabrielson KL, et al. The utility of contrast enhanced endoscopic ultrasound in monitoring ethanol-induced pancreatic tissue ablation: a pilot study in a porcine model. Endoscopy 2007;39:525–9.
41. Hermot S, Klibanov AL. Microbubbles in ultrasound-triggered drug and gene delivery. Adv Drug Deliv Rev 2008;60:1153–66.

Endoscopic Ultrasonography-Guided Tumor Ablation

Won Jae Yoon, MD[a], William R. Brugge, MD[b],*

KEYWORDS

- Endoscopic ultrasonography • Ablation • Tumor
- Radiofrequency • Photodynamic therapy • Laser • Ethanol

INTRODUCTION

When endoscopic ultrasonography (EUS) was first introduced in the 1980s, its primary role was a diagnostic tool.[1] With the introduction of curvilinear-array endosonoscopes, the ability of performing fine-needle aspiration (EUS-FNA) became possible. Recently, the introduction of EUS-guided fine-needle injection has made possible the introduction of interventional EUS.[2] The potential advantages of EUS-guided antitumor therapy are real-time imaging guidance, the ability to ablate tumor in poor surgical candidates, reduced morbidity compared with surgery, and the potential to be performed on an outpatient basis.[3] This review focuses on EUS-guided radiofrequency ablation (EUS-RFA), EUS-guided photodynamic therapy (EUS-PDT), EUS-guided laser ablation, and EUS-guided ethanol injection to solid tumors. EUS-guided pancreatic cyst ablation, injection of antitumor agents, fiducial marker implantation, and brachytherapy.

TECHNIQUES OF EUS-GUIDED TUMOR ABLATION
EUS-RFA

Radiofrequency ablation (RFA) uses electromagnetic energy to induce thermal injury to the target tissue. In monopolar RFA, a closed-loop circuit includes a radiofrequency (RF) generator, an electrode needle, a dispersive electrode (ground pad), and the patient.[4] The electrode delivers the energy to the tumor, resulting in a volume of high current density and localized heating. The ground pad closes the electrical current

Conflict of interest: None.

Financial support: None.

[a] Gastrointestinal Unit, Massachusetts General Hospital, Harvard Medical School, 55 Fruit Street, Boston, MA 02114, USA; [b] Gastrointestinal Unit, Massachusetts General Hospital, 55 Fruit Street, Boston, MA 02114, USA

* Corresponding author.

E-mail address: wbrugge@partners.org

Gastrointest Endoscopy Clin N Am 22 (2012) 359–369

doi:10.1016/j.giec.2012.04.017

1052-5157/12/$ – see front matter © 2012 Published by Elsevier Inc.

path; it is designed to disperse energy over a large area to reduce the possibility of thermal injury to the skin.[5] In bipolar RFA, current oscillates between 2 interstitial electrodes, obviating a ground pad.[6] It also confines current flow to the area between the electrodes and decreases the perfusion-mediated cooling, which results in faster and more focal heating of the target area.[5] RF energy is the most well-studied ablation source, and is one of the safest and most predictable techniques for thermal ablation.[5,7] Various EUS-RFA electrodes are shown in **Fig. 1**.

EUS-RFA was initially described by Goldberg and colleagues[3] in 1999. Under EUS guidance, a 19-gauge needle electrode with 1.0- to 1.5-cm tip was passed transgastrically to the pancreatic tail in 13 Yorkshire pigs. A 500-kHz monopolar RF generator supplied the electrosurgical current for 6 minutes, maintaining the electrode tip temperature of $90° ± 2°C$. During RF application, a hyperechoic region with diameter around 1 cm appeared around the distal needle tip within 1 minute of achieving of 90°C tissue temperature. EUS needle withdrawal revealed spherical or conical hyperechoic lesions 1 to 1.5 cm in diameter. Follow-up EUS was performed on 2 pigs. EUS 9 days later demonstrated a spherical and hypoechoic pancreatic lesion $1.9 × 2.0$ cm in diameter; the lesion was unchanged in size on EUS on day 14 but appeared more hypoechoic. EUS of the second pig on days 9 and 14 showed an elliptical, thick-walled fluid collection with a size of $2.7 × 2.8$ cm containing low-grade echoes (**Fig. 2**). Enhanced computed tomography (CT) scans in all pigs immediately after RFA revealed hypodense, nonenhancing foci measuring 8 to 10 mm in diameter with an enhancing rim. On CT scans from 6 pigs 14 days after RFA, 2 distinctive findings were noted. In

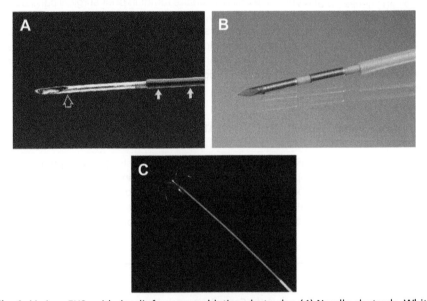

Fig. 1. Various EUS-guided radiofrequency ablation electrodes. (*A*) Needle electrode. White arrows indicate shrink tubing, open arrow indicates thermocouple embedded in tip. (*B*) Cool-tipped radiofrequency catheter. (*C*) Umbrella-shaped retractable needle electrode. (*Reprinted from* Goldberg SN, Mallery S, Gazelle GS, et al. EUS-guided radiofrequency ablation in the pancreas: results in a porcine model. Gastrointest Endosc 1999;50:392–401, with permission from Elsevier; and Brugge WR. EUS-guided ablation therapy and celiac plexus interventions. In: Hawes RH, Fockens P, Varadarajulu S, editors. Endosonography. 2nd edition. Philadelphia: Elsevier Saunders; 2011. p. 275–82; with permission from Elsevier.)

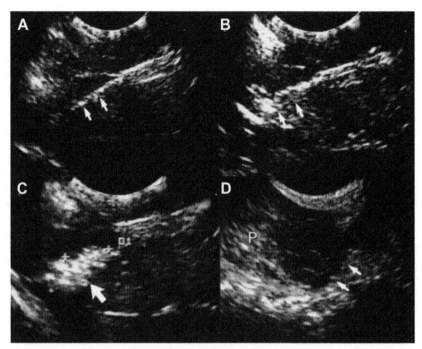

Fig. 2. EUS appearance of radiofrequency ablation. (*A*) Needle electrode (*arrows*) inserted into the pancreas. (*B*) Development of hyperechoic region (*arrows*) around the electrode during radiofrequency application. (*C*) Hyperechoic (*arrow*) region surrounding the electrode track immediately after ablation. (*D*) Hypoechoic focus seen 14 days after ablation (*arrows*). (*Reprinted from* Goldberg SN, Mallery S, Gazelle GS, et al. EUS-guided radiofrequency ablation in the pancreas: results in a porcine model. Gastrointest Endosc 1999;50:392–401; with permission from Elsevier.)

4 of 6 pigs, the previously visualized hypodense focus was not clearly delineated. In the other 2 pigs, a progressively enhancing rim 2 to 3 mm in thickness surrounding the coagulation focus of 1 to 1.2 cm could be seen. In pigs euthanized immediately after RFA, areas of treatment were visualized as 8- to 10-mm tan to brown lesions surrounded by normal pancreatic tissue; microscopic evaluation confirmed the presence of coagulation necrosis in treated tissues with sharp demarcation between treated and untreated tissue. In the 2 pigs euthanized 24 to 48 hours after the procedure, the gross findings were similar to those in pigs killed immediately. However, histopathology revealed a 1- to 2-mm watershed zone of an early inflammatory response surrounding the coagulated tissue. In the 6 specimens harvested 14 days after RFA, 2 patterns of tissue response were noted. In 2 pigs, a 1- to 1.2-cm cavity filled with necrotic tissue was identified; histology demonstrated an area of coagulative necrosis surrounded by a 2- to 3-mm fibrotic wall. In 4 pigs, a focus of brownish fibrotic tissue 5 to 8 mm long and 3 to 4 mm in diameter was seen invaginating the edge of normal-appearing pancreas. On histology, these foci were composed of fibrosis and scarring with residual areas of stromal and fat necrosis.

Correlation between imaging and gross pathology was excellent for lesions larger than 5 mm; the margin of difference was within 2 mm. Rim enhancement seen on CT images obtained immediately after RFA corresponded with interstitial hemorrhage. The rim enhancement seen at 14 days represented granulation tissue. Fours pigs showed resolution of previously visualized nonenhancing foci on CT; only residual fibrotic tissue was found in the ablated zone at pathology.

All pigs tolerated the RFA well, and no clinical evidence of distress was present in the surviving pigs. However, some complications were encountered. Three transmural gastric burns and one serosal small intestinal burn were attributed to improper electrode placement. There were no frank perforations of the gastrointestinal tract. One pig had elevated serum lipase, a focal pancreatitis, and a subsequent pancreatic fluid collection.

Modified RFA probes were tested subsequently. In 2008, Carrara and colleagues[8,9] reported their experience with a hybrid cryotherm probe that combines bipolar RFA with cryotechnology. The heated probe is cooled by cryogenic gas (CO_2 in this probe), which increases the RF-induced interstitial devitalization, and thus compensated the reduced efficiency of bipolar RFA compared with monopolar RFA. The investigators performed EUS-RFA of various solid organs, documented the size of the ablation lesion measured immediately after ablation (T0), before euthanasia (T1) using EUS and immediately after euthanasia macroscopically (T2), and described histologic findings and complications.

For pancreas, 14 ablations were performed in 14 pigs.[8] Energy input was 16 W, and cryogenic cooling was done by applying 650 psi of CO_2. Application time ranged from 120 to 900 seconds. Seven pigs were euthanized at week 1, and the other 7 at week 2. Ablation resulted in elliptic lesions. When compared with the lesion size at necropsy, the ablated area was always overestimated by EUS, with a correlation coefficient of 0.89. A positive correlation between T0 and the duration of RF application was demonstrated. In addition, the correlation between T2 and the application time demonstrated a fixed ratio of 2.3 ($P<.0001$) with a 1-week interval and 0.2 ($P = .01$) with a 2-week interval. Although all pigs tolerated the procedure well and there was no mortality, there was 1 clinically symptomatic and laboratory-proven necrotic pancreatitis with peritonitis, 1 histologically and histochemically proven pancreatitis without clinical symptoms, 1 gastric wall burn, and 4 adhesions between the pancreas and the gut. It should be noted that longer application time resulted in greater variation in the lesion size.

The hybrid cryotherm probe was also evaluated on the porcine liver and spleen.[9] For the liver, the histology after euthanasia revealed an area of liquefactive necrosis surrounded by coagulative necrosis and an inflammatory watershed zone composed of granulation tissue. The liver parenchyma surrounding the treated area was normal. The correlation coefficient for T1 versus T2 in the liver tissue was 0.71 ($P = .03$) after removal of one potential outlier. The EUS significantly overestimated the lesion area T2. A positive trend of T1 over application time was noted ($r = 0.51$, $P = .1$). For the spleen, the treated area showed a central hemorrhagic liquefactive necrosis surrounded by granulation tissue. The surrounding parenchyma was normal. The correlation coefficient for the correlation of T1 versus T2 in the spleen was 0.73 ($P = .04$). There was a clear correlation of T2 and application time ($r = 0.75$, $P = .01$). For both organs no complications, including the changes in laboratory tests, were observed.

Recently, an umbrella-shaped retractable electrode array, designed to provide a large area of coagulative necrosis, was investigated in pigs.[10] EUS-RFA was performed in 5 normal pig livers. There was no difficulty in the transgastric deployment and retraction of the umbrella-shaped electrode. The ablated area evaluated by EUS 15 minutes after ablation showed a spherical and hypoechoic area with a diameter of 2.3 cm in all 5 pigs. On gross analysis, the mean ablated zone in the liver was 2.6 cm (range 2.5–2.7 cm). Histopathology confirmed the presence of coagulation necrosis in the ablated area (**Fig. 3**). There was no evidence of a complication.

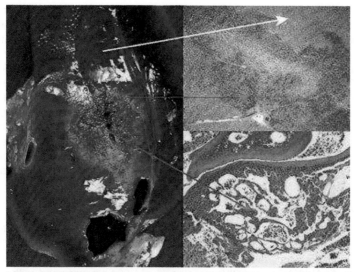

Fig. 3. Radiofrequency ablation of liver tissue with an umbrella electrode. The white arrow corresponds with unremarkable liver parenchyma. Cyan arrow indicates the zone of hyperemia. Green arrow designates the area of coagulative necrosis induced by radiofrequency ablation. (*Reprinted from* Brugge WR. EUS-guided ablation therapy and celiac plexus interventions. In: Hawes RH, Fockens P, Varadarajulu S, editors. Endosonography. 2nd edition. Philadelphia: Elsevier Saunders; 2011. p. 275–82; with permission from Elsevier.)

EUS-PDT

Photodynamic therapy (PDT) involves administration of a tumor-localizing photosensitizer, exposure of the target tissue to light of appropriate wavelength, and the generation of a highly cytotoxic oxygen species termed singlet oxygen.[11,12] Antitumor effects of PDT derive from direct cytotoxic effects, damage to the tumor vasculature, and induction of inflammatory reaction leading to the development of systemic immunity.[12]

A study with a porcine model evaluated the feasibility and safety of EUS-PDT.[13] Porfimer sodium was injected into 3 pigs as the photosensitizer 24 hours before EUS-PDT. Under EUS guidance, the liver, the pancreas, and the kidney were punctured with a 19-gauge fine needle. A quartz optical fiber with a 1.0-cm cylindrical light diffuser was inserted through the needle and into the tissue. The tissue was illuminated with a 630-nm light to a total light dose of 50 J/cm. The animals were euthanized and examined after 2 days of observation. No signs of complication were seen during observation period. On pathological examination, gross ecchymosis was noted on the surface of the pancreas in one pig. The mean area of necrosis induced by EUS-PDT in the pancreas, the liver, the kidney, and the spleen were 3.6, 3.3, 3.2, and 8.5 mm^2, respectively. The extent of complete necrosis was 100% only in the pancreas.

Another pilot study of EUS-PDT using the photosensitizer verteporfin on porcine pancreas was reported in 2008.[14] Verteporfin is a photosensitizer commonly used in PDT for choroidal neovascularization secondary to advanced age-related macular degeneration.[15,16] It has a shorter half-life of 4 hours and duration of photosensitivity of 5 days. In this study, 6 pigs were randomly divided into 3 groups with 2 pigs in each group; the first group was exposed to 10 minutes of 689-nm wavelength laser light at a light dose of 150 J/cm^2, the second group to 15 minutes, and the third group to 20 minutes. Serum amylase, lipase, and renal and liver function tests were obtained at baseline and 4 days after the EUS-PDT. An abdominal CT with contrast was performed on day 4 to evaluate the pancreas for tissue effect. The pigs were euthanized on day 7 and the pancreas tail was harvested for pathologic examination. On CT, the PDT-induced pancreatic lesion was a low-attenuation focus in the pancreatic parenchyma. The mean diameter of the lesion after 10, 15, and 20 minutes of laser-light exposure on CT was 6.6, 9.4, and 26.3 mm, respectively. On gross pathology, the treated area appeared as a localized necrotic lesion, and the mean diameter corresponded with the time of exposure (15, 24, and 30.5 mm for 10, 15, and 20 minutes, respectively). Histology revealed a well-defined, solitary lesion that included areas of fat necrosis, granulation tissue, inflammation, and fibrosis. Except for 1 pig in the 10-minute group with a mild increase in serum amylase without clinical evidence of pancreatitis, no complication was encountered.

EUS-Guided Laser Ablation

There is one pilot study of EUS-guided neodymium:yttrium aluminum garnet (Nd:YAG) laser ablation of porcine pancreas.[17] Under EUS guidance, a quartz optical fiber with a tip 300 μm in diameter was introduced to porcine pancreatic tail through a 19-gauge fine needle. An Nd:YAG laser with a wavelength of 1.064 nm was used, with an output power of 2 and 3 W and a total delivered energy of 500 and 1000 J on continuous mode. The pigs were followed up for 24 hours. For the same energy, the ablation area and ablation volume were increased when higher power was used. In detail, for the power setting of 2 W the mean ablation area was 49 and 67 mm^2 in cases of set energies of 500 and 1000 J, respectively. For the power setting of 3 W the mean ablation area was 59 and 80 mm^2 in the cases of set energies of 500 and 1000 J, respectively. For the ablation volume, the mean value was 314 and 460 mm^3 in cases with set energies of 500 and 1000 J, respectively, and a power setting of 2 W. For a higher power of 3 W, the mean ablation volume was 428 mm^3 in the cases with set energy of 500 J and 483 mm^3 for the case with set energy of 1000 J. There was no major complication defined as clinically symptomatic and chemistry-proven pancreatitis with peritonitis. In 6 of 8 pigs, small peripancreatic fluid collections on pathologic examination were identified, without clinical signs. Serum amylase levels were increased in 7 pigs, and serum lipase levels were increased in all animals.

Recently, a successful EUS-guided Nd:YAG laser ablation of a hepatocellular carcinoma in the caudate lobe was reported.[18] The optical fiber was inserted through a 22-gauge fine needle. Four needle insertions were performed to encompass the entire tumor, and for each illumination the laser was delivered at 5 W for 360 seconds and 1200 J per fiber. The total energy delivered was 7200 J in 36 minutes. The patient was discharged after 3 days uneventfully. CT obtained 24 hours after the procedure showed that the treated area was replaced by a homogeneous nonenhancing area. A subsequent CT 2 months after the procedure demonstrated uniform hypoattenuation without enhancement in the ablated zone.

EUS-Guided Ethanol Injection to Solid Lesions

The feasibility of EUS-guided ethanol injection of normal porcine pancreas was reported in 2005.[19] In this study, under EUS guidance 98% ethanol was injected to the pancreas of 4 Yorkshire pigs, and 50% ethanol to another 4 Yorkshire pigs. The first animal injected with 1.0 mL of 98% ethanol developed pancreatic pseudocyst; subsequently the amount of ethanol injected was reduced to 0.5 mL. No animals showed signs of distress. All animals had elevation of serum amylase. For animals receiving 50% ethanol, pathology revealed a 2- to 6-mm area of necrosis, inflammation, and

Table 1
Summary of EUS-guided tumor ablation techniques on porcine model

Technique	References	Year	N	Target Organ	Maximum Diameter of Ablated Area		Complications
					EUS (Immediately After Ablation)	Pathology	
RFA	Goldberg et al[3]	1999	13	Pancreas	15 mm	12 mm	Transmural gastric wall burns (n = 3) Intestinal serosal burn (n = 1) Pancreatitis with pancreatic fluid collection without symptoms (n = 1)
	Carrara et al[8a]	2008	14	Pancreas	~900 mm^2[2b]	~4000 mm^2[2b]	Necrotic pancreatitis with peritonitis (n = 1) Pancreatitis without symptoms (n = 1) Gastric wall burn (n = 1) Adhesion between the pancreas and the gut (n = 4)
	Carrara et al[9a]	2008	19	Liver (n = 10) Spleen (n = 9)	~500 mm^2 (liver)[bc] ~600 mm^2 (spleen)[bc]	~400 mm^2 (liver)[b] ~500 mm^2 (spleen)[b]	None
	Varadarajulu et al[10]	2009	5	Liver	23 mm	27 mm	None
PDT	Chan et al[13]	2004	3	Pancreas Liver Spleen Kidney	Results not given	14 mm^2 (pancreas)[b] 9 mm^2 (liver)[b] 20 mm^2 (spleen)[b] 11 mm^2 (kidney)[b]	Gross ecchymosis on the surface of the pancreas (n = 1)
	Yusuf et al[14]	2008	6	Pancreas	Results not given	30.5 mm[d]	None
Laser	Di Matteo et al[17]	2010	8	Pancreas	22 mm^2[2b]	87 mm^2[2b]	Peripancreatic fluid collection (n = 6) Elevated serum amylase (n = 7) Elevated serum lipase (n = 8)
Ethanol injection	Aslanian et al[19]	2005	8	Pancreas	11.7 mm[ce]	6 mm[e]	Pancreatic pseudocyst (n = 1)[f] Inflammatory colonic stricture (n = 1)[f] Elevated serum amylase (n = 8)[f]
	Matthes et al[20]	2007	6	Pancreas	35 mm	27 mm	None
	Giday et al[21]	2007	4	Pancreas	10 mm	10 mm	None

a RFA with cryotechnology.
b Only area was reported.
c Diameters measured by EUS immediately before euthanasia were reported.
d Mean diameter of the pigs that were exposed to 20 minutes of laser light.
e Results of pigs injected with 0.5 mL of 50% ethanol.
f Results of all pigs.

Table 2
Potential indications and limitations of EUS-guided tumor ablation

Target Organ	Indication	Human Reports/Type of Ablation	Limitations
Pancreas	Neuroendocrine tumors Isolated metastasis to the pancreas (eg, renal cell carcinoma)	Yes/Ethanol[24]	Size of the tumor Histologic evaluation of regional lymph nodes might be limited
Liver	Hepatocellular carcinoma Isolated metastasis to the liver (eg, colorectal carcinoma)	Yes/Laser,[18] ethanol[22]	Size of the tumor Anatomic limitation (approach to the right lobe difficult)
Adrenal gland	Isolated metastasis	Yes/Ethanol[25]	Size of the tumor Anatomic limitation (difficult to visualize the right adrenal gland)
Upper gastrointestinal tract	Subepithelial tumor (eg, gastrointestinal stromal tumor)	Yes/Ethanol[23]	Size of the tumor Histologic evaluation of regional lymph nodes might be limited

fibrosis. Two of those receiving 98% ethanol developed complication of pancreatitis: one developed pseudocyst and the other developed inflammatory colonic stricture. The mean diameter of treated pancreatic tissue after 98% ethanol injection was 18 mm. The investigators concluded that whereas 50% ethanol induces localized and self-limited changes, 98% ethanol causes more widespread and unpredictable pancreatitis.

A subsequent study was designed to determine the dose-response relationship of EUS-guided ethanol injection.[20] Under EUS guidance, the investigators injected 2 mL of ethanol with concentrations of 0%, 20%, 40%, 60%, 80%, and 100% to each porcine pancreatic tail, which all animals tolerated well. Abdominal CT obtained on day 4 showed a hypodense area with a mean diameter of 19.4 mm in the pancreatic tail of the pigs that received 40%, 60%, 80%, and 100% ethanol. The changes were confined to the pancreas, without inflammatory changes or peripancreatic necrosis in the rest of the pancreas. Euthanasia was performed on day 7. No lesion could be identified in the pancreatic tail of the pigs injected with 0% and 20% ethanol. The porcine pancreas injected with 40%, 60%, 80%, and 100% ethanol demonstrated a visible coagulation area, with an increasing diameter in correlation to the concentration of ethanol. Histology confirmed the presence of coagulation necrosis in pigs injected with 40%, 60%, 80%, and 100% ethanol. The area of the pancreatic necrosis estimated by CT, measured on gross findings, and histology correlated with the concentration of ethanol. No correlation was found between the diameter of EUS image change and ethanol concentration.

Giday and colleagues[21] evaluated the utility of contrast-enhanced EUS for visualization and monitoring of ethanol-ablated porcine pancreas, by modifying the injection technique described by Aslanian and colleagues[19] with the addition of purified carbon particle solution to facilitate visualization of the injected area on postmortem examination. Reevaluation of the pancreas with EUS and subsequent contrast-enhanced EUS using activated perflutren lipid microspheres intravenous bolus infusion was done at 24 hours (1 pig), 48 hours (2 pigs), and 7 days (1 pig). Injection of microspheres improved the visualization of the hypovascular necrotic lesion. In addition, the diameter of the area of pancreatic necrosis on histology correlated well with that of the area with altered microperfusion detected by contrast-enhanced EUS.

Human cases of EUS-guided ethanol injection to solid tumors has been reported in hepatic metastasis,[22] gastrointestinal stromal tumor,[23] pancreatic insulinoma,[24] and adrenal metastasis from non–small cell lung cancer.[25]

The results of EUS-guided tumor ablation techniques on porcine models are summarized in **Table 1**. The potential indications and limitations of the EUS-guided tumor ablation techniques are listed in **Table 2**.

SUMMARY

With the development of curvilinear EUS, clinicians have entered the era of interventional EUS. Various EUS-guided tumor ablation techniques using RFA, PDT, laser, and ethanol injection have been described. Most of the techniques described are experimental.

Development of dedicated devices such as modified delivery systems compatible with oblique EUS-needle delivery system and 3-dimensional mapping system are needed.[26] Precise indications for EUS-guided tumor ablation therapies should be defined. Potential curative indications would include pancreatic cystic neoplasms and neuroendocrine tumors of limited diameter. Meticulous evaluation using cross-sectional imaging, EUS and, if indicated, EUS-FNA, would be mandatory to safely exclude metastasis to the regional lymph nodes.

REFERENCES

1. Sreenarasimhaiah J. Interventional endoscopic ultrasound: the next frontier in gastrointestinal endoscopy. Am J Med Sci 2009;338:319–24.
2. Ashida R, Chang KJ. Interventional EUS for the treatment of pancreatic cancer. J Hepatobiliary Pancreat Surg 2009;16:592–7.
3. Goldberg SN, Mallery S, Gazelle GS, et al. EUS-guided radiofrequency ablation in the pancreas: results in a porcine model. Gastrointest Endosc 1999;50:392–401.
4. Brugge WR. EUS-guided ablation therapy and celiac plexus interventions. In: Hawes RH, Fockens P, Varadarajulu S, editors. Endosonography. 2nd edition. Philadelphia: Elsevier Saunders; 2011. p. 275–82.
5. Ahmed M, Brace CL, Lee FT Jr, et al. Principles of and advances in percutaneous ablation. Radiology 2011;258:351–69.
6. McGahan JP, Gu WZ, Brock JM, et al. Hepatic ablation using bipolar radiofrequency electrocautery. Acad Radiol 1996;3:418–22.
7. Verna EC, Dhar V. Endoscopic ultrasound-guided fine needle injection for cancer therapy: the evolving role of therapeutic endoscopic ultrasound. Therap Adv Gastroenterol 2008;1:103–9.
8. Carrara S, Arcidiacono PG, Albarello L, et al. Endoscopic ultrasound-guided application of a new hybrid cryotherm probe in porcine pancreas: a preliminary study. Endoscopy 2008;40:321–6.
9. Carrara S, Arcidiacono PG, Albarello L, et al. Endoscopic ultrasound-guided application of a new internally gas-cooled radiofrequency ablation probe in the liver and spleen of an animal model: a preliminary study. Endoscopy 2008;40:759–63.
10. Varadarajulu S, Jhala NC, Drelichman ER. EUS-guided radiofrequency ablation with a prototype electrode array system in an animal model (with video). Gastrointest Endosc 2009;70:372–6.
11. Dougherty TJ, Gomer CJ, Henderson BW, et al. Photodynamic therapy. J Natl Cancer Inst 1998;90:889–905.
12. Agostinis P, Berg K, Cengel KA, et al. Photodynamic therapy of cancer: an update. CA Cancer J Clin 2011;61:250–81.
13. Chan HH, Nishioka NS, Mino M, et al. EUS-guided photodynamic therapy of the pancreas: a pilot study. Gastrointest Endosc 2004;59:95–9.
14. Yusuf TE, Matthes K, Brugge WR. EUS-guided photodynamic therapy with verteporfin for ablation of normal pancreatic tissue: a pilot study in a porcine model (with video). Gastrointest Endosc 2008;67:957–61.
15. Houle JM, Strong A. Clinical pharmacokinetics of verteporfin. J Clin Pharmacol 2002;42:547–57.
16. Bylsma GW, Harper CA, Dutton F, et al. Australian angiogram review panel–monitoring the use of photodynamic therapy with verteporfin. Clin Experiment Ophthalmol 2006;34:550–6.
17. Di Matteo F, Martino M, Rea R, et al. EUS-guided Nd:YAG laser ablation of normal pancreatic tissue: a pilot study in a pig model. Gastrointest Endosc 2010;72:358–63.
18. Di Matteo F, Grasso R, Pacella CM, et al. EUS-guided Nd:YAG laser ablation of a hepatocellular carcinoma in the caudate lobe. Gastrointest Endosc 2011;73:632–6.
19. Aslanian H, Salem RR, Marginean C, et al. EUS-guided ethanol injection of normal porcine pancreas: a pilot study. Gastrointest Endosc 2005;62:723–7.

20. Matthes K, Mino-Kenudson M, Sahani DV, et al. Concentration-dependent ablation of pancreatic tissue by EUS-guided ethanol injection. Gastrointest Endosc 2007;65:272–7.
21. Giday SA, Magno P, Gabrielson KL, et al. The utility of contrast-enhanced endoscopic ultrasound in monitoring ethanol-induced pancreatic tissue ablation: a pilot study in a porcine model. Endoscopy 2007;39:525–9.
22. Barclay RL, Perez-Miranda M, Giovannini M. EUS-guided treatment of a solid hepatic metastasis. Gastrointest Endosc 2002;55:266–70.
23. Gunter E, Lingenfelser T, Eitelbach F, et al. EUS-guided ethanol injection for treatment of a GI stromal tumor. Gastrointest Endosc 2003;57:113–5.
24. Jurgensen C, Schuppan D, Neser F, et al. EUS-guided alcohol ablation of an insulinoma. Gastrointest Endosc 2006;63:1059–62.
25. Artifon EL, Lucon AM, Sakai P, et al. EUS-guided alcohol ablation of left adrenal metastasis from non-small-cell lung carcinoma. Gastrointest Endosc 2007;66:1201–5.
26. Wallace MB, Sabbagh LC. EUS 2008 Working Group document: evaluation of EUS-guided tumor ablation. Gastrointest Endosc 2009;69:S59–63.

EUS-Guided Anastomosis

Takao Itoi, MD[a],*, Kenneth F. Binmoeller, MD[b]

KEYWORDS

- Endoscopic ultrasonography • Pancreatic pseudocyst drainage
- Gallbladder drainage • Entero-entero anastomosis

INTRODUCTION

Surgical anastomosis using sutures and metal titanium staples between various parts of the gastrointestinal (GI) tract and biliary tract has been the standard method to restore continuity after resection or to bypass blockage in otherwise unresectable disease. The role of flexible endoscopy has been largely limited to restoring continuity within the GI tract. Methods to create a palliative endoscopic gastroenteric or bilioenteric anastomosis have been reported in animal studies and some clinical trials. These include use of a compression button,[1-3] compression coil,[4] magnets,[5-8] and a dedicated lumen-apposing metal stent.[9,10] The role of endoscopic ultrasonography (EUS) in guiding these minimally invasive treatments has gained importance. This article focuses on a review of experimental and clinical studies of the creation of EUS-guided anastomoses.

RATIONALE FOR EUS GUIDANCE

Surgical anastomosis primarily involves connecting 2 hollow organs originally not connected, such as the stomach and jejunum, stomach and bile duct, stomach and gallbladder, duodenum and bile duct, and duodenum and gallbladder. Adequate compression and closure is necessary to achieve anastomosis. Although a surgical anastomosis can be easily performed under direct visualization by a surgeon, an endoscopic anastomosis requires a series of coaxial interventions using multiple imaging modalities: endoscopy, ultrasonography, and fluoroscopy. Creation of an anastomosis under EUS guidance is attractive because it enables transenteric access to the target organ without having to cross an obstruction or surgically altered

Disclosures: Drs Binmoeller and Itoi are consultants for Xlumena Inc. Dr Binmoeller serves as Xlumena's Chief Medical Officer. Dr Itoi is a consultant and gives lectures for Olympus Medical Systems, Tokyo, Japan.

[a] Department of Gastroenterology and Hepatology, Tokyo Medical University, 6-7-1 Nishishinjuku, Shinjuku-ku, Tokyo 160-0023, Japan; [b] Paul May and Frank Stein Interventional Endoscopy Services, California Pacific Medical Center, 2351 Clay Street, 6th Floor, San Francisco, CA 94115, USA

* Corresponding author.

E-mail address: itoi@tokyo-med.ac.jp

anatomy. Initial access to the target organ is typically accomplished under EUS guidance with a fine-needle aspiration needle or cautery device (needle knife) followed by placement of a 0.035-in guide wire or a 0.025-in guide wire. The absence of intervening blood vessels between the 2 organs can be confirmed using Doppler imaging. The 19-gauge needle is removed and the tract dilated over the wire using a dilator catheter, balloon, and/or electrical cautery needle for bougie. Finally, stent and compression buttons are placed across the fistula.

ANASTOMOSIS DEVICES
Compression Buttons and Magnets

The first report on the use of a compression button by surgical insertion to create a sutureless anastomosis was described more than 100 years ago. Ischemic necrosis resulted in a leak-free anastomosis.[11] Swain and Mills[1] described the use of spring compression buttons and magnets to create a gastrojejunostomy in an animal study. Cope[12] described creation of a successful gastroenterostomy and cholecystogastric or cholecystojejunal anastomosis[13] using magnets surgically inserted in pigs.[12] Cope and colleagues developed a large-bore, covered yo-yo metallic stent, which yielded long-term patency after magnetic compression anastomosis.[9] Encouraged by the favorable outcomes of the experimental studies, Chopita and colleagues[5] created magnetic compression gastroenteric anastomoses followed by placement of the yo-yo stent in 15 patients with malignant obstruction. The success rate was 86.6% (13 of 15 patients). One perforation occurred and was attributed to manipulation of the recently formed fistula. Three stents migrated (2 distal and 1 proximal) without further complication. In a multicenter European study, Van Hooft and colleagues[14] evaluated the same technique, magnetic anastomosis device followed by the yo-yo stent. The yo-yo stent migrated in 3 of the first 7 patients (42.8%) and subsequently the investigators switched to a conventional 6-cm uncovered tubular duodenal stent design. The study was terminated after a fatal perforation in 1 patient for a total success rate of 66.7% (12 of 18 patients).

Creation of magnetic biliary anastomoses has been reported by several groups. Itoi and colleagues[6,7] reported creation of choledocho-choledocho anastomosis by magnetic compression using interventional radiologic and endoscopic techniques. Jamidar and colleagues[15] used a novel, hinged device comprising a 7F stent with a central ferrous magnet component. The metalloplastic device was inserted into the bile duct of pigs using a standard endoscopic retrograde cholangiopancreatography (ERCP) technique over a 0.035-in guide wire. A second magnet was then endoscopically positioned in the duodenum to mate with the bile duct magnet and exert compressive ischemic force. Anastomoses ranging from 5 mm to 10 mm were successfully accomplished in all survival animals. No clinical experience using this device has been reported to date.

Swain and coworkers were the first to develop and test a through-the-scope device for EUS-guided suturing and tissue approximation of the stomach with the gallbladder, and the stomach with the jejunum, in pigs.[2,3] A suturing device was constructed for suturing under EUS guidance to the desired depth, and sutures were placed into both hollow and solid organs up to 5 cm from the echoendoscope tip. The device allowed multiple sutures to be placed without withdrawing the echoendoscope. Stitching, knot tying, and thread cutting were achieved through the echoendoscope's 2.8-mm accessory channel. In that study, traction for the insertion of stents and other devices was provided through the lumens of both organs. Within 4 to 7 days, anastomoses had formed between the small intestine and the stomach and between the gallbladder and the stomach. The initial diameter of the anastomoses ranged from 3 mm to 9 mm, and no adverse events were reported.

Compression Coil

Chang reported the in vivo use of EUS-guided choledochoduodenostomy or chole-cystoduodenostomy using a prototype compression coil in dogs.[4] A prototype forward-viewing echoendoscope (Olympus Medical Systems, Tokyo, Japan) was advanced to the duodenum until the dilated common bile duct was visualized by EUS. The prototype coil delivery device (a 19-gauge needle preloaded with a stretched coil in the lumen and a screw-type stent over the needle) (Olympus) was passed through the channel of the scope. EUS-guided needle puncture into the common bile duct or gallbladder was followed by the deployment of 50% of the coil into the common bile duct or gallbladder, whereas the remaining 50% remained within the duodenal bulb to tightly secure the common bile duct or gallbladder and the duodenal walls by compressive force. Finally, a temporary stent was placed across the compression coil. As a result, in 1 of the 4 pigs in the EUS-guided choledochoduode-nostomy group, successful choledochoduodenostomy resulted in device-free relief of jaundice. Histologically, there was complete adhesion between the common bile duct and the duodenum. Based on this preliminary study, he examined compression coil and twin-headed needle for EUS-guided choledochoduodenostomy in 4 dog models.[16] Eventually, immediate drainage was successful in 3 of 4 dogs with overalll drainage successful in all 4 dogs. Creation of a chronic fistula between bile duct and duodenum was achieved in all 4 dogs. There was no evidence of bile leak or perforation.

Lumen-Apposing Metallic Stent

EUS-guided bile duct and gallbladder drainage using a self-expandable metallic stent (SEMS) has become an alternative treatment if ERCP fails.[17,18] Conventional tubular SEMSs, however, have several limitations when applied to transluminal drainage. First, they do not provide lumen-to-lumen anchorage. This may result in bile leakage and enteric contamination, because the lumens may become physically separated. Second, the stent may migrate because there is no stricture to hold it in place. Third, the exposed stent ends may cause tissue trauma, resulting in bleeding or perfora-tion.[10] In light of these limitations, a stent designed for enteric drainage of nonadherent

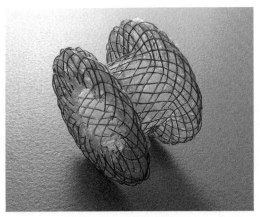

Fig. 1. Fully covered 10-mm × 10-mm–diameter AXIOS stent with bilateral flanges.

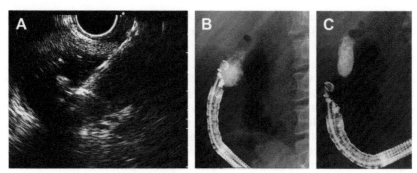

Fig. 2. EUS-guided cholecystoenterostomy for acute cholecystitis due to gallstones. (*A*) 19-gauge needle was advanced into the gallbladder under EUS imaging. (*B*) Cholecystography showed mutiple filling detect, suggesting gallstones. (*C*) Finally, the AXOS stent was placed between duodenum and gallbladder.

lumens is needed. Potential targets for anastomotic drainage include the gallbladder, bile duct, and adjacent bowel. Recently, Binmoeller and Shah[10] reported on a novel removable lumen-apposing stent designed for this purpose and reported the results of benchtop tests and experimental use in pigs. The AXIOS stent (Xlumena Inc., Mountain View, CA, USA) consists of a fully covered 10-mm–diameter stent with bilateral flanges (**Fig. 1**). Fully expanded, the flange diameter (20 mm) is twice that of the saddle section (10 mm). The collapsible braided stent is delivered through a 10.5F catheter. The stent was successfully deployed across the stomach and gallbladder lumens in all pigs to create a robust cholecystenterostomy without complications. Direct cholecystoscopy and contrast injections were used to confirm the absence of tissue trauma or leakage. Weekly follow-up gastroscopy showed the stents to be stable and patent, without dislodgment in any animals. The covering remained intact and there was no hyperplastic tissue ingrowth, overgrowth, or tissue injury. One stent was removed at 4 weeks. On necropsy, the gallbladders showed focal adherence to the stomach at the site of cystogastrostomy and a negative leak test. The AXIOS stent is currently undergoing clinical study for internal drainage of the gallbladder (**Fig. 2**) and pancreatic pseudocysts (**Fig. 3**).

The AXIOS stent may enable the creation of a bypass to the small bowel.[10] A gastrojejunostomy was created under EUS guidance in 5 animals (4 survival). The stents remained fully patent in all animals throughout the implantation period (up to 4.5 weeks) and were easily removed (**Fig. 4**).

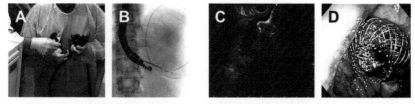

Fig. 3. EUS-guided cystenterostomy of the pancreatic cyst. (*A*) Appearance of equipment of the AXIOS. (*B*) A radiograph showed deployment of the dital flange of the AXIOS. (*C*) Deployment of the dital flange was easily detected under sonographic image. (*D*) Endoscopic image showed nicely deployment of the AXIOS.

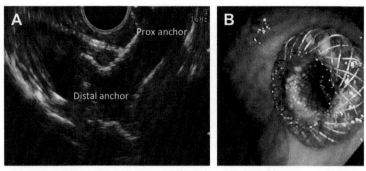

Fig. 4. EUS-guided gastrojejunostomy in a pig model. (*A*) EUS view of fully deployed AXIOS stent to create gastrojejunostomy. (*B*) Endoscopic view of fully deployed AXIOS stent to create gastrojejunostomy.

Future developments may include a catheter-based system that delivers multiple tools in a coaxial fashion without the need for device exchange. A prototype all-in-one device (AXT [Xlumena]) was evaluated in porcine survival studies with technical success in creation of a cholecystogastrostomy in 3 animals.[19–22] The AXT device Luer locks to the echoendoscope and is designed for single-operator, single-hand deployment. The exchange-free system is composed of a unique anchor needle that punctures the walls of the GI tract and bile duct and maintains continuous apposition of the 2 lumens to prevent leakage of contents during instrumentation. The AXIOS stent is then delivered and deployed directly over the anchor needle.

ROLE OF FORWARD-VIEWING ENDOSCOPES

The usefulness of prototype forward-viewing echoendoscopes has been described for diagnostic and therapeutic EUS.[23–26] Prototype forward-viewing echoendoscopes have 2 major advantages compared with oblique-viewing echoendoscopes. First, the use of forward-viewing devices facilitates the perpendicular puncture of the GI tract wall along the same axis as the echoendoscope, which makes monitoring of the procedure easy and reliable. Second, it is possible to confirm the exchange and deployment of devices under direct endoscopic visualization. In particular, when performing 1-step stent placement for anastomosis via echoendoscopy, an oblique-viewing echoendoscope does not always provide optimal endoscopic observation. Standard and ultraslim forward-viewing upper GI endoscopes for anastomosis are also useful for diagnosis and therapy, for instance, in tissue sampling or stone removal from the gallbladder by cholecystoenteric anastomosis.

LIMITATIONS OF EUS-GUIDED ANASTOMOSIS

Creation of a temporary EUS-guided anastomosis is useful, but the optimal method of maintaining permanent patency remains controversial. Large-scale prospective and randomized controlled studies of different methods and tools to create EUS-guided anastomoses are needed in the future.

SUMMARY

Although some technical challenges in the development of dedicated devices need to be overcome, creation of an EUS-guided anastomosis is promising as a minimally invasive technique for pancreatobiliary diseases.

ACKNOWLEDGMENTS

We are indebted to Mr Roderick J. Turner, Assistant Professor Edward F. Barroga, and Professor J. Patrick Barron, Chairman of the Department of International Medical Communications at Tokyo Medical University, for their editorial review of the English manuscript.

REFERENCES

1. Swain CP, Mills TN. Anastomosis at flexible endoscopy: an experimental study of compression button gastrojejunostomy. Gastrointest Endosc 1991;37:626–31.
2. Fritscher-Ravens A, Mosse CA, Mills TN, et al. A through-the-scope device for suturing and tissue approximation under EUS control. Gastrointest Endosc 2002;56:737–42.
3. Fritscher-Ravens A, Mosse CA, Mukherjee D. Transluminalendosurgery: single lumen access anastomotic device for flexible endoscopy. Gastrointest Endosc 2003;58:585–91.
4. Chang KJ. Endoscopic choledocho-duodenostomy (ECD) for the treatment of biliary obstruction using prototype compression coil and interventional endosonography (EUS): a "proof of principle" canine study. Gastrointest Endosc 2009; 69:S237–8.
5. Chopita N, Vaillaverde A, Cope C, et al. Endoscopic gastroenteric anastomosis using magnets. Endoscopy 2005;37:313–7.
6. Minuro A, Tsuchida A, Yamanouchi E, et al. A novel technique of magnetic compression anastomosis for severe biliary stenosis. Gastrointest Endosc 2003;58:283–7.
7. Itoi T, Yamanouchi E, Ikeda T, et al. Magnetic compression anastomosis: a novel technique for canalization of severe hilar bile duct strictures. Endoscopy 2005;37: 1248–51.
8. Jang SI, Kim JH, Won JY, et al. Magnetic compression anastomosis is useful in biliary anastomotic strictures after living donor liver transplantation. Gastrointest Endosc 2011;74:1040–8.
9. Cope C, Ginsberg GG. Long-term patency of experimental magnetic compression gastroenteric anastomoses achieved with covered stents. Gastrointest Endosc 2001;53:780–4.
10. Binmoeller KB, Shah J. A novel lumen-apposing stent for transluminal drainage of nonadherent extraintestinal fluid collections. Endoscopy 2011;43:337–42.
11. Murphy JB. Cholecysto-intestinal anastomosis, and approximation without sutures (original research). Med Rec NY 1892;42:665–76.
12. Cope C. Creation of compression gastroenterostomy by means of the oral, percutaneous, or surgical introduction of magnets: feasibility study in swine. J Vasc Interv Radiol 1995;6:539–45.
13. Cope C. Evaluation of compression cholecystogastric and cholecystojejunal anastomoses in swine after peroral and surgical introduction of magnets. J Vasc Interv Radiol 1995;6:546–52.
14. Van Hooft JE, Vleggaar FP, Le Moine O, et al. Endoscopic magnetic gastroenteric anastomosis for palliation of malignant gastric outlet obstruction: a prospective multicenter study. Gastrointest Endosc 2010;72:530–5.
15. Jamidar P, Cadeddu M, Mosse A, et al. A hinged metalloplastic anastomotic device: a novel method for choledochoduodenostomy. Gastrointest Endosc 2009;69:1333–8.

16. Chang KJ. EUS-guided choledocho-duodenostomy (ECD) for immediate and long-term treatment of biliary obstruction using prototype compression coil and twin-headed needle. Gastrointest Endosc 2011;73:AB326.
17. Itoi T, Coelho-Prabhu N, Baron TH. Endoscopic gallbladder drainage for management of acute cholecystitis. Gastrointest Endosc 2010;71:1038–45.
18. Itoi T, Sofuni A, Itokawa F, et al. Endoscopic ultrasonography-guided biliary drainage. J Hepatobiliary Pancreat Sci 2010;17(5):611–6.
19. Binmoeller KF, De La Mora-Levy JG. An exchange-free device for advanced translumenal therapy. Gastrointest Endosc 2010;71:AB349.
20. Binmoeller KF. A novel anchor guidewire to facilitate EUS-guided translumenal interventions. Gastrointest Endosc 2011;73:AB249.
21. Binmoeller KF, Weilert F, Marson F, et al. Self-expandable metal stent without dilatation for drainage of pancreatic fluid collection using the NAVIX access devices: initial clinical experience. Gastrointest Endosc 2011;73:AB253.
22. Binmoeller KF. EUS-guided gastrojejunostomy using novel tools designed for translumenal therapy. Gastrointest Endosc 2011;73:AB253.
23. Voermans RP, Eisendrath P, Bruno MJ, et al. Initial evaluation of a novel prototype forward-viewing US endoscope in transmural drainage of pancreatic pseudocyst drainage. Gastrointest Endosc 2007;66:1013–7.
24. De Lusong MA, Shah JN, Soetikno R, et al. Treatment of a completely obstructed colonic anastomosis stricture by using a prototype forward viewing echoendoscope and facilitated by SpyGlass. Gastrointest Endosc 2009;69:361–5.
25. Kida M, Araki M, Miyazawa S, et al. Fine needle aspiration using forward-viewing endoscopic ultrasonography. Endoscopy 2011;43:796–801.
26. Iwashita T, Nakai Y, Lee JG, et al. Newly-developed, forward-viewing echoendoscope: a comparative pilot study to the standard echoendoscope in the imaging of abdominal organs and feasibility of endoscopic ultrasound-guided interventions. J Gastroenterol Hepatol 2012;27(2):362–7.

Endo-Hepatology: A New Paradigm

Kenneth J. Chang, MD[a],*, Jason B. Samarasena, MD[a],
Takuji Iwashita, MD, PhD[b,c], Yosuke Nakai, MD, PhD[a,d],
John G. Lee, MD[a]

KEYWORDS

- Endoscopic ultrasound • Fine needle aspiration • Hepatology
- Liver disease • Portal hypertension • Liver biopsy
- Esophageal varices • Gastric varices

INTRODUCTION

Recent advances in hepatology have included new and effective treatments of viral hepatitis, with an increased need for the assessment of liver function and histology. At the same time, as demonstrated by these articles on interventional endoscopic ultrasound (EUS), there have been a growing number of endoscopic procedures that are pertinent to patients with liver disease. Ironically, although gastroenterology and hepatology are within the same specialty, these trends are not necessarily integrated and perhaps even disparate. Hepatologists increasingly turn to radiologists for liver imaging and interventional radiologists for liver biopsy and management of portal hypertension. However, it would be most ideal if the assessment and treatment of liver disease and portal hypertension could be performed and assimilated by the primary liver/gastrointestinal specialist. This integration among specialists is seen in esophageal and pancreaticobiliary diseases. It should be no different in hepatology. The authors like to consider this area of integration or overlap of endoscopic procedures within the practice of hepatology as endo-hepatology.

Consultant: Cook Medical, Inc, Olympus, Japan.
Research support: Cook Medical, Inc.
[a] Division of Gastroenterology and Hepatology, H.H. Chao Comprehensive Digestive Disease Center, University of California, Irvine, 101 The City Drive, Orange, CA 92868, USA; [b] Division of Gastroenterology and Hepatology, H.H. Chao Comprehensive Digestive Disease Center, University of California, Irvine Medical Center, 101 The City Drive, Building 22C, First Floor, Orange, CA 92868, USA; [c] First Department of Internal Medicine, Gifu University Hospital, Gifu, Japan; [d] Department of Gastroenterology, Graduate School of Medicine, The University of Tokyo, 7-3-1 Hongo Bunkyo-ku, Tokyo 113-8655, Japan
* Corresponding author.
E-mail address: kchang@uci.edu

CURRENT STATUS

Currently, most hepatologists perform either upper endoscopy[1] or capsule endoscopy[2] for detecting and assessing the severity of esophageal varices. In addition, endoscopic band ligation is the preferred technique for the treatment of active bleeding and for secondary prophylaxis.[3,4] For gastric fundal varices, practice guidelines from our societies (American College of Gastroenterology[5] and American Association for the Study of Liver Diseases[6]) recommend endoscopic-directed intravariceal injection of cyanoacrylate glue as the treatment of choice in the setting of acute bleeding.

POTENTIAL FUTURE ROLE OF EUS

Although the current role of endoscopy in hepatology practice is limited to the assessment and treatment of varices, there is a ground swell of emerging applications of EUS to patients with liver disease. These applications are summarized in the following section.

EUS LIVER ASSESSMENT

Transabdominal ultrasound (TUS) is routinely used in assessing the liver parenchyma for the degree of fibrosis/cirrhosis and detecting occult malignancy in high-risk individuals. Low-frequency gray scale imaging ($\leq$5 MHz) is typically used to assess the liver parenchyma, liver shape and size, spleen size, and hepatic vessel appearance. In contrast, high-frequency linear array gray scale imaging is used to assess the liver surface (>5 MHz). Doppler techniques, such as pulsed wave Doppler, are used to study the portal, hepatic, and splenic veins, and the hepatic artery, with the measurement of maximum or mean velocities. A recent meta-analysis showed that TUS was most useful (highest diagnostic accuracy) in assessing the liver surface as an indicator of chronic liver disease.[7] EUS is able to assess most of the liver parenchyma at frequencies between 5 and 10 MHz. Both the liver surface and parenchyma are well imaged, as well as Doppler studies of the portal vein, splenic vein, superior mesenteric vein, splenic artery, hepatic artery, celiac artery, and superior mesenteric artery. In addition, elastography (see article by Iglesias-Garcia) will likely become a standard option for EUS processors. With various types of elastography (especially transient elastography), the liver parenchymal stiffness can be measured; this has been shown to correlate well with the degree of liver fibrosis.[8–12] Elastography of the spleen may be useful in assessing portal hypertension.[13,14] Another EUS image enhancement is contrast-enhanced harmonic EUS (see article by Kitano).[15–18] This enhancement can also potentially help improve the detection of tumors in the liver.[19–22] Once tumors are detected, EUS-guided radiofrequency ablation (RFA) or cryotherapy may someday be available to treat appropriate lesions.[23,24]

EUS-GUIDED LIVER BIOPSY

Percutaneous liver biopsy is the standard procedure for obtaining hepatic tissue for histopathologic examination and remains an essential tool in the diagnosis and management of parenchymal liver diseases. The use of liver biopsy is increasing with the advent of liver transplantation and the progress being made in antiviral therapeutic agents. Although blind percutaneous needle biopsy has been the traditional technique, the use of ultrasound (US) guidance has increased considerably. A recent review of the literature indicates that the use of US-guided biopsy is superior to blind needle biopsy because of the higher risk for major complications, postbiopsy pain, and biopsy failure in the latter.[25] EUS-guided fine needle aspiration (FNA) has been reported to detect and biopsy focal lesions in the liver with high precision.[26–29] Preliminary reports using a spring-loaded core histology needle (Trucut, Cook Medical Winston-Salem, NC, USA) for random biopsy sampling showed the feasibility of obtaining core liver histology. DeWitt and colleagues[30] performed an EUS-guided Trucut biopsy using a 19-gauge needle in 21 patients with a median of 3 passes, a median core length of 9 mm, a median complete portal tract of 2 (range 1–10), with a specimen adequacy of 19%. Interestingly, a more recent study among 22 patients (including 5 with cirrhosis) using a standard 19-gauge needle (non-Trucut) with a median of 2 passes demonstrated a median core length of 36.9 mm, a median complete portal tract of 9 (range 1–73), and a specimen adequacy of 91%,[31] suggesting that a Trucut needle is not necessary to obtain core tissue. Most recently, a 19-core needle device (ProCore, Cook Medical, Winston-Salem, NC, USA) has been developed, which has a side notch (non-Trucut) that is designed to provide an additional cheese-grater action to obtain more specimen. The authors just reported a case of EUS-guided liver biopsy using this new needle device for the diagnosis of autoimmune hepatitis in a patient who was thought to be high risk for percutaneous or transjugular approaches (**Fig. 1**).[32] Thus, it seems that EUS-guided liver biopsy will become a viable option for core tissue acquisition, especially if done concurrently (under the same sedation) with surveillance endoscopy.

EUS ASSESSMENT OF ASCITES AND PARACENTESIS

EUS is has been shown to be sensitive in detecting ascites. If indicated, EUS-guided FNA can be used to perform diagnostic paracentesis.[33–35] In addition, any suspicious nodule in the peritoneum that can be imaged through the ascites fluid can be targeted

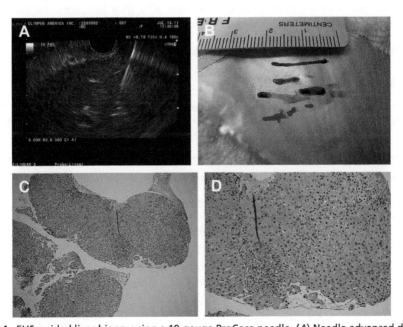

Fig. 1. EUS-guided liver biopsy using a 19-gauge ProCore needle. (*A*) Needle advanced deep within the liver parenchyma. (*B*) Gross image showing long core specimen. (*C, D*) Liver biopsy tissue showing moderate portal infiltration and interface hepatitis (hematoxylin-eosin, original magnification ×40 [*C*] and ×200 [*D*]).

by FNA for cytologic diagnosis.[36–38] Therapeutic paracentesis, although certainly possible via EUS-guided FNA, is more time consuming given the small caliber needles available and should be reserved for those who have failed percutaneous approaches.

EUS ASSESSMENT OF PORTAL CIRCULATION

There is now a growing number of EUS applications related to portal circulation and portal hypertension. A recent review by El-Saadany and colleagues[39] showed an impressive list of emerging EUS indications. These indications included EUS in the detection of esophageal varices and gastric varices, the study of esophageal and gastric variceal collaterals, the detection of perforating veins, the detection of portal hypertensive gastropathy, the assessment of the azygos vein, the study of the left gastric vein, the assessment of the thoracic duct, and the study of rectal mucosa and rectal venous changes. In addition, EUS can be used to study hemodynamic changes in portal hypertension, including portal vein flow, vessel dilation, and the development of collaterals. A prototype EUS catheter/pressure gauge transducer combination device was developed to assess intravariceal pressure in a varix model.[40,41] Even more intriguing is the idea of EUS-guided portal vein catheterization using a 22-gauge needle for direct portal vein pressure measurements in an animal model.[42]

EUS-GUIDED VASCULAR INTERVENTION

In this edition, Weilert and Binmoeller provide an exquisite overview of emerging EUS-guided vascular access and therapy procedures. These procedures include the EUS-guided cyanoacrylate injection of gastric varices, EUS-guided intravascular coil placement (alone or in combination with glue injection), intrahepatic portosystemic shunt, and microcoil embolization of vascular structures to occlude small and large vessels. These concepts are preliminary with limited data but, nonetheless, indicate an interesting and exciting growth area.

SUMMARY AND FUTURE DIRECTIONS

Table 1 summarizes the current and potential future roles of endoscopy in liver disease and portal hypertension. Among the emerging EUS procedures, perhaps

Table 1 Current and potential future roles of endoscopy in liver disease and portal hypertension		
	Diagnosis	**Therapy**
Current	Assess esophageal varices	Esophageal band ligation of esophageal varices
	Assess gastric varices	Intravariceal glue injection of gastric varices
Potential Future Role	Assess liver parenchyma and liver surface	Coil embolization of gastric varices
	EUS-guided liver biopsy	RFA or cryoablation of liver lesions
	Evaluate portal circulation	EUS-guided TIPS procedure
	Detect presence of ascites	Perform paracentesis
	Assess obliteration of esophageal varices	EUS-guided glue injection in combination with coils
	Assess obliteration of gastric varices	EUS-guided glue injection in combination with coils

Abbreviation: TIPS, transjugular intrahepatic portosystemic shunt.

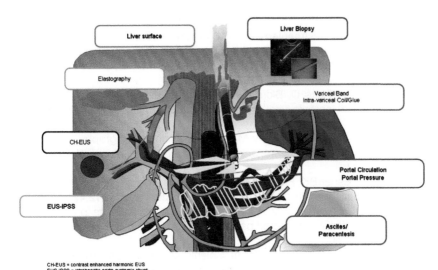

CH-EUS = contrast enhanced harmonic EUS
EUS-IPSS = intrahepatic porto-systemic shunt

Fig. 2. The concept of endo-hepatology.

the low-lying fruit may be EUS-guided liver assessment and biopsy. However, the authors think that many of the other possibilities will also become reality. As this intersection of endoscopy and hepatology (ie, endo-hepatology) expands, it will broaden interventional EUS to include proficiency in EUS assessment of the liver, peritoneum, and portal circulation, including EUS-guided liver biopsy and therapeutic vascular intervention (**Fig. 2**). Consolidating surveillance endoscopy (assessing varices) with a complete EUS evaluation into a single comprehensive procedure would optimize patient care.

REFERENCES

1. Moodley J, Lopez R, Carey W. Compliance with practice guidelines and risk of a first esophageal variceal hemorrhage in patients with cirrhosis. Clin Gastroenterol Hepatol 2010;8(8):703–8.
2. Guturu P, Sagi SV, Ahn D, et al. Capsule endoscopy with PILLCAM ESO for detecting esophageal varices: a meta-analysis. Minerva Gastroenterol Dietol 2011;57(1):1–11.
3. Khan S, Tudur Smith C, Williamson P, et al. Portosystemic shunts versus endoscopic therapy for variceal rebleeding in patients with cirrhosis. Cochrane Database Syst Rev 2006;4:CD000553.
4. Ravipati M, Katragadda S, Swaminathan PD, et al. Pharmacotherapy plus endoscopic intervention is more effective than pharmacotherapy or endoscopy alone in the secondary prevention of esophageal variceal bleeding: a meta-analysis of randomized, controlled trials. Gastrointest Endosc 2009;70(4):658–64, e655.
5. Garcia-Tsao G, Sanyal AJ, Grace ND, et al. Prevention and management of gastroesophageal varices and variceal hemorrhage in cirrhosis. Am J Gastroenterol 2007;102(9):2086–102.
6. Garcia-Tsao G, Sanyal AJ, Grace ND, et al. Prevention and management of gastroesophageal varices and variceal hemorrhage in cirrhosis. Hepatology 2007;46(3):922–38.

7. Allan R, Thoirs K, Phillips M. Accuracy of ultrasound to identify chronic liver disease. World J Gastroenterol 2010;16(28):3510–20.

8. Cardoso AC, Carvalho-Filho RJ, Stern C, et al. Direct comparison of diagnostic performance of transient elastography in patients with chronic hepatitis B and chronic hepatitis C. Liver Int 2012;32(4):612–21.

9. Fransen van de Putte D, Blom R, van Soest H, et al. Impact of Fibroscan on management of chronic viral hepatitis in clinical practice. Ann Hepatol 2011; 10(4):469–76.

10. Klibansky DA, Mehta SH, Curry M, et al. Transient elastography for predicting clinical outcomes in patients with chronic liver disease. J Viral Hepat 2012; 19(2):e184–93.

11. Lindvig K, Mossner BK, Pedersen C, et al. Liver stiffness and 30-day mortality in a cohort of patients admitted to hospital. Eur J Clin Invest 2012;42(2):146–52.

12. Merchante N, Rivero-Juarez A, Tellez F, et al. Liver stiffness predicts clinical outcome in HIV/HCV-coinfected patients with compensated liver cirrhosis. Hepatology 2012. [Epub ahead of print].

13. Hirooka M, Ochi H, Koizumi Y, et al. Splenic elasticity measured with real-time tissue elastography is a marker of portal hypertension. Radiology 2011;261(3): 960–8.

14. Llop E, Berzigotti A, Reig M, et al. Assessment of portal hypertension by transient elastography in patients with compensated cirrhosis and potentially resectable liver tumors. J Hepatol 2012;56(1):103–8.

15. Romagnuolo J, Hoffman B, Vela S, et al. Accuracy of contrast-enhanced harmonic EUS with a second-generation perflutren lipid microsphere contrast agent (with video). Gastrointest Endosc 2011;73(1):52–63.

16. Kitano M, Sakamoto H, Komaki T, et al. New techniques and future perspective of EUS for the differential diagnosis of pancreatic malignancies: contrast harmonic imaging. Dig Endosc 2011;23(Suppl 1):46–50.

17. Kitano M, Kudo M, Sakamoto H, et al. Endoscopic ultrasonography and contrast-enhanced endoscopic ultrasonography. Pancreatology 2011;11(Suppl 2): 28–33.

18. Xia Y, Kitano M, Kudo M, et al. Characterization of intra-abdominal lesions of undetermined origin by contrast-enhanced harmonic EUS (with videos). Gastrointest Endosc 2010;72(3):637–42.

19. Tanaka H, Iijima H, Nouso K, et al. Cost-effectiveness analysis on the surveillance for hepatocellular carcinoma in liver cirrhosis patients using contrast-enhanced ultrasonography. Hepatol Res 2012;42(4):376–84.

20. Nakano S, Tsushima Y, Higuchi T, et al. Contrast- and non-contrast-enhanced ultrasonography (US) findings of hepatic metastasis from malignant pheochromocytoma/paraganglioma. Jpn J Radiol 2012. [Epub ahead of print].

21. Strobel D, Bernatik T, Blank W, et al. Diagnostic accuracy of CEUS in the differential diagnosis of small (</= 20 mm) and subcentimetric (</= 10 mm) focal liver lesions in comparison with histology. Results of the DEGUM multicenter trial. Ultraschall Med 2011;32(6):593–7.

22. Kudo M. Diagnostic imaging of hepatocellular carcinoma: recent progress. Oncology 2011;81(Suppl 1):73–85.

23. Brugge WR. EUS-guided tumor ablation with heat, cold, microwave, or radiofrequency: will there be a winner? Gastrointest Endosc 2009;69(Suppl 2):S212–6.

24. Varadarajulu S, Jhala NC, Drelichman ER. EUS-guided radiofrequency ablation with a prototype electrode array system in an animal model (with video). Gastrointest Endosc 2009;70(2):372–6.

25. Al Knawy B, Shiffman M. Percutaneous liver biopsy in clinical practice. Liver Int 2007;27(9):1166–73.
26. DeWitt J, LeBlanc J, McHenry L, et al. Endoscopic ultrasound-guided fine needle aspiration cytology of solid liver lesions: a large single-center experience. Am J Gastroenterol 2003;98(9):1976–81.
27. Nguyen P, Feng JC, Chang KJ. Endoscopic ultrasound (EUS) and EUS-guided fine-needle aspiration (FNA) of liver lesions. Gastrointest Endosc 1999;50(3): 357–61.
28. Hollerbach S, Willert J, Topalidis T, et al. Endoscopic ultrasound-guided fine-needle aspiration biopsy of liver lesions: histological and cytological assessment. Endoscopy 2003;35(9):743–9.
29. Jagannath S, Puri K, Kantsevoy S, et al. Endoscopic ultrasound and fine needle aspiration for the diagnosis of hepatocellular carcinoma. Minerva Gastroenterol Dietol 2008;54(2):125–30.
30. Dewitt J, McGreevy K, Cummings O, et al. Initial experience with EUS-guided Tru-cut biopsy of benign liver disease. Gastrointest Endosc 2009;69(3 Pt 1):535–42.
31. Stavropoulos SN, Im GY, Jlayer Z, et al. High yield of same-session EUS-guided liver biopsy by 19-gauge FNA needle in patients undergoing EUS to exclude biliary obstruction. Gastrointest Endosc 2012;75(2):310–8.
32. Nakai Y, Samarasena JB, Iwashita T, et al. Autoimmune hepatitis diagnosed by endoscopic ultrasound-guided liver biopsy using a new 19-gauge histology needle. Endoscopy 2012;44(Suppl 2 UCTN):E67–8.
33. Wardeh R, Lee JG, Gu M. Endoscopic ultrasound-guided paracentesis of ascitic fluid: a morphologic study with ultrasonographic correlation. Cancer Cytopathol 2011;119(1):27–36.
34. DeWitt J, LeBlanc J, McHenry L, et al. Endoscopic ultrasound-guided fine-needle aspiration of ascites. Clin Gastroenterol Hepatol 2007;5(5):609–15.
35. Chang KJ, Albers CG, Nguyen P. Endoscopic ultrasound-guided fine needle aspiration of pleural and ascitic fluid. Am J Gastroenterol 1995;90(1):148–50.
36. Rial NS, Gilchrist KB, Henderson JT, et al. Endoscopic ultrasound with biopsy of omental mass for cholangiocarcinoma diagnosis in cirrhosis. World J Gastrointest Endosc 2011;3(6):124–8.
37. Rana SS, Bhasin DK, Srinivasan R, et al. Endoscopic ultrasound-guided fine needle aspiration of peritoneal nodules in patients with ascites of unknown cause. Endoscopy 2011;43(11):1010–3.
38. Rana SS, Bhasin DK, Srinivisan R, et al. Endoscopic ultrasound fine-needle aspiration of peritoneal deposits for diagnosis of tubercular peritonitis in a cirrhotic patient with ascites. Endoscopy 2010;42(Suppl 2):E306–7.
39. El-Saadany M, Jalil S, Irisawa A, et al. EUS for portal hypertension: a comprehensive and critical appraisal of clinical and experimental indications. Endoscopy 2008;40(8):690–6.
40. Miller ES, Kim JK, Gandehok J, et al. A new device for measuring esophageal variceal pressure. Gastrointest Endosc 2002;56(2):284–91.
41. Miller LS, Dai Q, Thomas A, et al. A new ultrasound-guided esophageal variceal pressure-measuring device. Am J Gastroenterol 2004;99(7):1267–73.
42. Giday SA, Ko CW, Clarke JO, et al. EUS-guided portal vein carbon dioxide angiography: a pilot study in a porcine model. Gastrointest Endosc 2007;66(4):814–9.

Index

Note: Page numbers of article titles are in **boldface** type.

Gastrointest Endoscopy Clin N Am 22 (2012) 387–399
doi:10.1016/S1052-5157(12)00043-8
1052-5157/12/$ – see front matter © 2012 Elsevier Inc. All rights reserved.

giendo.theclinics.com

Moving?

Make sure your subscription moves with you!

To notify us of your new address, find your **Clinics Account Number** (located on your mailing label above your name), and contact customer service at:

Email: journalscustomerservice-usa@elsevier.com

800-654-2452 (subscribers in the U.S. & Canada)
314-447-8871 (subscribers outside of the U.S. & Canada)

Fax number: 314-447-8029

Elsevier Health Sciences Division
Subscription Customer Service
3251 Riverport Lane
Maryland Heights, MO 63043

*To ensure uninterrupted delivery of your subscription, please notify us at least 4 weeks in advance of move.

Printed and bound by CPI Group (UK) Ltd, Croydon, CR0 4YY

03/10/2024

01040449-0005